Helping Adolescents Cope with Loss

Edited by Kenneth J. Doka and Amy S. Tucci

D1367532

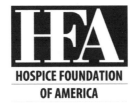

HOSPICE FOUNDATION OF AMERICA

This book is part of Hospice Foundation of America's *Living with Grief* series.

This book is part of HFA's *Living with Grief®* series.

Ordering information:

Call Hospice Foundation of America: 800-854-3402

Or write:
Hospice Foundation of America
1710 Rhode Island Avenue, NW #400
Washington, DC 20036

Or visit HFA's Web site:
www.hospicefoundation.org

Managing Editor: Lisa McGahey Veglahn
Layout and Design: HBP, Inc.

Publisher's Cataloging-in-Publication
(*Provided by Quality Books, Inc.*)

     Helping adolescents cope with loss / edited by Kenneth J.
       Doka and Amy S. Tucci.
         pages cm.—(Living with grief)
         Includes bibliographical references and index.
         LCCN 2013952644
         ISBN 9781893349179

        1. Grief in adolescence.   2. Bereavement in adolescence.
        3. Loss (Psychology) in adolescence.   4. Teenagers and death.
        5. Teenagers—Counseling of.
        I. Doka, Kenneth J.   II. Tucci, Amy S.
        III. Hospice Foundation of America.
        IV. Series: Living with grief.

       BF724.3.G73H45 2014   155.9'37'0835
                                      QBI14-600015

Dedication

*To Eddie Hodges
and
Bruce and Lynne Prochnik*

*For the pleasure of friendships begun in adolescence
and rediscovered in adulthood*

KJD

*To all adolescents whose lives have been shaped by the
pain of grief*

AST

Contents

Acknowledgments

We always begin by thanking the staff of the Hospice Foundation of America: Spencer Levine, Kristen Nanjundaram, Lindsey Currin, and Aziza Jones, as well as staff intern Justin Lewis. It truly is remarkable how much they accomplish. We applaud their devotion to our mission at the Hospice Foundation of America.

We also wish to recognize our outstanding managing editor Lisa McGahey Veglahn. Lisa frets over deadlines, keeps authors – and editors – on track, and carefully reviews all aspects of production.

Naturally we also need to thank all the authors who respond to our tight deadlines. We are extremely fortunate that we are consistently able to maintain an A-list of authors, and this year is no exception. As you peruse the Table of Contents, you will notice the names of many of the major researchers and writers in the field on adolescence and grief. We thank them for the contribution. We also thank the young authors of our *Voices* pieces. Ranging in age from their very early teens (13) to late adolescence, they have managed to tell their own stories their own way. We always see the *Voices* pieces as an unvarnished narrative that offers insight into the real experiences of grieving individuals. We thank this year's authors for their time and honesty.

We also thank the staff and the clients of Mourning Star, a community outreach program of VNA California that provides support for grieving children, teens, and their families. Adolescents from Mourning Star shared their personal and powerful artwork with us, one piece of which graces the cover of this book.

Both editors would like to thank their families and friends for their patience as we worked to publish a complex book in such a short time. Both editors benefit from the respite and grounding these family and friends offer.

As always, we wish to thank the Hospice Foundation of America's Board and all the organizations and individuals that support our efforts. We always remember the continuing legacy of the late Jack Gordon, founder and former chair of the Hospice Foundation of America and the counsel of David Abrams – former president, current board member, and friend.

Editor's Note: Readers of this volume will notice that authors may reference variations in age ranges when discussing the period of adolescence. There is no consensus on the exact age that correlates with the beginning of adolescence; and, of course, much is dependent on each individual's own cognitive, physical, and intellectual development. Generally, child development academicians and other experts define adolescence as the period between the onset of puberty and/or middle school and adult independence.

Introduction

Adolescent Encounters with Death: A Historical and Sociological Overview

Kenneth J. Doka

THE EMERGENCE OF ADOLESCENCE

Phillippe Ariès, a cultural historian, in his book *Centuries of Childhood* (1962), reminded readers that childhood was discovered in the Middle Ages. By that Ariès did not mean that some particularly observant peasant all of sudden noticed that three-foot tall people were working in the fields with him. Rather Ariès meant that, until that time, childhood was not viewed as a distinct phase of human development. Prior to that, children were often treated as miniature adults, dressing like adults and working and playing with them. In the Middle Ages childhood was now seen as distinct. Adults began to dress children differently, and there was greater recognition of their unique needs; the worlds of children and adults began to divide.

In a similar way, the concept of adolescence began to emerge around the time of the Industrial Revolution. Prior to that time there was little separation between the worlds of adults and adolescents. Once children reached puberty they often took on adult responsibilities – marrying, working, and even defending the home and hearth. Many religious and cultural rituals such as confirmation or bar mitzvah still reflect these rites of passage in which a child is seen to be symbolically moving from childhood into adulthood.

However, after the Industrial Revolution, societies began to acknowledge a transitional period between childhood and adulthood. This shift can be evidenced societally in the United States in mandatory school attendance and the passage of child labor laws. Organizations such as Boy and Girl Scouts and 4-H Clubs developed to serve this population, and these societal changes led to an increased academic interest in adolescent development.

ADOLESCENT DEVELOPMENT

Psychologists and developmental specialists began to recognize the unique developmental tasks encompassed in adolescence. Adolescents, they indicated, needed to gradually separate or differentiate from their parents in order to emerge as independent adults. As the adolescent struggles with this process, there is inevitably increased conflict with parents and other authority figures. However, this conflict can often be exaggerated in popular culture. Most adolescents adjust well throughout this period and maintain close, albeit sometimes ambivalent ties, with parents. Indeed, one aspect of the increased cognitive development in adolescence is the ability to understand other perspectives and points of view (Balk, 2009). So it is important not to overestimate the conflicts of adolescence, both external and internal, as many adolescents retain a sense of continuity with their past and maintain supportive relationships with their families and intimate networks.

Along with independence, adolescents need to develop their own identity. This identity formation affects every aspect of being, from what the adolescent believes, how he or she behaves and dresses, and even what the adolescent thinks.

Finally the adolescent has to deal with intimacy. This process is complex and includes developing both strong and sustained friendships as well as romantic relationships, perhaps even including a life partner.

The process of adolescence occurs at various levels. Biologically, adolescence encompasses puberty as the bodies of these young people experience multiple physical and hormonal changes that signify the physical emergence of adulthood and the emerging ability to reproduce sexually. There are emotional changes brought on by both hormonal changes and the aforementioned need to differentiate from parents. Cognitively, adolescents are now capable of more abstract thought. Socially, adolescents are expected to begin to develop clear career and life goals, even if they are tentative and subject to change. Given the extent of these physical, psychological, and social changes, it is little wonder that most societies marked this transition with varied rites of passage.

Adolescence is often divided into three distinct periods. Early adolescence is coterminous with the entry into middle school. Interestingly, while the grades, and therefore ages, of the beginning of middle school vary, adolescent behavior generally begins there. For example, adolescent friendships become more selective. While children will often form friendships on the basis of convenience, the young adolescent tends to see friendships as an aspect of identity; you are in part defined by those with whom you associate. Middle adolescence is generally linked with high school; late adolescence is associated with that period between the end of high school and the development of a fully differentiated and independent self.

In many Western societies, that period of late adolescence continues to lengthen, so much so that Arnett (2000) has suggested a new category of "emerging or young adulthood." Arnett notes that there is often a continuing and long process of emerging independence for people in their twenties. They have emerged from the school-based culture typical of adolescence but are not yet fully independent. Still living at home, many of them are delaying marriage, remaining childless, depending at least in part financially on parents, and not yet committing to careers. Arnett does note, however, that around 40% of individuals in this age span have made a full transition to adulthood, working, living independently, and raising families.

ADOLESCENCE: A GENERATIONAL PERSPECTIVE

In addition to acknowledging the development differences of adolescence, it is also important to acknowledge generational differences. Generational differences are often a hidden form of diversity. Yet each generation or age cohort is framed by its own set of historical, social, and demographic factors that differentiate that generation from other cohorts.

Middle and older adolescents are primarily from "Generation X," also called the Millennium Generation. While the birth years of each generation are somewhat debated, this generation refers to those born around between 1982 and 2000 (Strauss & Howe, 1991). This generation was born in a time when there was a deep interest in youth. At a time when abortion and contraceptive services were very available, this was a wanted and nurtured generation. Governments, both federal and state, passed programs designed to address the health, education, and safety of this generation. Parents too were very concerned about both safety and self-esteem; often children in this generation had comparatively limited free time as many were enrolled in supervised activities and social promotion was supported. Strauss and Howe (1991) suggest that this generation's high and perhaps unrealistic expectations may be dashed as they enter a highly competitive world in adulthood, in the sense that their experiences may have created "work-life unreadiness."

An increased emphasis on, and respect for, diversity has tended to make this a more tolerant generation. Societally, this generation has been exposed to the quick and constant stimulation of television and other media. Some see that constant stimulation as leading to the high diagnostic rate of Attention Deficit Disorder and Attention Deficit Hyperactivity Disorder. These diagnoses may be exacerbated by parental concerns that have often focused on any perceived divergence from performance norms. Research shows that this has become one of the more medicated generations.

This was also, especially in the younger members of this cohort, the first generation of *digital natives,* growing up with computers and the Internet as well as cell phones. These technological advances have had significant impacts, and have also spurred a fault line along social class, widening a distinct between the *haves* and *have nots* into the *knows* and *know nots.* While many of this generation have grown up with easy access to computers, the poorer members of this generation may have much more limited access.

The youngest adolescents are part of "Generation Z," born after the beginning of the millennium. Like most age cohorts born on the cusp, they share many characteristics with middle and older adolescents. They are even more technologically connected, growing up in a world with not only computers and the Internet but smartphones, tablets, and massively multiplayer online role-playing games (MMORPG).

Yet these young adolescents have also grown up in a world post 9/11. They have experienced the Great Recession as well as numerous incidents of horrific school violence. This then is a cautious generation. They have learned early that information on the Internet cannot always be trusted and even the most seemingly benign sites may harbor destructive computer viruses. Unlike the earlier generation, they are not as drawn to escapist literature like *Harry Potter,* veering more toward dystopian, post-apocalyptic books such as *The Hunger Games.*

In addition to being digital natives, Generation Z does share some characteristics with adolescents of Generation X. Like prior generations, Generations X and Z grew up in a world where guidance counselors and social workers were common in school and many large corporations had robust EAP programs. These are generations that have grown up in a world where information is freely exchanged. Still, they may not realize the potential consequences of the lack of privacy and confidentiality inherent in the online world. Counselors working with this population can expect that they will be "googled" and may need to develop policies in their consent forms regarding social networking sites ("to friend or not to friend"). They may also have to address the use of cell phones and texting in group and individual sessions. In addition, since adolescent members of both generations who are grieving may use the Internet for a variety of functions including memorialization, support, and information about grief, it is critical to maintain an ongoing dialogue about Internet use.

ADOLESCENT ENCOUNTERS WITH DEATH

We often speak of adolescence as a time when strength, energy, and health peak. It is not much of an exaggeration. Adolescence is a period of great growth and development – physically, cognitively, and emotionally. Today it is also one of the healthiest periods of life. Less than one percent of deaths in the United States are experienced between those in the adolescent demographic. Adolescents, for the most part, have survived the genetic or congenital diseases of birth without falling yet to the degenerative diseases of older age. Less than 12% will die each year from such illnesses. Here the leading causes of death are cancer (6%), heart disease (3%), and then other genetic or congenital conditions such as muscular dystrophy or cystic fibrosis (Miniño, 2010).

The large majority of adolescents die of largely preventable causes, such as accidents, suicides, and homicides. Forty-eight percent of adolescent death is accounted for by accidents, and nearly three-quarters of those are due to automobile accidents. Homicide and suicide account for another near quarter of deaths, with homicide being the leading cause of death among African American male adolescents. Gender and age also play a role. Male adolescents are more likely to die than females and the death rate increases as one ages in adolescence. This means that adolescents are likely to die traumatic deaths that are both sudden and preventable, two factors likely to complicate loss in adolescents as they grieve the loss of a peer from such causes.

In addition to these peer losses, other losses experienced by adolescents, such as the death of a parent or sibling, are likely to be out-of-order deaths that may be sudden as well. Harrison and Harrington (2001) found that over 77.6% of their sample of British adolescents had experienced the death of someone close to them by that point in their life. The intrusiveness of the death, that is, how much the death changed their lives, was a critical factor in how they viewed and coped with that loss.

Finally, adolescents are likely to experience not only direct but indirect experiences with death. Given the traumatic nature of the deaths that most adolescents experience, it is not unusual that such deaths are reflected in the video games, films, and music that appeal to adolescents. While Anderson and Bushman's analysis suggested that playing such games habituated violence, desensitizing players to violence and increasing anti-social behavior, others have found that participation in such games calms violence by offering symbolic catharsis (Kestenbaum & Weinstein, 1985).

ADOLESCENCE AND LOSS, DEATH, AND GRIEF

Despite the comparatively low death rate of adolescents, death is very much part of the adolescent world. As mental health professionals, clinicians, educators, end-of-life specialists, volunteers, and, most importantly, parents, we do adolescents little good by ignoring that reality. This book, arising from and accompanying our annual program, focuses on ways to assist adolescents as they encounter loss, grief, and death. Here we invited some of the foremost experts in the field to share their insights on this critical topic.

Subsequent sections delineate the variety of losses adolescents encounter as well as the ways to support adolescents with life-threatening illness as well as grieving adolescents. Because of the unique developmental issues inherent in adolescence, it is critical for organizations such as hospices, palliative care units, schools, and other counseling programs to develop services and programs that are specifically tailored to the unique needs of adolescents who are dying or bereaved. For example, ethical issues can be complicated with adolescents experiencing a life-threatening illness; younger adolescents, while not legally of age to offer consent, should be full participants in their treatment and assent to medical decisions in keeping with their individual ability, and family and cultural context. In addition, due to the unique developmental issues of adolescents, grief support such as individual counseling or group support should be carefully tailored, understanding factors that can complicate an adolescent's grief. Interventive strategies that build on the developmental strengths of adolescents are essential. And throughout this book, we intersperse the voices of adolescents, for adolescents are best able to articulate both their losses and the sources of their support.

Kenneth J. Doka, PhD, MDiv, is a professor of gerontology at the Graduate School of the College of New Rochelle and senior consultant to the Hospice Foundation of America (HFA). Dr. Doka serves as editor of HFA's Living with Grief® book series, its Journeys newsletter, and numerous other books and publications. Dr. Doka has served as a panelist on HFA's Living with Grief® video programs for 21 years. He is a past president of the Association for Death Education and Counseling (ADEC) and received an award for Outstanding Contributions in the field of Death Education. He is a member and past chair of the International Work Group on Death, Dying, and Bereavement. In 2006, Dr. Doka was grandfathered in as a mental health counselor under New York's first state licensure of counselors. Dr. Doka is an ordained Lutheran minister.

REFERENCES

Anderson, C. A. & Bushman, B. J. (2001). Effects of violent video games on aggressive behavior, aggressive cognition, aggressive affect, physiological arousal, and prosocial behavior: A meta-analytic review of the scientific literature. *Psychological Science, 12,* 353-359.

Ariès, P. (1962). *Centuries of childhood: A social history of family life.* New York, NY: Vintage Books.

Arnett, J. (2000). Emerging adulthood: A theory of development from the late teens through the twenties. *American Psychologist, 55*(5), 469-480.

Balk, D. (2009). Adolescent development: The backstory to adolescent encounters with death and bereavement. In D. Balk & C. Corr (Eds.), *Adolescent encounters with death, bereavement, and coping* (pp. 3-20). New York, NY: Springer.

Bowen, M. (1978). *Family therapy in clinical practice*. New York, NY: Aronson.

Harrison, L. & Harrington, R. (2001). Adolescents' bereavement experiences. Prevalence, association with depressive symptoms, and use of services. *Journal of Adolescence, 24,* 59-69.

Kestenbaum, G. & Weinstein, L. (1985). Personality, psychopathology, and developmental issues in male adolescent video game use. *Journal of the American Academy of Child Psychiatry 24,* 325-337.

Miniño, A.M. (2010). Mortality among teenagers aged 12-19 years: United States, 1999-2006. NCHS data brief, no 37. Hyattsville, MD: National Center for Health Statistics.

Strauss, W. & Howe, N. (1991). *Generations: The history of America's future, 1584-2069*. New York, NY: Quill.

Adolescence and Loss

Adolescence is a time of both emerging strength and good health. Few adolescents actually die. However this does not mean adolescents are immune from loss. Adolescents do die, both from diseases as well as from largely preventable causes such as accidents, suicides, and homicide. Older adolescents, or emerging adults, may die in combat. Adolescents also may experience the loss of others close to them, including parents, siblings, or peers.

This section explores the losses encountered in adolescence. Kenneth Doka begins this section with a chapter on adolescents encountering life-threatening illness. He notes that the very nature of life-threatening illness deeply challenges some of the key developmental tasks of adolescence – independence, intimacy, and identity. Yet Doka also acknowledges that the invulnerability that many adolescents experience is a developmental strength. Part of the strength of Doka's chapter is a model that acknowledges life-threatening illness is a process involving many phases. In each phase, Doka reviews the particular issues that might arise for the adolescent with a life-threatening illness and his or her family, as well as ethical and legal circumstances that may be encountered by adolescents and their parents.

Bruce Jennings further explores these unique ethical quandaries in his chapter. Jennings notes research that supports the idea that by 14 (middle adolescence), most adolescents have functional capacity to make decisions, but not – except in rare situations – legal capacity. He emphasizes the need to recognize the relational nature of ethical decisions and the need to make medical decisions *with* rather than *for* the adolescent patient.

David Balk offers a chapter that not only neatly illustrates these principles but offers a transition to the adolescent grieving a death. Balk begins by demonstrating, in the case of Helene, the ways that developmental factors influence her response to living with Graves Disease. In exploring the reactions that Helene has to the disease, Balk neatly draws the parallels with grief reactions that follow a death. It is a cogent reminder that grief encompasses reaction to death and illness but that it can also include losses frequently experienced by adolescents, such as parental divorce or break-ups of romantic relationships or friendships (Doka, 2002).

Adolescents, of course, do experience death. J. William Worden considers the effects of parental loss on the adolescent summarizing results from the influential Harvard Child Bereavement Study where he was one of the principal investigators. Worden makes a number of cogent points that have clinical importance. Chief among these is that often the effects on the adolescent may not be evident until the second year. Worden notes that one of the best predictors of adolescent outcomes is how well the surviving parent functions, thus emphasizing the importance of family-based therapy (Hayne, Ayers, Sandler, & Kolchak, 2008). Worden also calls for the use of screening techniques to identify the 20% of adolescents at risk for more complicated reactions.

Evan Brohan, a 13-year-old, offers the first of the *Voices* chapters, reflecting on the loss of his dad. His *Voices* piece reminds us of Worden's affirmation of the continuing bonds that remain even after a loss. Evan also projects the strengths and strategies often used by adolescents as they cope with loss.

Nancy Hogan reflects upon a different kind of familial loss, that of a sibling. The sibling bond is unique. Siblings are family but the relationships are more equal, less hierarchical than they are in the parent-child bond. Siblings are part of our identity. Our place in the constellation of siblings – older, younger, or middle – deeply influences development. Siblings also share unique perceptions, such as the smell of Mom's perfume or the taste of Grandma's biscuits. While Hogan primarily focuses on the death of a sibling through illness, her points can be taken more generally. The loss of a sibling is by very nature traumatic. However, an illness creates additional issues as children live in houses of chronic sorrow, where the families are often coping with the effects of life-limiting illness. In addition, the lives of siblings are contingent, always affected by the ill sibling's condition (Bluebond-Langner, 1997). Yet while there are possible negative effects, Hogan affirms the continuing bond that siblings retain as well as opportunities for growth (Calhoun & Tedeschi, 2012).

Alivia Seay recounts her experience with the death of her grandmother, a not uncommon loss in adolescence. Alivia illustrates a point often made by Hogan's chapter as well as by Calhoun and

Tedeschi (2012) that grief can be an impetus to growth. In Alivia's case, her grandmother's death influenced not only her interest in volunteering with hospice but also her decision to major in nursing.

Carlos Torres, Nicole Alston, and Robert Neimeyer address a not uncommon but often neglected and disenfranchised loss in adolescence – that of perinatal loss. The authors recognize the multiple challenges that adolescent mothers experience in a perinatal loss. They compare the perinatal loss of an adolescent to that of an adult. While noting many commonalities, the authors recognize the stigma of the adolescent unwed mother that discourages support. They also acknowledge this as a nonfinite loss, one that is ongoing as the adolescent constantly reconstructs "what could have been."

The leading causes of death in adolescence are accidents, suicide, and homicide. Illene Cupit and Karissa Meyer begin by reviewing the impact of accidents on adolescents. They root the effects of an accidental death both in the internal and external worlds of adolescence. Cupit and Meyer explore both the deaths of family and of friends, emphasizing that those reactions are similar. As the authors comment, such a result is not unusual given the strong role that peers play in adolescent life. Cupit and Meyer recommend a strength-based approach – noting the considerable resources adolescents retain even as they deal with loss, including both their own physical prowess and their sophisticated use of technology. The technological world of adolescence is reflected in a number of chapters and explored more fully by Carla Sofka in the next section.

Lillian Range discusses adolescent suicide, another leading cause of adolescent death. Range offers a comprehensive view that encompasses prevention, intervention, and postvention. Prevention can offer particular challenges for two reasons. First, while we often think that suicide is an act *sui generis*, suicide can be the result of many different conditions. For example, it may be an act arising from depression. It could be a response to a crisis – a failing grade or a break-up in a romantic relationship, or even a psychotic episode, perhaps induced by drugs. Second, the risk factors associated with adolescent suicide, such as isolation from peer support or lack of involvement is school or community activities, yield many false positives. What this means is that many of the factors associated with adolescent suicide, such as poor academic performance, family difficulties, less active peer life, low involvement in school, and fears of sexuality (to name a few), are relatively common among adolescents and thus are not very predictive about an adolescent's actual level of risk. This inability to offer strong evidence-based criteria for prevention can complicate intervention and postvention.

This inability to predict is evidenced by Dylan Rieger who offers a *Voices* piece in which he recounts his reaction to the suicide of his friend, Zach. Dylan confesses the profound emotions of guilt that many survivors of suicide experience. Only after a long process is he able to acknowledge that Zach – and Zach alone – is responsible for that fatal choice.

Tashel Bordere describes another all too common form of adolescent grief, grief that is a reaction to homicide. Bordere reminds us that in African American communities, homicide is the leading cause of death for young men. Bordere offers an exceptional review, noting the factors that complicate such a loss while offering sage suggestions for clinicians. Noting the scarcity of literature connecting grief to violence and violent death, especially among adolescents, Bordere draws from contemporary examples and personal accounts of young people grieving a death by homicide. Bordere's advice for clinicians reminds us that one of the major costs of homicide is that it challenges both the sense of safety and the sense of fairness, so both have to be addressed in counseling.

The final chapter in this section, by Heather Campagna, Tina Saari, and Jill Harrington-LaMorie, considers combat deaths. The authors note that many of these deaths leave a host of adolescent grievers in their wake, including children, siblings, and sometimes peers. Campagna, Saari, and Harrington-LaMorie offer an insightful overview of military culture and rituals and the ways both can complicate and facilitate grief. They note the range of losses that adolescents may experience, including the separation of deployment as well as a possible relocation following a death. The authors also note the rising rate of military deaths by suicide – one that creates distinct issues for disenfranchised grievers. Sensitive to both the issues of adolescent development and military culture, Campagna, Saari, and Harrington-LaMorie provide sound advice both to clinicians and educators.

REFERENCES

Bluebond-Langner, M. (1987). Worlds of dying children and their well siblings. *Death Studies, 11*, 279-295.

Doka, K. J. (Ed.). (2002). *Disenfranchised grief: New directions, challenges, and strategies for practice.* Champaign, IL: Research Press.

Haines, R., Ayers, T., Sandler, I., & Wolchik, S. (2008). When a parent dies: Helping bereaved children and adolescents. In K. J. Doka & A. S. Tucci (Eds.), *Living with grief: Children and adolescents* (pp 141-158). Washington, DC: Hospice Foundation of America.

—

CHAPTER 1

Living with Life-Threatening Illness: An Adolescent Perspective

Kenneth J. Doka

Adolescence remains one of the healthiest periods in the lifecycle. Adolescents have survived, for the most part, any congenital or childhood diseases. They have not yet suffered the debilitating conditions that occur with advancing age. In fact, adolescents account for less than one percent of all deaths in the United States.

Yet, adolescents do die. Nearly half die of accidents and another quarter die due to suicide and homicide. The remaining deaths are due to life-threatening illnesses, with cancer and heart disease the two leading causes of death. In addition, some adolescents will die of congenital or genetic conditions first encountered in childhood, such as muscular dystrophy or cystic fibrosis. Each year about 3,000 adolescents die from these varied chronic conditions (Freyer, 2004).

This chapter focuses on the needs of adolescents with life-threatening illness. Life-threatening illness in adolescence presents a paradoxical situation. As many of their peers are coping with emerging strengths, physical maturity, and independence, adolescents with life-threatening illness see their strengths, world, and independence diminish. The chapter begins by reviewing the unique developmental challenges posed when adolescents experience life-threatening illness; it then reviews the sensitivities and issues, including ethical issues that can arise in counseling adolescents with life-threatening illness.

ADOLESCENT DEVELOPMENT AND
LIFE-THREATENING ILLNESS

Identity

In many ways, the development or continuation of a life-threatening illness becomes extremely difficult in adolescence since it so severely complicates the normal processes associated with this phase of development. For most adolescents, identity emerges as a key concern. Adolescents will often experiment and redefine their sense of self at various periods of this life stage. The adolescent is constantly seeking and examining the issue of personal identity. This process also involves a sense of differentiation from significant others in their lives. *How am I alike and how am I different from my parents?*

A life-threatening illness complicates the quest for identity in a number of ways. First it affects body image, a key attribute of identity. Most adolescents are extremely concerned about whether they are the right height and weight; they worry about how they look and how they dress or if they are developing too quickly or too slowly. Adolescence can be a cruel time for those whose dress or body image does not conform to accepted norms. For the adolescent with life-threatening illness, body image issues can loom large. Depending on the treatment, adolescents may lose hair, gain or lose weight, or have obvious physical manifestations of disease such as amputations. This altered body image can affect the sense of identity in a number of ways. First it might result in a sense of stigma, or a sense of spoiled identity (Goffman, 1963). Here the adolescent copes with a marred sense of self – a sense that he or she is both different and deficient when compared to his or her peers, perhaps contributing to a sense of isolation. In some cases the ill adolescent may withdraw out of embarrassment by his or her appearance. In other cases, peers, discomforted by the ill adolescent's appearance, may exclude such an adolescent from interaction.

There is another issue with identity. Part of identity formation involves a critical assessment of spiritual issues. As adolescents struggle with identity issues, the question arises of *What do I believe?* Here adolescents know the values and beliefs taught by their parents, clergy, and other spiritual influences. Yet adolescents need to determine what beliefs they now have as their own. As Barra et al. (1993) indicate, this process can be a long and painful struggle. In this time when beliefs are questioned, beliefs about God and the afterlife that were very comforting in childhood may provide less support to the adolescent.

Intimacy

Another developmental issue in adolescence is that of intimacy. As adolescents develop they begin to experiment with intimate relationships outside of the family. In early adolescence, this would be manifested in sharing confidences with best friends. In middle adolescence, this would mean exploring romantic relationships. In later adolescence, it might involve the search for a life partner.

The experience of illness may offer challenges to the adolescent's search for intimacy. The adolescent may be limited in his or her ability to establish ties with a peer group. Frequent hospitalizations and time-consuming treatments may interrupt opportunities to interact with peers. The limitations and disabilities caused by the illness may preclude participation in, and acceptance by, more socially or athletically-oriented peer groups. In addition, both the treatment and illness may retard academic progress, thereby limiting association with and acceptance by more intellectually inclined groups (Easson, 1988). Easson (1988) also notes that these issues, as well as the impaired physical image of the adolescent, may inhibit development of peer relationships as well. Here two aspects of adolescent development interact. As part of identity, adolescents form peer groups of like-minded individuals. That is, the adolescent is very conscious that the friends they associate with are part of their own presentation of self. The younger child will often associate with whatever children are available; adolescents are more selective in their relationships. When adolescents with life-limiting illness find their opportunities to interact and identify with peers more difficult, opportunities to develop intimacy are thwarted. Opportunities for developing sexual intimacy may likewise be limited. The adolescent with life-limiting illness may face considerable barriers in developing romantic and sexual partnerships. These include the limitations for peer interaction, physical changes and residues of the illness that impair attractiveness, and the stigma of the disease. In addition, the sense of a limited future might discourage commitment.

Independence

For most young people, adolescence is a time of slowly emerging independence, of making more choices and continuing to differentiate from parents. Illness is likely to complicate this quest for independence. If the illness begins in adolescence, the adolescent may be forced into a more dependent role just at the time in the life cycle when he or she is trying to achieve a degree of independence. If the illness extends from childhood into adolescence, the adolescent may have already experienced a history of overprotectiveness. This in turn may result in a lack of early maturing experiences that increase passivity and impair the assumption of a more independent role. This situation may generate increased ambivalence toward and conflict with parents and other authority figures. Very traditional experiences of adolescence such as driving or getting a part-time job may be precluded by the constraints and limitations posed by the illness.

In addition, adolescence is a time when adolescents look forward and plan their future. Will they go on to college? What career or job do they aspire to obtain? When an adolescent has a life-threatening illness, the uncertainty of the disease impairs the ability to do such planning, further precluding the possibility of independence.

There may be other difficulties as well. While adolescent conflict with parents is often exaggerated, relationships with parents can be wrought with some ambivalence. This ambivalence, as well as the adolescent's quest for independence, may complicate the adolescent's ability to seek or to accept support from parents and other adults.

This can emerge in a number of different ways. First, adolescents and their caregivers may conflict over adherence to the medical regimen. Often these conflicts are a sign of the adolescent's need for independence and control. These conflicts can be mitigated if the adolescent feels like a full partner in treatment, and is kept informed about the need for adherence. As much as possible, the treatment regimen should be adjusted to conform to the adolescent's lifestyle (Doka, 2014).

A second area where conflicts can arise that reflect the adolescent's need for independence is over treatment issues within end-of-life care. Adolescence is a gray area ethically. Adolescents may have decisional capacity; the adolescent can understand the medical information offered; assess the consequences of varied decisions; demonstrate reasoning in making a decision; and express a decision consistent with his or her beliefs and priorities (Meade & Freibert, 2012). However, while the adolescent may have decisional capacity, he or she does not have legal capacity to make such decisions. That power is invested in their surrogate, generally a parent or guardian. Ideally the situation should be one of shared decision making, one where the young person makes a decision that is supported by both parents and medical professionals.

While this is the ideal, it may not always be the case. In situations where there are profound disagreements between the parent and the child over the course of treatment, Meade and Friebert (2012) offer a number of principles. First and foremost, the adolescent's opinion should not be solicited unless there is a commitment that it should be seriously considered. Second, even prior to that, the adolescent's intellectual capacity, as well as emotional and spiritual maturity, needs to be assessed. This not only involves understanding whether the adolescent can really understand the medical information underlying any decision but also to what extent the adolescent can appreciate how fears and insecurities may be influencing any decision, as well as if he or she has the spiritual maturity to assess issues of meaning and suffering. Third, Meade and Friebert (2012) argue that decisions of adolescents who have lived with a chronic condition for a long time should be given greater weight than those just coping with the new reality of a life-threatening illness. Finally Meade and Friebert (2012) assert that proximity to the end of life means that the adolescent's decision be offered more weight. For example, the wishes of a 16-year-old with osteogenic sarcoma to refuse an amputation that offers a reasonable chance for recovery would have less weight than such an adolescent, now in the terminal phase, receiving experimental chemotherapy that has little probability of meaningfully extending life.

Invulnerability

While identity, intimacy, and independence are often called the *3 I's* of adolescence, there is actually a fourth *"I"* – invulnerability. Most adolescents have a sense of indestructibility, as adolescents have not fully encountered their own personal awareness of mortality (Doka, 2002). That sense of invulnerability underlies many of the risky behaviors often seen in adolescence, such as experimentation with drugs or other reckless activities such as driving at high speeds. Yet, in many ways, that same sense of invulnerability can be a source of strength as the adolescent copes with illness. The adolescent may retain a sense of hope that he or she can still overcome the disease, allowing him or her to actively participate in treatment. In addition, the adolescent can draw from cognitive abilities and coping skills that now are more developed.

COUNSELING ADOLESCENTS WITH
LIFE-THREATENING ILLNESS

Meeting developmental needs

Since the developmental issues arising in adolescence can complicate the experience of illness, parents, guardians, and health professionals need to be sensitive to meet the developmental concerns of adolescents. Many of the negative effects of illness can be mitigated if those around the adolescent support his or her emerging individuality, independence, and intimacy needs.

First, this means respecting the adolescent's need for privacy. All adolescents, as part of emerging independence, often spend less time with parents and demand privacy and autonomy. This need can be challenged by the constraints of an illness where the adolescent may require careful monitoring and assistance with more intimate tasks. Acknowledging and accommodating privacy concerns are critical to maintaining trust. Similarly, body image is an important aspect of identity. Adolescent concerns about body image are often expressed in concerns about clothes and appearance. Supportive adults will acknowledge and assist the adolescent in maintaining and projecting a positive body image and normalcy.

Second, it is important to meet the normal needs of adolescence for bonding with peers. Creating and encouraging opportunities for peer interaction, including online interaction, can be critical. For example, one family developed a web page for friends to show support and communicate with their teenage daughter as she underwent treatment for her illness out of state.

Finally, as mentioned earlier, respect for the emerging autonomy and independence of the adolescent means allowing them a role in making decisions about care. This entails involving the adolescent in decisions about care such as educating them about pain control options (Selove, Cochran, & Cohen, 2008) and gaining assent to ethical decisions that may need to be made (Jennings, 2008).

Understanding the illness experience

While this chapter focuses on end-of-life care, it is important to understand that experience in the context of what has likely been a long process of coping with life-threatening illness, whether the illness was congenital or developed earlier in the life course. In prior work, I have found it useful to understand life-threatening illness as consisting of a series of phases that may or may not be experienced in an individual's experience with disease (see Doka, 2014). These phases include the *prediagnostic, diagnostic, chronic, recovery,* and *terminal* phases. Understanding issues that had arisen in these earlier phases will often influence behaviors and reaction in the terminal phase.

The *prediagnostic phase* refers to the period of health-seeking that often begins with the recognition of symptoms and ends with a definitive diagnosis. It is worthwhile to explore this process as it can offer an unguarded window that casts light on underlying issues that might be influencing the way the family is coping with the illness. For example, in one case, a young adolescent boy complained of persistent pain in his leg. Given the boy's age and active athleticism, his mother dismissed the complaints as "growing pains." As the pain continued to worsen, the mother finally took the boy to a physician. The diagnosis was osteogenic sarcoma or bone cancer, in a relatively late stage. Though the boy's leg was amputated and he went through a regimen of chemotherapy, the cancer soon metastasized to his lung. The prognosis was poor and both her son and his father, as well as the physician, suggested palliative care. The mother, however, was insistent on additional treatment, even though the medical team agreed that further treatment was likely to be futile. Through counseling, the mother acknowledged her sense of guilt over the delayed diagnosis and began to understand how that fueled her request for further treatment.

The *diagnostic phase* revolves around the time when the diagnosis is clear and the adolescent patient and family now experience an existential crisis, recognizing the possibility of death. Throughout this time, a family has to deal with a series of tasks that include:

- understanding the disease;
- examining and maximizing health and lifestyle;
- maximizing one's coping strengths and limiting weaknesses;
- developing strategies to deal with issues created by disease;
- exploring the effect of illness on one's sense of self and relationships with others;
- ventilating feelings and fears; and
- incorporating the present reality of the diagnosis into one's sense of past and future (Doka, 2014).

These tasks may involve complications for the preadolescent (depending on time of onset) or adolescent patient. The adolescent may not fully understand either the diagnosis or prognosis. This may be due to the limited cognitive or emotional maturity of the adolescent; a sense of invulnerability that can fuel denial; or the overprotectiveness of parents who carefully control and filter information.

Critical to these tasks is fully involving the adolescent. For example, adolescents are more likely to adhere to medical regimens if tailored to their life style and sensitive to their concerns. In one case an adolescent girl with leukemia was able to arrange sessions of chemotherapy that allowed her to continue to participate in her high school band, an important activity in her life and a source of peer support.

Similarly, adolescents may benefit from peer support groups, as ventilating feelings and fears to parents may compromise a sense of independence. Peer support groups can also assist in meeting intimacy needs, particularly in cases where there is a sense of isolation from prior peer relationships.

Adults also need to have sensitivity to the concerns about the future that might arise in the crisis of diagnosis. Plans about attending college or other future activities may need to be revisited. For example, one high school senior decided he needed to attend a community college closer to home to continue treatment at a major cancer center in his area rather than go to a more distant college.

The *chronic phase* of illness is that long period in which the patient continues treatment in hopes of extending life or finding a cure for the illness. Here the crisis of diagnosis has abated, yet there is not the urgency aroused by impending death. Individuals struggle with the disease and treatment along with all the normal stress adolescents are likely to experience. Tasks here include:

- managing symptoms and side effects;
- carrying out medical regimens;
- preventing and managing medical crises;
- managing stress and examining coping;
- maximizing social support and minimizing social isolation;
- normalizing life in the face of disease;
- dealing with financial concerns;
- preserving self-concept;
- redefining relationships with others throughout the course of the disease;
- ventilating feeling and fears; and
- finding meaning in suffering, chronicity, uncertainty, or decline.

The issues and sensitivities emerging from these tasks are similar to those addressed earlier. The adolescent needs to be actively involved in directing care, encouraged to maintain peer relationships and, as much as possible, normalcy of life, and supported as he or she deals with the fears and emotions aroused by both the disease and uncertainty of a future.

The quality of life in this chronic phase will be in large part defined by the particular symptoms of the underlying disease. In diseases where the adolescent is asymptomatic or only experiences minor symptoms and little pain, the effect of the disease on the sense of self may be minor. In other cases, where symptoms are persistent, recurring, and disruptive, and pain is chronic, life may be seriously disrupted.

The trajectory or pattern that the illness takes often shapes the experience of the chronic phase. For example, in diseases that show a slow but steady or relentless pattern of decline, individuals and their families may have to cope with the psychological distress of constant and continued deterioration. "Every night," one young man with muscular dystrophy told me, "I go to bed knowing I will wake up weaker." Diseases such as leukemia, marked by remissions and relapses, may create a sense of constant uncertainly and anxiety.

Even given that the focus of this chapter is on end-of-life care, a few comments ought to be made about recovery. Obviously, and in increasing numbers, more adolescents survive life- threatening illness. Yet it is important to recognize that the experience of the disease may leave physical, psychological, spiritual, or social residues that will continue to influence the adolescent's life and development. For example, one adolescent survivor of cancer decided that given the extensive radiation and chemotherapy he experienced, he would choose not to have children. In other cases the residues of prior illness may have increased significance in adolescence. In one case, an adolescent had extensive heart surgery as a young child, leaving the scar of a large incision across his chest. While this scar was largely ignored when the boy was a child, he became extremely self-conscious of it in adolescence.

It is worthwhile to continue to explore the issues that have emerged in earlier phases of the illness. Not only will this allow a sense of family dynamics, it may uncover issues still unresolved that emerge as the adolescent faces death.

The adolescent in the terminal phase

The *terminal phase* begins when the goal of care becomes palliative; little can be done to cure or meaningfully extend life. There is much that might be done, however, to make the adolescent comfortable and his or her life meaningful. It may be very difficult for the parents and guardians as well as the adolescent, and sometimes the medical staff, to acknowledge that the goal of care is now palliative. Given the high value placed on youth as well as the relative rarity, in contemporary developed societies, that children predecease parents, the reluctance is understandable. However, the failure to recognize that the goal of treatment is now palliative may inhibit effective pain management, delay appropriate referrals to hospice or palliative care services, and create ethical issues around futile care (Selove, Cochran & Cohen, 2008; Jennings, 2008).

This transition can become particularly complicated when parents try to protect the adolescent from the fact that he or she is dying. This is not likely to be effective as most adolescents can respond to external and internal cues and are likely to have multiple sources of information including the Internet (see Bluebond-Langner, 1965; Doka, 1982). Such a strategy is likely to impede trust and complicate the adolescent's coping.

In the terminal phase, the adolescent who is dying must cope with a variety of tasks, including:

- dealing with symptoms, discomfort, pain, and incapacitation;
- managing health procedures and institutional procedures;
- managing stress and examining coping;
- dealing effectively with caregivers;
- preparing for death and saying goodbye;
- preserving self-concept;
- preserving relationships with family and friends;
- ventilating feelings and fears;
- finding meaning in life and death.

Some of these tasks may intersect with the developmental tasks of adolescence and complicate coping in this phase of illness. And again, the adolescent needs to be actively involved in all discussions and choices in end-of-life care. At this phase, it is also still important to encourage peer relationships. In one case, an adolescent dying of muscular dystrophy developed critical peer support through participation in a massively multiplayer online role-playing game

(Hensley, 2009). Websites such as Caring Bridge and Care Pages are specifically designed to support families struggling with life-threatening illness. These sites allow patients and families to post medical updates and blogs and allow others opportunities for support.

Spiritual support can be essential here as well. In adolescence, the emergence of critical thinking, continued development of identity, and new experiences such as college can cause adolescents to question their prior beliefs (Barra et al., 1993). This is likely to be exacerbated by an abbreviated life span that may raise doubts about the fairness of the world and the goodness of a deity. Adolescents then may need spiritual support that cannot only tolerate but support that spiritual struggle.

It is critical too in this terminal phase that adolescents are supported in their presentation of self. Appearance may remain important in preserving self-concept.

Because of an abbreviated life span, the issue of finding a sense of meaning in life and leaving a legacy may become important. As Selove, Cochran, and Cohen (2008) note, journaling and expressive arts such as painting, poetry, or music can offer valued opportunities to leave a mark. Given the fact that adolescents are *digital natives,* having grown up with the Internet, there may be opportunities online as well as through blogs or personal websites. Adolescents will take comfort in knowing that their life, however brief, had impact.

The adolescent indirectly affected by illness

During the HIV crisis, a distinction was made between children *infected* by HIV and those *affected* by HIV, often the children of HIV-infected women soon to be orphaned by the disease. In many ways, that is shared in all illnesses. Life-threatening illnesses are inevitably family diseases. Even if the adolescent is not directly suffering from the disease, the fact that someone in the family is struggling with illness will impact the adolescent. Bluebond-Langner (1987), for example, found that the well siblings of children with chronic diseases often experienced living in "houses of chronic sorrow." In addition, these adolescents reported they lived "contingent lives"; any plans were always contingent on the health of their ill sibling. Living in the shadow of illness often meant that their own crises were discounted. This was stated by the sister of a sibling with cancer: "Nothing that happens to me seems important. If I am worried about a grade, or having fights with friends, it always go back to be thankful you don't have cancer." It is little wonder that Bluebond-Langner found siblings struggling with difficult affect aroused by the illness including guilt, ambivalence, and anger. Similarly, well siblings often felt isolated, over-achieved in an attempt to please, or acted out (Burton, 2010).

CONCLUSION

While few adolescents actually die of life-threatening illness, those who do, as well as those affected by a life-threatening illness, may need support and counseling. Often the fact that these illnesses affect the whole family means that such support will need to come from outside of the family system. That support will be much more effective if health professionals and counselors acknowledge both the unique challenges and strengths of adolescents as they stare in the face of illness or death.

Kenneth J. Doka, PhD, MDiv, is a professor of gerontology at the Graduate School of The College of New Rochelle and senior consultant to the Hospice Foundation of America (HFA). Dr. Doka serves as editor of HFA's Living with Grief® book series, its Journeys newsletter, and numerous other books and publications. Dr. Doka has served as a panelist on HFA's Living with Grief® video programs for 21 years. He is a past president of the Association for Death Education and Counseling (ADEC) and received an award for Outstanding Contributions in the field of Death Education. He is a member and past chair of the International Work Group on Death, Dying, and Bereavement. In 2006, Dr. Doka was grandfathered in as a mental health counselor under New York's first state licensure of counselors. Dr. Doka is an ordained Lutheran minister.

REFERENCES

Barra, D. M., Carlson, E., Maize, M., Murphy, W., O'Neal, B., Sarver, R. & Zinner, E. S. (1993). The dark night of the spirit: Grief following a loss in religious identity. In K. Doka with J. Morgan (Eds.), *Death and Spirituality,* (pp. 291-308). Amityville, NY: Baywood Publishing Co.

Bluebond-Langner, M. (1965). *The private worlds of dying children.* Princeton, NJ: Princeton University Press.

Bluebond-Langner, M. (1987). Worlds of dying children and their well siblings. *Death Studies, 11,* 279-295.

Burton, M. (2010). Supporting adolescents who have a sibling with life-threatening illness: An exploratory study. *Counseling and Psychotherapy Research, 10*, 316-321.

Doka, K. J. (1982). The social organization of terminal care in two pediatric hospitals. *Omega: Journal of Death and Dying, 12*, 347-356.

Doka, K. J. (2002). Death in life. In K. J. Doka (Ed.), *Living with grief: Loss in later life*. Washington, DC: Hospice Foundation of America.

Doka, K. J. (2014). *Counseling the individual with life-threatening illness* (2nd Edition). New York, NY: Springer.

Easson, W. (1988). The seriously ill or dying adolescent: Special needs and challenges. *Postgraduate Medicine, 8*, 183-189.

Freyer, D. (2004). Care of the dying adolescent: Special considerations. *Pediatrics, 113*, 381-385.

Goffman, E. (1963). *Stigma: Notes on the management of spoiled identity*. New York, NY: Prentice-Hall.

Hensley, L. (2009). Death and disenfranchised grief in virtual communities: Challenges and opportunities. Paper presented at the Annual Conference of the Association for Death Education and Counseling. Dallas, TX. April.

Jennings, B. (2008). Dying at an early age: Ethical issues in pediatric palliative care. In K. J. Doka and A. S. Tucci (Eds.), *Living with grief: Children and adolescents* (pp. 99-119). Washington, DC: Hospice Foundation of America.

Meade, K. & Friebert, S. (2012). Informed decision making and the adolescent patient. In K. J. Doka, A. S. Tucci., C. A. Corr & B. Jennings (Eds.), *End-of-life ethics: A case study approach* (pp. 231-241). Washington, DC: Hospice Foundation of America.

Selove, R., Cochran, D., & Cohen, I.T. (2008). Management of end-of-life pain and suffering in children and adolescents. In K. J. Doka and A. S. Tucci (Eds.), *Living with grief: Children and adolescents* (pp. 75-98). Washington, DC: Hospice Foundation of America.

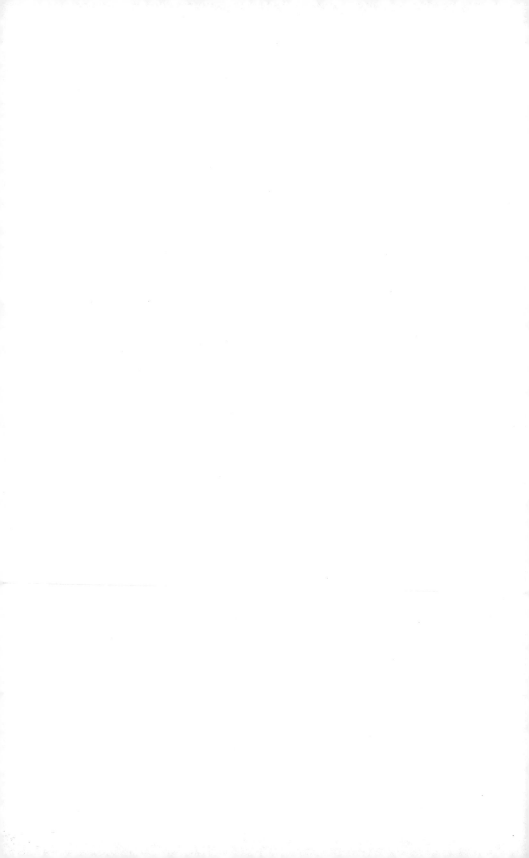

CHAPTER 2

Rights of Passage: Ethical Aspects of Adolescent End-of-Life Care

Bruce Jennings

T his chapter reviews salient ethical issues that arise in the context of adolescent health care and decision making. It pays special attention to decision making near the end of life by those adolescents in the terminal phase of an incurable illness for whom palliative and hospice care services offer important benefit. The discussion will proceed in three steps.

First, I discuss the values and psychosocial assumptions that underlie the category of adolescence in our culture. I note significant differences between an age-graded categorical approach to rights and decision-making autonomy and a functional and developmental approach. The former is still largely operative in the law, while the latter is more common in clinical practice settings.

Second, I consider the current developmental viewpoint concerning adolescent capability in relation to common standards of decision-making capacity, informed consent, and reasonable judgment. These standards are not solely empirical or operational in character; they are also value-laden. A focus on the special features of adolescent reasoning suggests that neither the standard bioethics account of individualistic autonomy nor the account of objective, paternalistic best interests (beneficence) fits well with the health care situation of most adolescents. A more relational and contextualized concept of autonomy and patient rights is needed.

Finally, I address decisions to forgo life-sustaining medical treatments and to adopt palliative and hospice care plans in light of an expanded ethical role for relational autonomy for adolescent patients. The emerging consensus holds that end-of-life care decision making should be *decision making with* adolescents, rather than *decision making for* them by others. Adolescents with chronic or life-threatening illness can and should have a central voice in the health care decision-making process, in partnership with their physicians and other health professionals and in cooperation with their parents and families. Moreover, when disease-modifying treatments reach a stage where they are unavailing and more burdensome than beneficial, the personal values and preferences of the adolescent individual should be the touchstone of palliative care planning and decision making.

CATEGORICAL AND DEVELOPMENTAL RIGHTS

American society has one set of rules for the care and governance of typical children and another set for typical adults (Scott, 2000; Hartman, 2000). The dividing line between these sets of rules is chronological age, and the legal age of majority (adulthood) is 18. In the case of children, including adolescents (defined in this chapter as those between 14 and 18), custodial adults (usually biological or adoptive parents) are entrusted to guide and control the child in accordance with that child's safety and long-term best interests. Children are not permitted to autonomously govern themselves. Adults, on the contrary, are granted the presumptive legal and moral right to be self-directing and autonomous. In virtually all sectors of society, professionals and officials give considerable deference and latitude to adult autonomy and virtually none at all to the autonomy of children, including adolescents.

One exception to this is in the system of criminal justice, where some stress the autonomy and hence the responsibility of juvenile offenders as a rationale for placing them in the adult criminal justice system. (Those who advocate for a separate juvenile justice and court system, aimed more at rehabilitation than at punishment, do stress the lack of competency, autonomy, and responsibility of juvenile offenders.)

However, this pattern is very well illustrated in health care. In the health care system adults are granted autonomy to make their own decisions and may not be treated (except in some emergency situations) without their informed consent. Adults have a legal and ethical right to forgo any and all forms of medical treatment, even life-prolonging medical treatment. (In a few states, terminally ill adults have the additional right to actively enlist the assistance of physicians in ending their life in accordance with their informed decision and at a time of their own choosing.) The autonomy of adults may also be exercised indirectly through the actions of health care proxies and surrogate decision makers, who have been authorized by the patient ahead of time or by state statute. Only as an ethical and legal last resort, when the autonomous preferences and choices of the patient are not knowable, is an objective best interest standard applied to adult health care near the end of life. With children, on the other hand, the best interest standard is the ethical gold standard at all times, including in decisions concerning life-sustaining medical treatment (Mutcherson, 2005; Scott, 2000; Hartman, 2000).

Categorical groupings such as grading by chronological age often encounter problematic cases at the margins of the categories and by individuals or groups who seem to require treatment and assessment that goes beyond chronological age alone. Categorical ways of thinking are also in tension with thinking that sees human capabilities as developing over time along a spectrum or a functional continuum. This developmental approach does not make capacity, autonomy, and certain rights an all-or-nothing proposition, but admits of degrees of capacity based on contextual and task-specific situations. Categorical approaches are quite general and undifferentiated, and they are therefore efficient and equitable when it is very costly or difficult to make individuated assessments on a case-by-case basis. But categorical approaches also make mistakes of overinclusion and underinclusion precisely because they are not fine-grained enough to discern individual differences that may be ethically relevant to fair and appropriate treatment.

Adolescents reside at the margins of our age-graded legal and ethical system. What shall we do with them? The way adolescents are viewed and the degree of rights and autonomy granted to them are changing in medicine, ethics, and, more slowly, in the law. Developmental thinking is challenging categorical thinking.

Human beings in their teenage years both inspire and trouble the societies in which they live. Their vitality and promise provide hope and renewal. Teaching, working with, and caring for them are surely among the most fulfilling adult vocations. Their tastes and fashions play an important role in our consumer economy, and they drive popular media and entertainment. On the other hand, they indulge in risky behavior and pose many public health and law enforcement problems. When they make serious mistakes, the long-term ramifications can be costly and severe. Intelligent and physically capable, yet impulsive and clumsy; wanting to be accepted and aloof at the same time; needing the haven of familiarity and family yet seeking novelty and independence—teens both challenge social norms and represent the future continuity of those norms. It is little wonder that ethics has trouble fitting these dynamic persons into its frameworks and categories. Especially when it comes to the ethical standards of medical care and decision making, the second decade of life presents a number of dilemmas and enigmas.

ADOLESCENT DECISION-MAKING CAPACITY AND CAPABILITY

The passage from childhood to adulthood is significant in every society, although its prescribed forms and rituals vary greatly in different cultures and historical periods. The significance of adolescence is both biological and social. Biologically the years of puberty represent one of the two major developmental and growth surges of the human lifespan. (The other surge takes place in the first three years of life.) A hormonal cascade rapidly develops the reproductive system and changes body size and shape. Accelerated development takes place in the brain, affecting emotional intensity and executive function. Concomitantly, behavioral capabilities and cognitive skills become more extensive and complex. Socially, the second decade of life is a time of a widening world of groups and relationships outside the immediate family and a time of deepening self-awareness and emerging individuated self-identity. The biological and the social must be fit together in the second decade, but there is no single right or best way to do that.

In its most general sense biology and society coexist with a system of rules, roles, and relationships, and every society categorizes and classifies individuals in certain ways. Life-stage concepts such as infancy, childhood, adolescence, adulthood, and old age do have an underlying biological rationale, but ultimately they are conventional and shift over time.

It is important to bear in mind the distinction between how persons at different ages are classified in terms of their autonomy or rights of choice and self-direction, on the one hand, and rules concerning what kinds of treatment and social activities are allowable for persons in certain age groups, on the other. The age at which a person may drive a car, legally marry, quit school, join the military, vote, or consume alcoholic beverages are all examples of the age-based classifications of autonomy. Child labor laws, rules concerning endangering a minor, corporal punishment, and the like are examples of the latter. Both of these kinds of rules vary tremendously cross-culturally and historically.

As noted earlier, childhood and adulthood (the age of minority and the age of majority) are the core functional categories of the classification system traditional and widespread in the law. Contemporary societies have elided adolescence from childhood as a kind of transitional or liminal zone. And this makes sense from a physical, sexual, cognitive, and social perspective. The law presumes competency on the part of those over age 18 and bestows autonomy rights on them despite manifest functional or capability differences among adults. The law presumes incompetency for those under 18 and denies autonomy rights to them. However, a functional, developmental focus on capability rather than competence is changing some of our norms and practices. Today adolescents may be permitted to do many of the things that adults do regarding their health care, provided that they have demonstrated the ability to do so safely to the satisfaction of either the parents or the state.

Three important innovations in American law should be noted (Scott, 2000; Hartman, 2000; Rosato, 2002). The first is the passage of the 26th Amendment to the United States Constitution, changing the voting rights age from 21 to 18. This was the result of a decade-long grassroots movement that generally disseminated new scientific information about the true cognitive capacities of individuals in the age group between 18 and 21. The cognitive and reasoning abilities necessary for responsible decision making as democratic citizens are clearly in place by age 18. As it has turned out, research since the 1960s has actually extended those findings to an earlier age, roughly 14 to15, in many, perhaps most minors. If adolescents are permitted to make adult decisions and judgment on a par with adults in the political realm, they should be permitted to do so in other realms of life and choice as well, including medical decisions that affect the person's future prospects and quality of life. In addition to a capability argument, however, lowering the voting age was motivated by a fairness argument brought to the fore by the context of military conscription and the war in Southeast Asia. If 18-year-olds can be drafted and sent into combat in Vietnam, they should also be democratically enfranchised. Only in this way can they have an influence on public policies that greatly affect their lives and perhaps even their deaths.

In lowering the voting age to 18 as a matter of constitutional right, the 26th Amendment changed the legal age of majority and turned former children ages 18 to 20 into legal adults. Two other legal innovations did not move some former children into the group of adults, but rather created special rights for a particular class of children who remained minors, but who now have increased protection, authority, and freedom through their parents.

One of these is the notion of the "emancipated minor." Life situations such as living independently and being financially independent, marrying, and bearing a child take the person out of the childhood situation of dependency on the nuclear family and the custodial parent(s). These special circumstances place the emancipated minor, who is virtually always an adolescent, in a situation that functionally resembles adulthood, and therefore in many states the law recognizes the adult rights of those minors to make autonomous decisions in many areas of life, including health care.

The second innovation that carves out special rights and freedoms for minors is the notion of the "mature minor." This innovation has arisen largely in the context of reproductive health care and in the context of public health concerning sexually transmitted diseases and drug abuse. In these settings, the normal presumption that the custodial parents will act in the best interest of the child is called into question by the extremely controversial and sensitive nature of the health care at issue. Adolescent girls seeking to obtain a legal first trimester abortion may be dangerously delayed or blocked altogether by dissenting parents if prior parental notification and consent are needed. And these adolescents may be subject to reprisals after the fact for accessing health care services. This may deter them from seeking an abortion, contraception, counseling for drug problems, or medical treatment for a sexually transmitted disease in the first place. In cases of conflict such as these, a judicial mechanism has been created for mature minors that can bypass parental notification and consent.

Mature minors do not meet the criteria of emancipation; they are a distinct group. The mature minor doctrine singles out some adolescents of demonstrated capacity and grants to them decisional autonomy to give informed consent to medical treatment. It represents a shift from an age-graded system of rights to a more functional and situational approach. In this regard the law in some cases resembles the process of capacity assessment and communication that takes place in good clinical settings, and indeed the law largely defers to the clinical process. In the judicial bypass mechanism, however, judges themselves, not health professionals, must directly determine the maturity or capacity of the individual before the minor is granted a special kind of autonomy.

Generally speaking then, adolescence is not currently a privileged category that grants substantial autonomy rights in the eyes of the law. However, adolescence is of considerable interest as a distinct social, functional, and developmental category in the eyes of the social and behavioral sciences and the clinical professions. Social scientists, more interested in questions of psychosocial development and behavior than in social order and protection, have described adolescence in some detail.

It is generally agreed that around age 14 individuals have reached a level of reasoning and understanding, and have the ability to compare options and consequences, on a par with that of adults. Some see adolescence as the period between achieving adult-equivalent decision making capacity and reaching the legal age of majority: roughly ages 14 to 18. Others define adolescence as a decade-long developmental continuum beginning roughly at the onset of puberty and concluding with complete physical and neurological maturation in the early 20s. This continuum has been divided into three phases: early adolescence (10 to 14), middle adolescence (15 to 17), and late adolescence (18 to 20+). The early phase typically shifts attachment from family to peers. The middle phase develops self-image and a sense of self-efficacy. The late phase consolidates confidence and the ability to form lasting attachments (Hamburg, 1998; Klopfenstein, 1999).

It is important to note that this developmental view does not define distinct thresholds but sees instead a more gradual transformation taking place in the adolescent years that varies in pace and extent from person to person. This is particularly important for the adolescent role in health care decision making because individuated assessments of the elements of informed consent, although complex and time-consuming, can be practically made in clinical settings and in the context of an ongoing physician-patient relationship (Leikin, 1993).

For any person, adult or adolescent, a functional demonstration of the capability to make informed medical decisions involves several cognitive elements. One must have the ability to reason and to consider many elements in forming expectations about future consequences of a decision. One must be able to comprehend essential medical and factual information that has a bearing on the consequences of a given decision. One must be able to appreciate the seriousness of a given choice in terms of its permanent or long-lasting effects on the individual and on others. Finally one must have achieved sufficient self-esteem and self-confidence to act independently of other authority figures, family, and friends (Faden & Beauchamp, 1986).

Another important factor is the person's understanding of death. Younger children tend to see death as temporary, reversible, and as something happening outside their world and only to others, or as something caused by some previous thoughts or actions. Adolescent development brings about an awareness of death as something permanent and universal (Freyer, 2004). The threat of death gradually comes to be seen as a danger against which one can take precautions. Many researchers have found that even preteens (8 to 10 years old) are capable of attaining this attitude toward death (Foley & Whittam, 1990). Life experience with death (or the prospect of death) is a key factor in this cognitive development, and it is a particularly important factor among children who have lived with serious chronic illness and life-threatening illness.

Today there is a broad consensus among experts that by about age 14 (or middle adolescence) most teens do in fact have those cognitive capabilities (Freyer, 2004; Freyer, 1992). Reflecting this consensus, new ethics guidelines from The Hastings Center on end-of-life care propose the following standard:

> From fourteen years of age onward, the decision-making capacity of adolescents should be respected. As appropriate based on individual assessment, they should be offered opportunities to make informed choices and to participate with their parents or guardians in decisions about their treatment and care (Berlinger, Jennings, & Wolf, 2013, p. 85).

Therefore, the presumption of clinical practice and decision making should be that middle and late adolescents are capable of giving informed consent or informed refusal concerning their medical care. Although until the child reaches age 18 the parents will be the legally authorized health care decision makers of record, they should be strongly guided by the preferences and judgments of their adolescent children. Failure to do so is to overlook the insight that adolescents often have concerning their own illness and medical care (Traugott & Alpers, 1997). It is to deny individuals with solid capabilities autonomy rights that are well recognized in the world today and that deserve respect from parents and professionals (Rosato, 1996). And it is to deprive the child of a significant opportunity to benefit from the experience of participation in one's own health care decision making as a way of furthering the process of maturation and development that is a requisite part of adolescence itself (Smetana, Campione-Barr, & Metzger, 2006). Adolescents who will survive the medical care in which they have been empowered to participate as an agent, and not merely as a passive patient, will benefit from this experience in many ways that go beyond their successful medical care and rescue itself.

DISTINCT ISSUES IN ADOLESCENT END-OF-LIFE CARE

The considerations mentioned above pertain to health care decision making generally, regardless of the etiology of the illness or its prognosis. When we enter the realm of decision making concerning the use of life-sustaining treatments and technologies, however, additional considerations come into play. Death is an intruder at all ages, but it is especially unseemly during childhood and adolescence. In developed societies pediatric deaths are infrequent and make up a small part of all annual deaths. Between 2000 and 2010 the U.S. death rate among those aged 1 to 24 years went down from 72.1 per 100,000 population to 60.7. The leading causes of death in this age group were unintentional injuries (38%), homicide (13%), suicide (12%), cancer (7%), and heart disease (3%). All other causes accounted for 25 percent of deaths (Miniño & Murphy 2012). Total deaths for adolescents are difficult to determine because of the ways age classes are defined in Census data. In 2010 it is estimated that there were approximately 5,271 deaths in the 5 to14 age group and 29,519 among those age 15 to 24 (Murphy, Xu, & Kochanek, 2012). The leading causes of adolescent death—accident, homicide, and suicide—are directly related to psychosocial factors, physicality, and risk taking. Nonetheless, a decade ago it was estimated that approximately 3000 adolescents die each year following a prolonged illness (cancer, heart disease, AIDS, pulmonary disease) and metabolic disorders and congenital anomalies (Freyer, 2004).

One factor that has a special bearing on the autonomy and decision-making capacity of adolescents in end-of-life care is the experience of chronic illness itself. Various forms of medical treatment, frequent hospitalizations for procedures or acute episodes, disruptive medical regimens of diet, restricted physical and social activity, drug therapy with its untoward side effects, and many other similar experiences may have punctuated the entire childhood of the individual will color his or her outlook on self-identity, body, and illness. By the time the child reaches adolescence—and as the chronic illness progresses and becomes seriously life-threatening—this background will be a salient factor in the teen's attitudes and capability. Clinical experience suggests that life experience with chronic illness enhances the adolescent's decision-making capacity by giving him or her a realistic and more mature outlook on treatment options, prognosis, and quality of life. And, as was mentioned earlier, the experience of chronic illness tends to give the child and adolescent a more mature attitude toward death than one might expect previously healthy teens to have if suddenly faced with the prospect of a terminal illness.

Another crucial factor is suggested by the fact that those adolescents who face end-of-life treatment decisions and who may benefit from hospice and palliative care almost all have long experience with a chronic condition. As a result, their parents' knowledge, emotions, and attitudes have been shaped by that chronic illness experience as well. Also affected are the dynamics of their family's communication and decision-making style. The learning curve of chronic care and the common bonds forged in coping with chronic illness can form a powerful and constructive platform for good communication and respectful treatment of adolescents near the end of life.

These considerations do not suggest that end-of-life decision making for adolescents will be easy or trouble free (Traugott & Alpers, 1997). Nor does long experience with chronic illness necessarily guard against errors of overtreatment or undertreatment near the end of life. Parents may continue to seek disease-modifying treatments, even experimental treatments, as a result of this experience, and may be reluctant to relinquish control. Likewise, the experience of serious chronic illness may have induced in the adolescent a dependency and passivity that is in contrast to normal adolescent development. Thus even if their autonomy is recognized and respected, it does not follow that all adolescents will welcome it or use their role in medical decision making to express their own voice in all cases (Lyon, McCabe, Patel, & D'Angelo, 2004).

Advance directives (durable powers of attorney for health care or "proxies" and explicit treatment directives or "living wills") have been devised to deal with adult decision making in the face of the loss of decision-making capacity. Current laws do not permit minors to execute advance health care directives. One suggested approach to deal with some of the possible pitfalls of a breakdown of agreement between adolescent patients and their parents is to extend the notion of an advance directive, from situations of lost adult competence to the situation in which adult competence has not yet been attained (Weir & Peters, 1997). While the parents will remain the legal surrogate decision makers for dying adolescents, they should be guided by specific indications of their adolescent child's own values and preferences rather than by some impersonal standard of best interests. Adolescents who are capable of participating in their own health care decision making are also capable of creating an "advance directive" in this sense (McCabe, Rushton, Glover, Murray, & Leikin, 1996). It is simply a way of clearly recording, for the benefit of both parents and third parties, what they should be talking about and discussing with their parents at home and at the bedside.

The empowerment of adolescent patients in end-of-life decision making is based on their putative cognitive capabilities and maturity. But this rationale remains controversial, often heatedly so. Consider the widely publicized case of a 15-year-old boy named Starchild Abraham Cherrix who in 2005 was diagnosed with Hodgkin disease, a form of lymphoma that often responds well to treatment (Associated Press, 2006). After an initial round of chemotherapy was not successful, in 2006 Abraham refused additional chemotherapy or radiation due to the side effects and opted instead to undergo alternative therapy. His parents agreed, but the state accused them of medical neglect and a lower court ruled against the parents, ordering conventional treatment to resume for Abraham (who was then 16), over the objections of both him and his parents. However, that decision was overturned on appeal and a compromise was reached in which Abraham would undergo alternative therapy under the supervision of a board certified oncologist and the court would monitor his condition until he turned 18.

Inspired by this dispute, the following year the Virginia legislature enacted a statute that has come to be known as "Abraham's Law." It establishes the right to refuse medically recommended treatment for adolescents 14 and older who have a life-threatening illness, if the following conditions are met: the parents and the adolescent make this decision jointly; the patient is capable of making an informed choice; a range of treatments have been considered; and the parents are acting in the best interest of their child. If these conditions are fulfilled the parents are protected from charges of medical neglect if they concur in the decision to forgo medically recommended treatment (Mercurio, 2007).

Affirming the rights of adolescents in medical decision making involving life-threatening conditions has also been controversial within the field of bioethics. It has been challenged in the clinical and the bioethics literature in two ways (Ross, 1997). First, it has been argued that adolescents do have a tendency to prioritize (and they seek unduly to avoid) short-term problems related to their social acceptance, physical appearance, and treatment side effects over the long-term benefits of disease-modifying and life-prolonging treatment. Greater empowerment of their autonomous perspective may risk decision making that is not in the best interests of the adolescent from an adult point of view. It may not reflect a reasonable assessment of treatment benefits and burdens. These arguments conclude that while adolescents do have autonomy rights, they also have a right to an open future that should not be cut short on the basis of not yet fully-formed values and preferences.

A second line of argument critical of adolescent autonomy in end-of-life care is that it is overly individualistic. Framing the dynamics of end-of-life decision making in terms of clashing rights and separate interests among individuals is both ethically and psychosocially mistaken. It will undermine the important protective and nurturing role of the parents in many individual cases, and it may more generally undermine the integrity of the family unit in society and culture.

Clearly, each of these arguments deserves to be taken seriously, especially from the perspective of hospice. Hospice and palliative care have no interest in depriving anyone of efficacious life-sustaining treatment with the prospect of return to a meaningful quality of life, and doing so would be in conflict with fundamental hospice values. Moreover, hospice has a long-standing concern for the well-being of entire families, and it approaches the dying individual in the context of a family system. The understanding of autonomy that comports best with hospice and palliative care is not a notion of highly individualistic and adversarial negative liberty, but rather a relational notion of care and a recognition of the dignity of the human person and the respect owed by others for that dignity (Eccles et al., 1991). In the literature of bioethics, this conceptual distinction is marked by the terms, "individualistic autonomy" and "relational autonomy" (Mackenzie & Stoljar, 2000; Jennings, 2009; Nedelsky, 2011).

There is an important distinction between short-term quality of life judgments of the kind that adolescents may be prone to make and longer-term adult judgments about open futures. One factor that complicates matters when adolescents have reached the point where further disease-modifying therapy is unavailing is the fact that this distinction tends to break down. When adolescents and their parents are deciding to implement a palliative care plan, there need be no stark conflict between adolescent autonomy and adult paternalism. The future offered by hospice and palliative care is the open future in these cases.

The central point to take from the current understanding of the role of the adolescent in end-of-life care decision making, however, is the importance of good communication and a realistic and trusting relationship among the adolescent, the parents and other family members, and the health care professionals. From this point of view, one of the best advantages of the chronic illness experience is that there may be a well-functioning physician-patient-family relationship already established. This can be built on as the decision-making process moves into the end-of-life-care phase.

THE CRUCIAL ROLE OF HOSPICE PROFESSIONALS

Recognizing and respecting the rights of passage for dying adolescents is not easy in our culture and health care system. It faces many legal, cultural, emotional, and institutional barriers. Those who study adolescent development, and work closely with this population, see the exciting achievements and growth that this remarkable time of life represents. Unfortunately, our dominant cultural images of adolescence are often otherwise. So the empowerment of adolescent autonomy continues to be an uphill battle despite the progress that has been made in the past decade in the law and especially in ethics and in the changing clinical practice in pediatrics and adolescent medicine.

The time is right for physicians, nurses, and other health care professionals in hospice and palliative care to join in this creative new clinical environment on behalf of those relatively small numbers of teens who come to the final chapter in lives. Those lives will not be of normal length, but they nonetheless can be complete, if they receive good hospice or palliative care. Taking the dying adolescent's voice more seriously and giving it a more prominent role in the end-of-life care decision-making process requires the tact, patience, and skill of those whose profession is healing and finding meaning. Those in adolescent medicine, pediatric oncology, and other specialties, who have been caring well for these patients earlier, sometimes for many years, can benefit from the cognate communication and trust building skills of their colleagues in palliative care (Himelstein, Hilden, Boldt, & Weissman, 2004).

The ambivalence of the elderly dying and their families is powerful and challenging, but no more so than how torn people tend to be when death comes to an adolescent (or a younger child). If it is a unique caregiving challenge, and I think it is, then it may be because the passage in question is two-fold.

One passage is the passage of the dying process, of course. But in the midst of this, another passage is taking place, a passage from being one who is always guided to being one who is self-directing; from being one who is shaped by others to being one who has taken shape and can now act to impress his or her own mark on the world. This is important even when one's remaining time in the world is very limited. Terminal illness will foreshorten a life, but it need not always deprive the last times of that life of the experience of finding one's own voice and of experiencing the recognition of effective personhood.

Each of these two passages has rights of self-determination, recognition, agency, and dignity that must be respected as a matter of justice. Dying adolescents must receive these rights at the same time, instead of having them separated by many decades in the life span. One of the great challenges in the years ahead for hospice and palliative care is to function effectively in partnership with dying adolescents and their families. The value on sensitivity, the holistic practice orientation, the experience of orchestrating effective communication and sustaining relationships during the hard times of life—each of these hallmarks of hospice and palliative care expertise will serve the field well as it rises to the occasion of this challenge.

Bruce Jennings is director of bioethics at the Center for Humans and Nature and holds faculty appointments at the Yale School of Public Health and the New York Medical College. He is also a Fellow and Senior Advisor at The Hastings Center. He is author of many works on end of life and palliative care, including Access to Hospice Care: Expanding Boundaries, Overcoming Barriers *(2003) and* The Hastings Center Guidelines for Decisions on Life-Sustaining Treatment and Care Near the End of Life *(2013). His new book,* Hospice Ethics, *co-edited with Timothy W. Kirk, will be published by Oxford University Press in 2014.*

References

Associated Press. (2006). *Teen, court reach agreement over cancer care.* Retrieved from www.nbcnews.com/id/14371567

Berlinger, N., Jennings, B., and Wolf, S. M. (2013). *Hastings Center guidelines for decisions on life-sustaining treatment and care near the end of life*, Revised and Expanded Second Edition (pp. 67-88). New York, NY: Oxford University Press.

Eccles, J. S., Buchanan, C. M., Flanagan, C., Fuligni, A., Midgley, C., & Yee, D. (1991). Control Versus Autonomy During Early Adolescence. *Journal of Social Issues, 47*, 53-68.

Faden, R. R. & Beauchamp, T. L. (1986). *A history and theory of informed consent.* New York, NY: Oxford University Press.

Foley, G. V. and Whittam, E. H. (1990). Care of the child dying of cancer: Part 1. *CA: A Cancer Journal for Clinicians, 40*, 327-354.

Freyer, D. R. (2004). Care of the dying adolescent: Special considerations. *Pediatrics, 113*, 381-388.

Freyer, D. R. (1992). Children with cancer: Special considerations in the discontinuation of life-sustaining treatment. *Medical and Pediatric Oncology, 34*, 532-536.

Hamburg, B. A. (1998). Psychosocial development. In S. B. Friedman, M. M. Fischer, S. K. Schonberg, and E. M. Alderman (Eds.), *Comprehensive Adolescent Health Care*, 2nd ed. (pp. 38-49). St. Louis, MO: Mosby.

Hartman, R. G. (2000). Adolescent autonomy: Clarifying an ageless conundrum. *Hastings Law Journal, 51*, 1265-1362.

Himelstein, B. P., Hilden, J. M., Boldt, A. M., & Weissman, D. (2004). Pediatric palliative care. *New England Journal of Medicine, 350*, 1752-1762.

Jennings, B. (2009). Public health and liberty. *Public Health Ethics, 2*, 123-134.

Klopfenstein, K. J. (1999). Adolescents, cancer, and hospice. *Adolescent Medicine, 10*, 437-443.

Leikin, S. (1993). The role of adolescents in decisions concerning their cancer therapy. *Cancer, 71*, (Supplement): 3342-3346.

Lyon, M. E., McCabe, M. A., Patel, K. M., & D'Angelo, L. J. (2004). What do adolescents want? An exploratory study regarding end-of-life decision-making. *Journal of Adolescent Health, 35*, 529.e1-529.e6.

McCabe, M. A., Rushton, C. H., Glover, J., Murray, M. G., & Leikin, S. (1996). Implications of the Patient Self-Determination Act: Guidelines for involving adolescents in medical decision making. *Journal of Adolescent Health, 19*, 319-324.

Mackenzie, C. & Stoljar, N. (Eds.). (2000). *Relational autonomy: Feminist perspectives on autonomy, agency, and the social self.* New York, NY: Oxford University Press.

Mercurio, M. R. (2007). An adolescent's refusal of medical treatment: Implications of the Abraham Cheerix case. *Pediatrics, 120, 6* (December), 1357-1358.

Miniño, A. M. & Murphy, S. L. (2012). Death in the United States, 2010. NCHS Data Brief, No. 99, (July) Retrieved from http://www.cdc.gov/nchs/data/databriefs/db99.htm

Murphy, S. L., Xu, J., & Kochanek, K. D. (2012). Deaths: Preliminary Data for 2010. National Vital Statistics Reports, *60, 4* (January 11), 1-52. doi: 198.246.124.22

Mutcherson, K. M. (2005). Whose body is it anyway? An updated model of health care decision-making rights for adolescents. *Cornell Journal of Law and Public Policy, 14*, 252-325.

Nedelsky, J. (2011). *Law's relations: A relational theory of self, autonomy, and law.* New York, NY: Oxford University Press.

Rosato, J. L. (2002). Let's get real: Quilting a principled approach to adolescent empowerment in health care decision-making. *DePaul Law Review, 51,* 769-803.

Rosato, J. L. (1996). The ultimate test of autonomy: Should minors have a right to make decisions regarding life-sustaining treatment? *Rutgers Law Review, 49,* 3-105.

Ross, L. F. (1997). Health care decisionmaking by children: Is it in their best interest? *Hastings Center Report, 27,* 41-45.

Scott, E. S. (2000). The legal construction of adolescence. *Hofstra Law Review, 29,* 547-598.

Smetana, J. G., Campione-Barr, N., & Metzger, A. (2006). Adolescent development in interpersonal and societal contexts. *Annual Review of Psychology, 57,* 255-284.

Traugott, I. & Alpers, A. (1997). In their own hands: Adolescent's refusals of medical treatment. *Archives of Pediatric Adolescent Medicine, 151,* 922-927.

Weir, R. F. & Peters, C. (1997). Affirming the decisions adolescents make about life and death. *Hastings Center Report, 27,* 29-40.

CHAPTER 3

Adolescence and Emerging Adulthood: A Developmental Perspective

David E. Balk

The anticipated life crises that shape adolescents form a triad of developmental transitions youth are expected to traverse in their passage to young adulthood. Mastering these developmental transitions, adolescents gain increased maturity. Operationally, society expects young persons to become adults by achieving individual autonomy, a clear sense of direction in how to make a living, and intimate friendships.

Unanticipated life crises, the types of challenges that ambush persons at any stage of development, occur for adolescents as they cope with the developmental transitions we expect them to master. Two clear examples of unanticipated life crises are being stricken with a life-threatening illness and being left bereft over the death of a family member or friend. This chapter will examine the overarching developmental transitions which shape the journey into young adulthood and which form the back story for any adolescent grappling with a life-threatening illness or bereavement.

I have organized the chapter according to the three life phases into which scholars divide adolescent development: early, middle, and later adolescence. Then I have presented the case of a young woman's adolescent journey. I have made use of the holistic conceptual framework as a perspective for understanding the richness of the changes that mark adolescent development, particularly when coping with an illness or with bereavement.

THREE LIFE PHASES

Peter Blos (1979) introduced distinctions regarding three separate phases that distinguish changes over time during adolescence. These three phases are early, middle, and later adolescence. The age ranges for the phases are somewhat arbitrarily set as 10 to14 for early adolescence, 15 to17 for middle adolescence, and 18 to 23 for later adolescence. Entrance into early adolescence is marked by the onset of puberty. Hard and fast boundaries between these phases are elusive. The demarcations between early and middle adolescence and between middle and later adolescence coincide with the traditional ages when youth in the United States begin certain forms of schooling: the movement into middle adolescence coincides with entering high school, and the movement into later adolescence coincides with entering college. Of course a large proportion of youth never goes to college but rather enters the work force or enlists in the military, and some never finish high school. So basing the three phases of adolescent development upon ages of schooling is at best heuristic. A much more critical set of criteria encompasses developmental issues youth are expected to grapple with and master in these three phases of growing up.

At the beginning of this chapter I mentioned the overarching developmental transitions contemporary society expects young people to master on the journey to becoming productive adults: establishing an autonomous self-identity, forging a sense of purpose and direction, and achieving fidelity in intimate interpersonal relationships. These three fundamental transitions form the primary crucible within which individual maturity is shaped.

Within the early adolescent phase of development, the central challenge facing youth, at least in Western developed countries, involves separating emotionally from the security of parental authority. Two ways early adolescents show they are engaging in separating emotionally from their parents are (a) preferring to spend increasing amounts of time with peers and (b) resisting, in fact practically abhorring, any public parental displays of affection for them.

Within the middle adolescent phase of development, the central challenge facing youth builds on the efforts to achieve emotional independence from parents, and now the challenge accentuates gaining increased autonomy and self-efficacy. Parents still need to enforce limits, but when parents have been shaping their children to accept greater responsibility, these limits relax some. There is a growth in belief in one's self-efficacy, which occurs almost tacitly, as middle adolescents act on this expression of trust.

Within the later adolescent phase of development, the central challenge builds on the growth in emotional separation from parents and in the self-confidence that one can achieve things that matter. The central challenge for later adolescence involves entering into and maintaining relationships of intimacy and love. In addition, building on mastery of the central challenges in early and middle adolescence, the individual has a greater repertoire of knowledge and skills to become her or his own person and to select a specific direction whereby earning a living will be possible and fit the young adult's self-concept.

These musings on the developmental transitions, issues, and challenges faced in the three phases to adolescent development are guideposts. They remain notional until given specific, existential examples with an individual's life. Further, the transitions do not occur overnight but emerge gradually as the adolescent makes choices in the early, middle, and later phases of adolescence. The choices involve judging the predictability of existence, belonging to a specific human group, developing a viewpoint about fairness and justice, believing in one's self-efficacy, and forming an integrated self-concept. The decisions an adolescent makes about these five choices, superimposed on decisions made about personal autonomy, self-direction, and interpersonal relationships, form the adolescent's assumptive world.

An adolescent's decisions obviously will be shaped by dilemmas the youth faces. Adolescents coping with a life-threatening illness or grieving the death of a family member or friend will very likely be forced to adjust her or his assumptions about reality. To understand grappling with assaults on an adolescent's assumptive world, I have used a case of a late adolescent female coping with various pressures that test individuals. The case will be used to examine developments in light of issues defining growth into young adulthood.

A CASE OF AN ADOLESCENT BECOMING A YOUNG ADULT

Helene was finishing her baccalaureate in the late 1990s at one of the state universities, located in her home town. When we pick up this story, Helene is a senior studying history. She is a good student. First, we will move back in time to look at some earlier experiences in her life.

Helene's maternal grandfather died after an extended illness when Helene had just entered early adolescence. She responded resiliently and gave no indications over the coming months and years that the death troubled her. She was grateful to be in a family in which people talked about death and grief. She was particularly grateful for a mother who had a keen intuitive grasp of what was the right thing to do and acted on that knowledge.

A difficult transition occurred when, a few weeks prior to her grandfather's death, her family had moved across the country so her father could take a new job. Helene had left several good friends, and the changes encountered in her new school were not always easy. Particularly galling was the clique of privileged students who basically ran social life at the elementary school.

Things got much better when in two years she moved to the town's middle school. There were many more students at the middle school than were in her elementary school, and the school was not dominated by the small clique of privileged youth whom Helene did not care for. She gravitated to persons she liked, did well in her studies, and moved on to high school.

In high school Helene continued to do well. Her friends were non-conformists and definitely none was a member of the elite clique of "preppies" and "jocks." She took advanced placement courses, graduated, and then moved on to the university. She loved history and liked the environment of a university. Following her undergraduate program, she worked on campus for a racial diversity project and for a university program whose mission is to help students at risk of dropping out.

While in college, Helene was infected with mononucleosis, strep throat, and tonsillitis. It is plausible that her medical complications as a young adult can be attributed to after-effects of a weakened immune system caused during this cascade of illnesses, specifically by mononucleosis. In her middle twenties she began to have sudden, unpredictable episodes of vomiting. She would be fine, suddenly say, "You'd better take me home," and then within five seconds be vomiting violently. Eventually medical tests identified she had Graves disease, an immune system disorder causing an excessive production of thyroid hormones. The medical decision was to use radioactive iodine therapy to inactivate her thyroid and then find a regimen of medication to supply the needed hormones a healthy thyroid produces. Finding this medication dosage can be tricky. At one test her hormone levels were so compromised that her physician told her, "You should be dead."

Developmental transitions and life choices

Let's look at Helene in terms of the three major developmental transitions and five choices that mark the adolescent journey to young adulthood. In short, we will look at how Helene engaged these elements of growing up: (a) becoming an autonomous person, (b) gaining self-direction, (c) investing in interpersonal relationships, (d) assessing the predictability of existence, (e) gaining a sense of belonging to a specific human group, (f) developing a viewpoint about fairness and justice, (g) believing in one's self-efficacy, and (h) forming an integrated self-concept.

Helene and autonomy

Helene's parents acknowledge that from early childhood she had manifested a sense of independence. She was not willful, but rather chose activities that appealed to her regardless whether other children joined in. Thus, often during her free time as a young child in day care, Helene would be seen on her own reading books while the rest of the children would be engaged in other activities.

As an early adolescent she had appreciated rides with her father to middle school, but she was adamant that he would not kiss her goodbye in front of her friends or any of the other middle school students. This near repulsion over visible signs of affection from her parents mellowed in Helene's high school days. By the time she was ready to attend college, she gladly walked about campus with her arm entwined in her father's and gave him a kiss on the cheek when meeting up with her friends and thanked him for going to lunch with her.

As a high school student she had burned over a teacher's response to an assignment Helene had finished regarding *The Odyssey*. Helene's teacher had said, "Write your opinion of Odysseus." Helene wrote that she thought he was, in effect, a male chauvinist, a bully, and a cheat. She used episodes from the book to support her claims. The teacher chastised Helene for being wrong. Helene thought the teacher cautious, prejudiced, and chained to convention. She also said to her dad, "She asked me for my opinion, and then she tells me I am wrong because I don't have the same opinion as her."

Helene and self-direction

Helene always enjoyed learning, and particularly liked reading well-written histories that examined how values were put into practice in different times and places. At one point she had thought of becoming a high school history teacher, but had to admit she would have found it difficult dealing with so many students who disliked school. Now she has decided to complete a graduate degree in adult education and land a job as a faculty member in a community college. Part of this self-direction comes from her commitment to help students who face barriers in succeeding in higher education.

Helene and interpersonal relationships

As a child Helene had entered new social situations with caution and some reluctance. The more experience she gained with adults and with school children, her hesitancy and caution disappeared. She manifests today a confidence in being with others. Her middle school years were ripe with strong attachments that could crumble unexpectedly; one such episode involved someone she thought of as a good friend who told other girls thoughts and feelings Helene had confided in her and considered private. This betrayal hurt Helene and made her more circumspect in trusting others. She has remained in contact with several friends since middle school, and she feels especially close to one of her roommates and to another young woman who was in her high school class. She prefers spending her free time either with her roommate or reading quietly on her own.

Helene and the predictability of existence

Helene is an empiricist, but she also knows that there are complexities to reality that cannot be reduced to whatever can be observed. She was not raised in a religious tradition. While not yet settled on her religious stance, she has accepted that there is a God, that evil seems to be beyond God's power to stop, and that miracles are implausible. She finds naïve the belief that God interferes with the order of events in the world. She has learned about the rosary, and enjoys saying it as a kind of meditation but not in any sense that she expects divine intervention to occur. She accepts that randomness can emerge and change people's lives; however, she believes that for the most part she can count on life being governed by probability rather than randomness. Part of this trust in predictability spills over into (a) trusting her judgment about the reliability and character of persons she meets and into (b) believing that working to make a difference in the lives of persons matters.

Her physical condition has been a considerable concern to Helene and the persons who love her. She feels confident in the realization that should her Graves disease get out of control, it is quite predictable what the outcome can be; and in her trust in good medical practice and proper self-maintenance to prevent such conditions from occurring.

Helene and belonging to a specific human group

While strong in her sense of personal autonomy, Helene realizes that part of her trust in herself comes from being accepted by others. She has a distinct group of friends. Since her days in elementary school, Helene has gravitated toward others her age who are non-conformists. She was thrilled to be in middle school because it got her out of the confines of a small elementary school dominated by preppies. The preppies were very conformist, but also elitists. As she put it, "they think they're better than everyone else just because their parents have lots of money." One day she wore an outfit to middle school that today she admits was "radical." A preppie came up to her and said, "I really hate that outfit you're wearing." To which Helene replied, "Then I suggest you not get one." She has volunteered at the community food bank and at the zoo. She now works at the university in a special program designed for retaining incoming students who likely will fail if left without guidance and structure. She has decided to write a master's thesis evaluating the program.

Helene and justice

Helene gravitates naturally, it would seem, to the underdog. As a middle school student, she organized a protest against U.S. involvement in the first Gulf war. In high school she vehemently protested to school administrators about an English teacher who, in front of the whole class, made fun of an exchange student from India who did not know what a Christmas tree was. In college she filed sexual harassment charges against a professor who had been suspected for years but against whom no student had been willing to take a stand.

Helene and self-efficacy

Helene has learned that she can accomplish things that matter to her. Further, she has resisted pressure to be mediocre. In elementary school she did well on a spelling test, and another student advised her to ease off "because then people won't expect much of you." Her elementary school sponsored a contest for students to draw the school mascot; the winning drawing would be used on school banners. Helene was in second grade at the time and was the only student that young to submit a drawing. She has learned she can help students who lack study skills learn how to study. She is confident she has the grades and experience and life goals that will interest graduate programs to accept her. She definitely has an internal locus of control.

Helene and self-concept

Self-concept is a multi-dimensional phenomenon. Each topic discussed directly above forms part of Helene's understanding of herself. Her success has helped her to recognize her gifts and to realize she has considerable promise. In addition to her sense of autonomy, self-direction, trust in the predictability of life, success in interpersonal relationships, being an integral part of several human groups, beliefs about fairness and justice, and attributions about self-efficacy, Helene has a wickedly funny sense of humor. Once when she had made a mistake, she joked about it and then said, "Remember, if you can't laugh at yourself, there are always others."

ANOTHER PERSPECTIVE TO CONSIDER

We have looked at two main aspects of adolescent development, each selected in the hopes of providing an enlightened framework for understanding the back story within which an adolescent copes with either a life-threatening illness or bereavement. The study of adolescent development is so diverse and deep that several salient features rightfully could be examined. To name a few, there are the dramatic physical and cognitive changes that occur during early, middle, and later adolescence. In addition, building on the cognitive changes that occur during adolescence, we could examine brain development, social perspective taking, interpersonal relations, constructivism, and faith consciousness. However, I've chosen to use a perspective that has particular bearing for understanding persons coping with life crises and apply the perspective to Helene, who is coping with her illness and to Phyllis, Susan, Sarah, and Tara, college students coping with deaths of family members and friends. This perspective is the holistic framework.

Holism

The holistic framework emphasizes the importance of the whole person and identifies six dimensions of particular importance for understanding human existence. These six dimensions are the (a) physical, (b) emotional, (c) cognitive, (d) behavioral, (e) interpersonal, and (e) spiritual. The hospice movement uses this framework to organize services for a terminally ill person and the person's family. I think the framework has considerable power for understanding persons coping with life crises, particularly the prototypical life crisis, bereavement over the death of a family member or friend. Of considerable import for this part of my argument is that all of the dimensions identified in the holistic framework were identified decades ago in Lindemann's (1944) landmark paper on acute grief.

The physical dimension

Helene's various illnesses, most particularly Graves disease, have had severe physical impacts. Of greatest concern is that her medication be tuned appropriately lest she fall victim to hypothyroidism. When her medication is not working properly, Helene has serious night sweats, headaches, trouble sleeping, and many aches and pains. She becomes tired more easily than before the onset of Graves disease.

Bereavement has several effects on people physically in the first few weeks and months following a death. Common physical reactions include problems sleeping, trouble eating, chills, diarrhea, exhaustion, and vulnerability to opportunistic diseases due to a compromised immune system. Here is what two students told me (See Balk, 2011b, pp. 120-130).

> Physically bereavement is feeling ill in my stomach, headaches and trouble eating. I can't eat because I feel sick to my stomach and when I don't eat I get headaches. I think about the death and go over and over it in my mind and then I get bad headaches. I cry at times and it can be disturbing to others because I am usually a very happy person. (Phyllis, 21 years old, is a social work major. Her best friend committed suicide nearly eight years ago. In addition to her friend's suicide, a man who became like a second grandfather to her died of respiratory ailments shortly before Phyllis went to college).

I really haven't had too many physical problems. At first I did have trouble eating when my Mom was in the hospital and she was about to die. I couldn't swallow or keep anything down. There have been nights when I miss my Mom so much that I can't sleep well. I remember one night I had a dream with my Mom in it and I was crying in my sleep. That was the first time ever I had cried in my sleep, and never knew that was possible before. (Susan, 19 years old, is a chemistry major. Her mother died two years ago after complications from a hiking accident. Her grandmother died five years ago from breast cancer.)

The emotional dimension

Helene's emotions are fairly stable, but there is a mercurial quality to her emotional makeup, particularly when job stresses pile up. Complications with her medication can impact her emotionally; for instance, one emotional impact is frustration over her lack of energy.

Emotions commonly reported by grieving individuals include anger, guilt, sadness, yearning, confusion, and shock. Some grievers surprise themselves and others that all is not replete with sorrow. Some memories prompt laughter over humorous episodes from the life of the person who died. The two students introduced above shared these experiences.

Bereavement has been confusion and loneliness for me. I felt guilty when my friend committed suicide because I did not see that he was depressed or unhappy with himself. I was also angry because he left me rather than fighting to live. The losses I have had have made me feel uncertain about the future. I don't know how to move on or I am having trouble keeping up with life because I am frazzled and forget things. (Phyllis)

Bereavement has been a rocky experience. It took me about a year and a half to move forward and accept that the people I loved are no longer physically in my life. There were times when I felt guilty thinking, "Could I have been more helpful so that she could have recovered?" or "If I was just looking out for her she probably would be alive today." I have been afraid of not knowing what will happen to my family next week or a year from now. Though, there is this feeling of appreciation of how amazing the people I have lost are to my life. I gained so much knowledge of how the world is and how to be a good friend to others. (Susan)

The cognitive dimension

Helene's job makes many demands that call for planning, thinking ahead, and being decisive. She has many students' papers to read and grade and courses to prepare. She develops courses and remains current with the latest developments in digital technology. She makes sure credits received by students at the community college transfer to four-year programs. She knows, inside and out, the nuances of Graves disease.

Among the cognitive issues commonly attributed to bereavement are problems remembering things, intrusive thoughts and images of the death, and trouble concentrating. Students' grades typically suffer in the semester following a death. Planning can be particularly difficult. Here is what Phyllis and Susan said about the cognitive impact of bereavement in their lives.

I have had many problems thinking and remembering school work because I keep going over and over the deaths in my life. I also worry about other people I love dying or me dying. I worry about forgetting the good times with my loved ones and how they smiled or laughed. (Phyllis)

When I think about how my mother died, it does distract me school wise. I would continuously run all the events that happened within the two days that led to her passing away. It is lessened as time passes, but if something triggers the fact that she is gone, many times I am unable to do school work and can't focus. Just recently was my Mom's death anniversary and I was in summer school studying for a final a few days before. I got a call from my sister saying that they will be having a memorial service for her a day before she died, and it was the same day as my exam and I broke down. They were able to change the day so I could make it, but I was not the same for the rest of the day. I couldn't focus and emotionally I was overwhelmed. In the end I didn't do as well on the exam as I could have. (Susan)

The behavioral dimension

Helene at times must simply call in ill. It is the new normal for her, although she has been able, for the most part, to maintain a regular schedule. Setting aside time to relax has proven invaluable, as has finding time to meditate.

Agitated restlessness and loss of patterns of conduct are two behaviors reported by many persons in the first few months after a death. Crying is a common behavior for grievers. Keeping to a regular schedule can present a challenge.

> When I am feeling particularly bereaved I have to keep moving. I'm restless so I go out to do stuff with friends, but when I'm with those friends I want to be alone. I like to get my school work and other stuff done to pass my time and to get my mind off things. (Phyllis)

> I have become more independent in my decision making. When my Mom was alive I would go to her for advice, but since she is not physically in my life, most of the time I have to problem solve on my own. (Susan)

The interpersonal dimension

Helene is a person of consequence in her college. She is recognized by many for her talents, and is in high demand from students as an advisor. She has been singled out for awards, and received the college's Difference Maker award twice. Several students she advises have received awards: five have been members of the all academic team for the entire state, several have won various scholarships, and six were named outstanding graduates upon completing their degrees. There have been some problems with persons who do not understand the complications Graves disease causes.

Many persons become uncomfortable when learning someone in their presence is grieving. An incident that a college student related captures this discomfort that others convey when grief enters the room.

> Sarah was in the middle of her junior year when her younger brother was killed in a car accident. It was now ten months later, and Sarah had just landed a job at a popular bar near the campus. It was her first day at the job, and she was helping set up for the influx of customers around 5 p.m.
>
> She was working with two male college students she had met at her job. They were getting to know one another as they set up the place. "What are you studying?" "Do you live in the dorms or off campus?" "Where are you from?" "Do you have any brothers or sisters?" When asked that last question, Sarah said "I had a younger brother Jimmy. He died in a car wreck about ten months ago." And the two young men simply left the room. (Balk, 2011, p. 5)

Both high school and college students have told me that to keep a social life, they must camouflage their grief. Sarah learned this lesson.

The spiritual dimension

Transcending self, searching for meaning, expressing hope, and finding purpose in existence are all primary signs of the human being's spirituality. For some persons spirituality and religion are intertwined, but for a growing number of persons religion seems implausible but spirituality possesses value. For Helene, spirituality encompasses a deeply-felt link to animals. Organized religion holds little sway in her life (probably none, in fact). She does make use of a religious artifact (a rosary) as a means to meditate.

For some grievers, a death so shakes their assumptive world that they must reconstruct their sense of the spiritual in order to cope well with their loss. For some grievers, hope is absent because the future does not beckon with any promise. For some grievers, the loss of spirituality means a descent into the abyss of absurdity. Here is what two bereaved college students said when asked how bereavement had affected them spiritually. For them spirituality and religion are closely intertwined.

> Since I have never been religious I have kept mainly indifferent to going to churches for funerals and such. Other than that, I have not really thought about it. (Phyllis)

It has actually strengthened my faith more than before. Having faith in God gives me a reason to believe that she is watching over me, still affecting my life. I get out of losing my Mom and grandmother a greater unknown understanding of why they died. I constantly think their life on this earth is over and God felt it was their time. (Susan)

Here are the words of Tara, a 20-year-old physics major whose father died of prostate cancer 18 months ago.

Mainly I wonder how God could have let this happen. I wonder why it had to be my father. I wonder if it would have been different if my father had a stronger relationship with God. I wonder if it was meant to happen so that I would accomplish certain things in college. Sometimes I even wonder if God really exists.

CONCLUSION

This chapter's material presents some fundamental ways of looking at adolescent development as the back story for understanding adolescent coping with bereavement or a life-threatening illness. Individuals are expected to master three developmental transitions as they journey through early, middle, and later adolescence toward young adulthood. These transitions are (a) becoming an autonomous individual, (b) gaining a direction for making a living, and (c) entering into and maintaining intimate friendships. Other topics germane to adolescent development are five crucial choices that adolescents face in various guises during the early, middle, and later adolescent years: (a) the predictability of existence, (b) belonging to a definite human group, (c) justice, (d) self-efficacy, and (e) self-concept. I looked at these five choices in terms of a case study of a young female named Helene who was not coping with bereavement, but who had some serious encounters with illness in later adolescence and young adulthood. Finally, the holistic perspective was employed to examine the responses of Helene and some college students regarding the impact, respectively, of illness and bereavement in terms of six dimensions of human existence.

Editor's Note: Student quotes are reproduced from Helping the Bereaved College Student *(Balk, 2011b). Reprinted with permission of Springer Publishing Company, LLC ISBN: 9780826108784*

David E. Balk, PhD, MC, MA, is a professor at Brooklyn College where he directs Graduate Studies in Thanatology and is chair of the Health and Nutrition Sciences Department. He earned a Bachelor of Arts in philosophy from Immaculate Conception Seminary, an MA in theology from Marquette University, an MC in counselor education from Arizona State University, and a PhD in counseling psychology from the University of Illinois at Urbana-Champaign. He is the author of the book Helping the Bereaved College Student (Springer Publishing Company, 2011). *His newest book is* Dealing with Dying, Death, and Grief during Adolescence (Routledge, 2014).

REFERENCES

Arnett, J. J. & Tanner, J. L. (Eds). (2006). *Emerging adults in America: Coming of age in the 21st century.* Washington, DC: American Psychological Association.

Balk, D. (2011a). Adolescent development and bereavement: An introduction. *The Prevention Researcher, 18*(3), 3-9.

Balk, D. E. (2011b). *Helping the bereaved college student.* New York, NY: Springer Publishing.

Blos, P. A. (1979). *The adolescent passage: Developmental issues.* New York, NY: International Universities.

Bonanno, G. A. (2009). *The other side of sadness: What the new science of bereavement tells us about life after loss.* New York, NY: Basic Books.

Doka, K. J. & Martin, T. L. (2010). *Grieving beyond gender: Understanding the ways men and women mourn.* New York, NY: Routledge.

Fleming, S. J. & Adolph, R. (1986). Helping bereaved adolescents: Needs and responses. In C. A. Corr & J. N. McNeil (Eds.), *Adolescence and death* (pp. 97-118). New York, NY: Springer Publishing.

Kauffman, J. (Ed.). (2001). *Loss of the assumptive world: A theory of traumatic loss.* New York, NY: Routledge.

Lindemann, E. (1944). Symptomatology and management of acute grief. *American Journal of Psychiatry, 101*, 141-148.

Lindholm, J. A. (2007). Spirituality in the academy: Reintegrating our lives and the lives of our students. *About Campus, 12*(4), 10-17.

Servaty-Seib, H. L. & Hamilton, L. A. (2006). Educational performance and persistence of bereaved college students. *Journal of College Student Development, 47*, 225-234.

CHAPTER 4

Adolescents Coping with Parental Death

J. William Worden

In this chapter we will look at the impact of parental death on adolescent children who were 12 through 17 at the time of the death. These adolescents were part of the Harvard Child Bereavement Study based at the Massachusetts General Hospital; Co-principal Investigators for this study were Drs. J. William Worden and Phyllis R. Silverman.

The Harvard study was unique in several ways. It was *longitudinal in design*. Bereaved children and their families were followed for two years after parental death. A longitudinal study is desirable to a cross-sectional study since mourning is a process and children are growing and changing over time. The study involved a *community-based sample*. Communities in the Greater Boston area were selected based on their varying demography, including economic, racial, and social class makeup. An effort was made to include all families from these communities where there had been the death of a parent leaving children from 6 to 17 years of age. *Non-bereaved control children* were also included in the investigation. Without following controls it is difficult to be sure if the behavior exhibited is the result of losing a parent to death or just being a 15-year-old boy. Controls were matched on the basis of age, gender, grade in school, family religion, and community. *Children were interviewed* along with their surviving parent to give the fullest picture of what was happening in the lives of the children and their families. In addition to open-ended interview protocols, standardized measures were used. This process enables the findings to be compared with findings from other studies. Finally, this was a *descriptive study not an intervention study*. A descriptive study enables one to follow what happens in the normal course of mourning and then to use these findings to develop interventions for children and adolescents.

The Harvard Child Bereavement Study had three aims: a) to do a descriptive study of parentally bereaved school-age children (6-17); b) to identify children most at-risk for poor adaptation during the first two years after the death; and c) to develop a screening instrument for early identification of at-risk children. Assessments of the children and their families were done at four months (T-1), one year (T-2), and two years (T-3) after the death.

The Harvard Child Bereavement Study followed 125 children from 70 families for two years after parental death. In this group of 125 children there were 65 adolescents ranging in age from 12 to 17 at the time of death. These teenagers serve as the basis for the findings discussed in this chapter. These 65 adolescents came from 46 of the 70 families. In the 46 families, 28 had one teenager, 17 families had two teens, and one family had 3 teens.

DEMOGRAPHY

In this group of 65 adolescents there were 37 boys (57%) and 28 girls (43%). There were 47 (72%) teens who lost a father to death and 18 (28%) who lost a mother. Most of the deaths were from natural causes (92%), while 6% were from accidents and there was one suicide. Of the natural deaths 40% were sudden and 60% were expected.

Family demography is as follows: The average age of the surviving parent was 42 and the average age of the dead parent was 44. Seventy-two percent of the families were Catholic in family religion with 23% of them being Protestant and 5% Jewish. Family income ranged from under $10,000 to over $50,000 with the modal income ranging from $20,000 to $29,000. These incomes represented the range of incomes in the communities selected.

ASSESSMENTS

In addition to assessing the teens through a semi-structured interview, teens completed the Perceived Competence Scale for Children (Harter, 1985); the Locus of Control Scale for Children (Nowak & Strickland, 1973); and the Smilansky Death Questionnaire (Smilansky, 1987). For each adolescent, at every assessment point, the surviving parent completed the Achenbach Child Behavior

Checklist (CBCL) (Achenbach, 1991). The CBCL is a widely used and well-normed instrument for assessing emotional/ behavioral problems in children and adolescents.

To assess the surviving parent and family a semi-structured instrument was also used. Three instruments assessed family structure and functioning: Family Adaptability and Cohesion Evaluation Scale (FACES III) (Olsen, 1985); Family Inventory of Life Events (FILE) (McCubbin, Patterson, & Wilson, 1979); and Family Crises Oriented Personal Evaluation Scales (F-COPES) (McCubbin, Larson, & Olson, 1987). Depression was assessed with the CES-D (Radloff, 1977) and trauma with the Impact of Events Scale (IES) (Zilberg, Weiss, & Horowitz, 1982).

WHAT IS THE IMPACT OF PARENTAL LOSS?

To assess the impact of parental loss on these adolescents, we compared their responses to the preadolescents in the study and also compared them with the matched non-bereaved adolescents who served as controls.

Comparison with preadolescents

Adolescents were more likely than preadolescents to know that their parent was going to die, and to know it for a longer period. They were more likely to attend the funeral, to be prepared for the funeral, to see the body of their dead parent, and to remember what was said at the funeral. Two years after the death they were more likely to remember the date of the death than their younger counterparts.

Adolescents, especially males, were the most likely to receive explicit messages from family members to act more grown up because of the loss. Although they were no more or less attached to the dead parent throughout the two years of follow-up, they did place more value on objects belonging to the dead parent, and kept such objects close at hand. Bereaved adolescents had lower levels of self-esteem than bereaved preadolescents at each of the three assessments, perhaps related in part to the admonition to "grow up." Unlike preadolescents, adolescents rated their conduct as less good than their peers. However, in spite of this, they also reported at each assessment that they felt more mature because of the death.

Peer relationships are very important to adolescents, and they were more likely than preteens to feel like an "odd kid" because of the loss. "When people I meet ask me about my mother and I tell them she died, I kinda feel different with one parent," said a 17-year-old boy. However, despite this, teens were twice as likely as preteens to talk to their friends about their dead parent.

Comparisons with non-bereaved controls

During the first year following the death, bereaved adolescents were more likely to experience health problems and sleep difficulties than their matched non-bereaved counterparts. By the second year sleep problems and health problems had dropped to match those of the controls. In the first year there were no differences in learning problems, difficulty with concentration, or in frequency of accidents. Levels of anger and delinquent behavior were also not significantly higher for bereaved than controls.

With regard to self-perception, bereaved adolescents saw themselves as doing less well in school and being less well-behaved than their non-bereaved counterparts saw themselves. These differences continued into the second year. In addition, by the second anniversary of the death, bereaved adolescents reported lower self-esteem than the non-bereaved and believed they had less ability to affect and change what was happening to them as opposed to feeling controlled by outside influences (self-efficacy).

A greater number of differences between the bereaved and non-bereaved adolescents began to appear two years after the death. During the second year the bereaved exhibited more withdrawn behavior, experienced more anxiety and depression, and were more worried about how their families were functioning than the controls. In addition, they were also more likely to be experiencing social problems as assessed on the CBCL, though not necessarily having fewer friends.

Impact on adolescent development

Fleming and Adolph (1986) have identified five core issues that the adolescent needs to grapple with as part of his or her adolescent development. These are 1) the predictability of events; 2) the development of self-image; 3) a sense of belonging; 4) a sense of fairness and justice; and 5) increased mastery and control. We wanted to see how the death of a parent might affect the adolescent's negotiation of these key core issues for these teenagers.

With regard to the first core issue, *predictability of events*, we found that the increased levels of anxiety and fear found in these teens is directly related to the issue of predictability, or lack thereof, stemming from the death of a parent. Fearing for the safety of their surviving parent and for their own personal safety was high for some of these teens and remained high into the second year. It is interesting that self-efficacy or the ability to affect what happens to oneself started to go down during the first year of loss and was significantly lower than the non-bereaved teens by the second year.

With regard to *self-image*, the second core issue, bereaved adolescents were more likely than bereaved preteens to feel like the "odd kid" and were more likely than non-bereaved adolescents to believe that their conduct and school performance were not as good as that of their peers. By the second year the self-esteem of the bereaved teens was significantly lower than that reported by the non-bereaved controls.

Bereaved adolescents showed less of a sense of *belonging*, the third core issue, than their non-bereaved counterparts. They had more social problems and were more withdrawn socially. We did not look at the fourth core issue, *fairness and justice*, but we did look at the fifth issue of *mastery and control*. During the second year the effect of parent loss on mastery took its toll. It was at that point that bereaved adolescents believed they had significantly less control over what happened to them than their non-bereaved counterparts and were controlled by fate or other outside influences.

It becomes clear that the impact of parental death is greater for these teens during the second year of bereavement than it was during the first year. During the second year the bereaved teens showed more social problems and withdrawn behavior than the non-bereaved teens. They saw themselves as behaving less well and doing less well in school than other teens they knew. Low self-esteem and lower self-efficacy were more prominent in the second year than the first.

Is it Worse to Lose A Mother or A Father?

It is not good for an adolescent to lose either parent to death. However, one can look to see which type of death had the most impact on the teen. We looked at the total impact on the child using the Achenbach CBCL that measures emotional and behavioral problems in the child. For both teen boys and teen girls, those experiencing the greatest number of emotional or behavioral problems at each time point were the children who *lost their mother to death*. This was true for both genders of teens but the greatest impact was for the girls whose mother died and were left with fathers as single parents.

When a father dies there may be financial set-backs for the family but greater than these are the emotional set-backs after a mother dies. Mothers, for the most part, are the emotional caretakers of the family. When a mother dies the loss of this role leaves a big gap. One dimension of this caretaker role is the promotion of discussions and the expression of feelings about the dead parent. Fathers had more difficulty in doing this. This was a frustration to some of the children who wanted to talk about their dead mother but whose fathers inhibited such conversation. This was the case in one family with three kids, and they expressed this frustration to the interviewer at four months. Over the next eight months they found that they could speak with each other about their mother, even if dad did not want to. By the second year anniversary the father had come "on board" and was more open in participating in such conversations about their mom, which pleased the teens very much.

Dads in general had a much more difficult time being a single parent. Minimizing daily life changes is important in helping bereaved teens to move forward through their grief; fathers did this less well than mothers. It was more difficult for dads to get on-time meals to the table, and to push for regular schedules in such things as completing homework assignments, curfews, and bedtimes than it was for moms in our study.

WHO IS AT-RISK FOR SERIOUS EMOTIONAL AND BEHAVIORAL PROBLEMS?

One of the aims of the study was to identify the number of children who experienced serious emotional and behavioral problems after parental death. To assess this we used the child's Total (T) score on the Achenbach CBCL. Professor Achenbach and colleagues have determined that total CBCL scores exceeding a T-score value of 64 indicate that those children are seriously disturbed and should be singled out for further psychological evaluation. We used this conservative criterion to identify those bereaved children we call "at-risk."

Four months after the death a fifth of the teens (22%) fell into this risk group. Over the following eight months this percentage had dropped to 18% by the first anniversary of the death. Keep in mind that this decrease occurred without any special intervention. How does this compare with their matched control counterparts? At the same time point only 10% of the controls fell into the risk group, significantly fewer than their bereaved counterparts. The percentage of bereaved teens falling into the risk group remained steady at 20% at the second anniversary (25 months) following the death of a parent. For the control group, only 7% of the control teens fell into the risk group at the 25 month period. One could generalize that approximately a fifth of bereaved teens are experiencing serious emotional or behavioral problems at any time point over the first two years. These are the children that we should target specifically for our bereavement interventions.

Not every teen at risk fell into that category at each assessment point. Out of the total group of teens, 31% fell into the risk group at one or more of the three time points. This compares to the lower number of 12% for the control group being at risk at one or more time points. Clearly the death of a parent contributes to putting some teens at risk.

What was the influence of the gender of the child and the gender of the parent who died on placing the child in the risk group? The gender of the dead parent and the gender match (boys who lose fathers, girls who lose mothers) of the teens did not contribute to their risk status. However gender played an important role at the second year assessment for girls. At one year only 15% of the girls were in the risk group. This rose to 27% at 2 years. At the same time points the boys with risk status had dropped from 20% to 15%.

What were the factors that contributed to children being in the at-risk group? Risk factors related to the child, the surviving parent, and to family dynamics. The greatest influence on the adjustment of bereaved teens was the functioning of the surviving parent. Parents with high levels of depression, trauma, and stress scores had less well-functioning children. These parents tended to be younger and with more children under 12 years of age. They received less support from friends, neighbors, extended family, and religion to help them deal with more family life stressors on the FILE. Their personal coping style tended to be more passive and they lacked the coping skill to redefine and reframe problems. Tensions and argument within these families ran high.

Child factors related to at-risk status were a greater number of daily life changes and inconsistent discipline, both of these making them feeling less safe. They had less peer support than the teens not at-risk. Feeling less good about themselves (self-esteem) and feeling less able to control circumstances in their lives (self-efficacy) also contributed to their having high levels of emotional and behavioral problems.

Resilience in Parentally Bereaved Adolescents

Although approximately 20% of the adolescents fell into the at-risk group at any one point in time, this still left 80% of them who never showed a high level of emotional and behavioral disturbance. This larger group of not at-risk teens could be further divided into two sub-groups. The first group was a large group of teens who were "slugging it through" and "making do" with their lives while adapting to the death of their parent. The second and smaller group was those we call the *resilient teens*. These were the kids who were making a very good adaptation to the loss and for whom the loss led to reported personal growth. We identified several protective factors that discriminated these resilient kids from the others.

- Resilient teens were more *socially active* than the less well-functioning children. They tended to have more friends and spend more time with these friends than the less resilient children.
- On the *self-esteem* measure they reported significantly higher self-esteem than did the others.
- Their sense of *self-efficacy* was also higher than the less resilient; they felt that they had a lot of control over what happened to them versus being a victim of circumstances.
- These adolescents experienced *fewer daily life changes* than the less adjusted teens. Keeping daily life as consistent as possible is a protective factor for adjusting to the death of a parent. These include such things as consistent discipline, consistent mealtimes, bedtimes, homework assignments, etc.
- At each assessment point adolescents were asked about their personal safety on a standardized scale. Resilient teens reported *higher personal safety scores* than did those not in the resilient group.
- These teens in the resilient group reported that they were *well prepared for the funeral*. This was a strong empirical finding and suggests that they came from families more tuned into the children and their needs.
- These resilient teens had a *surviving parent who was functioning well* in coping with the death of their spouse. This included managing feelings, ability to garner support when needed, and utilizing more effective coping strategies such as active versus passive coping and the ability to reframe and redefine problems.

The question arises as to whether these protective factors preexisted the death or were forged in the context of the loss. I see them as mostly preexisting the loss but there were some skills and self-perceptions that were developed in families that were less dysfunctional. These resilient teens tended to have a surviving parent who was well tuned into their needs and able to help them with these needs despite being bereaved themselves.

Continuing Bonds and Relationship To Deceased Parent

We were interested in the kind of relationship that these teens had with the parent who died both before the death and after the death. Unlike Freud (1917), who posited that ties to the deceased should be broken over time so that the mourner could be free to invest this emotional energy into new relationships, these teenagers did not do this. Many of them went on to keep a tie with their deceased parent and we called these ties continuing bonds.

Bonds with the deceased parent were maintained through several different activities. They maintained a connection by a) speaking to the dead parent, b) feeling watched by the parent, c) thinking about the parent, d) dreaming about the parent, e) locating the parent in a specific place, f) keeping objects that belonged to the parent, and g) by identifying with the dead parent when asked which parent they were most alike.

The teens in the study maintained the following bonding activities at four months (T-1); one year (T-2); and two years (T-3).

Table 1

	T-1	T-2	T-3
Speaking	52%	34%	34%
Being watched	77%	71%	65%
Thinking	80%	66%	57%
Dreaming	48%	34%	36%
Locating parent	71%	72%	67%
Keeping objects	80%	88%	89%
Identifying with dead parent	n/a	72%	75%

Over the two-year period we found that the teens spoke less to their deceased parent; they felt less watched by the parent; and also thought about the deceased parent less frequently. There were no significant changes in dreaming or locating the deceased parent; objects belonging to the deceased parent continued to be important to them. They continued seeing themselves as more like the deceased parent than the living parent.

What do we know about these highly connected teens? Gender of the child or gender of the lost parent was not significant. However, there was a slight trend for these connected teens to be female. In addition to seeing themselves as most like the dead parent (regardless of their gender or the gender of the deceased parent), they found it easier to talk about the death and to show emotional pain within the family as well as to their friends. They were likely to come from more cohesive families (FACES III) and they were able to accept support from others. They reported that their relationship with their dead parent was good before the death and they were aware of wanting to please their dead parent, even two years after the death. They would be more conscious of wanting to show the dead parent what they were currently doing to please them than the less connected children. Several of these more connected children reported sharing the same vocational and avocational interests that their deceased parent had.

DEVELOPING A SCREENING INSTRUMENT

The third aim of the Harvard study was to develop a screening instrument for the early identification of at-risk children. There are three different philosophies for intervening with bereaved children and adolescents. The first is to intervene with all children who lose a parent to death. However this is not necessary nor is it cost effective. Our study shows that not all bereaved children need intervention. Most do well over the first two years after loss without a special intervention.

The second approach is to wait and see which bereaved children have emotional or behavioral problems and refer those children to professional resources. This approach is followed in many communities. The downside is that one must wait until the child is experiencing difficulty before reaching out to him or her. Many of the teens in the Harvard study did not experience emotional and behavioral difficulties until two years after the death of a parent.

Screening and early intervention is the third approach and comes out of a preventative mental health approach espoused by the department of psychiatry at Harvard Medical School. We used information collected on the adolescents and their family four months after the death to develop a screening scale that would predict which teens would be in the risk group two years later. Although some teens were showing emotional and behavioral difficulties four months after parent death, many were not. Their difficulties showed up much later. If we can identify early the children who will have later difficulties then we can offer them early intervention to preclude a later negative sequlae.

Editor's Note: The screening instrument which identifies at-risk children with a high degree of accuracy can be found in the Appendix of Children & grief: When a parent dies *by J. William Worden, Guilford, 1996.*

Conclusion

- Most adolescents who lose a parent to death do well during the first two years without special intervention.
- There is a group of approximately 20% who are not doing well at one or more of the assessment points and we call these at-risk teenagers.
- A combination of factors put these children at risk. The strongest risk predictor is the functioning of the surviving parent. Parents who are young, with younger children, whose families experience a large number of concomitant stressors, and who have less well-developed coping skills will have bereaved children who show higher levels of emotional and behavioral problems.
- The emotional and behavioral impact of parental death shows up stronger at two years than it does at one year when bereaved children are compared with their non-bereaved matched counterparts. At two years the bereaved were more withdrawn, experienced more anxiety and depression, and had lower self-esteem and self-efficacy than their matched controls.
- There are three implications of these findings for intervention with bereaved teens:
  — Follow them for a longer time period than the traditional one year follow-up post death.

- — Use a screening instrument to do early identification of at-risk children so being identified they can be offered intervention to preclude a later negative sequelae.
- — Identify the group of parents who are not functioning well so that intervention can be offered to them as well as to the at-risk children.

- Pay attention to adolescent girls after the death of their mother. This group of girls showed particularly high scores after their mother's death that included high levels of aggression and some delinquent behavior. As the oldest female in the family they may have been given responsibility for chores and meals, and caring for younger siblings, something that was accepted closer to the death but very much resented by the second year.
- Many of the bereaved adolescents stayed connected to their dead parent by speaking to, thinking of, dreaming, feeling watched, locating the parent in a specific place, and keeping objects that belonged to the dead parent. They also saw themselves as more like the dead parent than the surviving parent. For the most part these continuing bonds were a salutatory experience.

J. William Worden, PhD, ABPP, is a fellow of the American Psychological Association and holds academic appointments at the Harvard Medical School and at the Rosemead Graduate School of Psychology in California. He is also Co-Principal Investigator of the Harvard Child Bereavement Study, based at the Massachusetts General Hospital. Recipient of five major NIH grants, his research and clinical work over 40 years has centered on issues of life-threatening illness and life-threatening behavior. He was a founding member of the Association for Death Education and Counseling (ADEC) and the International Work Group on Death, Dying, and Bereavement (IWG). Dr. Worden was on the advisory board for the first U.S. hospice in Branford, CT as well as the Hospice of Pasadena, CA. His book Grief Counseling & Grief Therapy: A Handbook for the Mental Health Practitioner *(Springer Publishing, 2009), now in its fourth edition, has been translated into 14 languages.*

REFERENCES

Fleming, S. & Adolph, R. (1986). Helping bereaved adolescents. In C. A. Corr & J. McNeil (Eds.), *Adolescents and death* (pp. 97-118). New York, NY: Springer.

Freud, S. (1917/1967). Mourning and Melancholia. In J. Stachey (Ed.), *The Standard Edition of the Complete Psychological Works of Sigmund Freud*. London, England: Hogarth Press.

McCubbin, H., Larson, A., & Olson, D. (1987). F-COPES: Family crisis oriented personal scales. In H. McCubbin & A. Thompson (Eds.), *Family assessment inventories for research and practice*. Madison, WI: University of Wisconsin.

McCubbin, H., Patterson, J., & Wilson, L. (1979). Family inventory of Live Events. St. Paul, MN: University of Minnesota.

Olson, D. (1986). Circumplex model VII: Validation studies and FACES III. *Family Process, 25*, 337-351.

Radloff, L. (1977). The CES-D Scale: A self-report depression scale for research in the general population. *Applied Psychological Management, 1*(3), 385-401.

Sandler, I., Ayers, T. Wolchik, S., Tein, J., Kwok, O. M., Haine, R. A.,… Griffin, W. A. (2003). The family bereavement program. Efficacy evaluation of a theory based prevention program for parentally bereaved children and adolescents. *Journal of Counseling and Clinical Psychology, 71*, 587-600.

Silverman, P. R. (2000). *Never too young*. New York, NY: Oxford.

Worden, J. W. (1996). *Children & grief: When a parent dies*. New York, NY: Guilford.

Worden, J. W. (2008). Grieving children and adolescents: Lessons from the Harvard Child Bereavement Study. In K. J. Doka & A. S. Tucci, *Living with grief: Children and adolescents* (pp. 125-137). Washington, DC: Hospice Foundation of America.

Worden, J. W. (2009). *Grief counseling & grief therapy: A handbook for the mental health professional*. New York, NY: Springer.

Worden, J. W. & Silverman, P. R. (1993). Grief and depression in newly widowed parents with school-age children. *Omega, 27*, 251-160.

Zilberg, N., Weiss, D., & Horowitz, M. (1982). Impact of Events Scale (IES): A cross-validation study. *Journal of Counseling and Clinical Psychology, 50*, 407-414.

Editor's Note: The Child Bereavement Study was funded by a grant from the National Institute of Mental Health (MH-41791) and by grants from the National Funeral Directors Association and the Hillenbrand Corporation.

CHAPTER 5

Voices
When Dad Died

Evan Brohan

I t's been two years since my dad died. He was a good man and I miss
him a lot. I still remember the day he died and how sad I was, but
I usually don't think about him a lot anymore. When I do think of
him I think about all the good times we used to have when we hung
out.

Sometimes I just sit down and wonder about what my life would
be like if he was still alive. Would I behave better? Would I get better
grades in school? Would I still be doing the same sports and activities
I do now? I always think about that type of stuff and how my life might
be different. My life could also be exactly the same as it is now. I mean,
it is not like I am doing poorly. My grades are good and I pretty much
stay out of trouble. I don't know, and I guess I never will know.

I also feel like I have unfinished business with my dad. One thing
still bothers me. The last time I saw him in the hospital, I was 11 years
old. I didn't give him a hug. For whatever reason, I did not want to
hug. Maybe it was just growing up, or maybe I was scared that I would
be saying goodbye forever. Whatever it was, I didn't do it. Now I wish
I did.

I wish he was here today so he could support me with my hobbies
and tell me how proud of me he is. I feel like I'm missing out on a
father-son bond. There are so many things I want to do and say to my
dad, like spend more time with him and tell him I love him. I'm sure
my brothers and sister also think of him all the time and miss him a
lot. I know my mom especially misses him. She cried just reading my

chapter. My mom still has his ashes on his nightstand in her room. The point is my whole family misses and loves him still. We wish he was here with us.

I wonder sometimes what he would think of my sports. My dad was into football and baseball, two sports I really do not do or even like. But I am into skating, track and field, wrestling, and basketball. I even spent the last two summers going to a basketball camp with my kid brother and a good friend. It was fun. I know my dad would still be proud. He wasn't one of those dads who only wanted you to play *his* sports. I think he would even be proud that I followed my own interest.

Skating (skate boarding) is important to me. Sometimes when I feel down, it gets my mind off things and lets off steam. I am thinking I might even start snowboarding.

There have been changes since my dad died. My mom works really hard. That means we all have to be more responsible. I keep an eye out for my kid brother Jesse. He can be a pain at times but most of the time he's cool. I watch him sometimes, help him choose clothes (so they actually match), and let him hang out with me and my friends—sometimes.

We still have a lot of Dad's old stuff around in the basement, in the closet, in my mom's room, everywhere, so we always know he is with us. He will always be with us in our hearts. We went through a rough time, everyone does, but trust me it does get better. It did for me and it will for others who have lost someone special to them.

Evan Brohan is 13 years old and an 8th grade student in middle school.

CHAPTER 6

When a Sibling Dies

Nancy S. Hogan

The death of a sibling is one of the most traumatic losses that an adolescent may experience. For adolescents whose sibling dies due to an illness, suffering is compounded because of the multiple traumatic events they experience, often over an extended time span. The family's life changes irrevocably with the news that a child has a life-threatening disease. This may be followed by months and often even years of medical and surgical treatments with hopes for a remission, only to experience another exacerbation with all of the attendant stressors. Then, at some point, the family learns that more curative treatment is futile and the child dies. This multiplicity of losses is followed by the deep despair of grieving the loss of the sibling and facing the day-to-day reality that their brother or sister will be forever physically missing in their life. Yet, in time, the young person becomes aware that while their sibling is physically absent from their life, he or she is now an existential presence. They sense an ongoing attachment, a continuing bond to their dead sibling.

This chapter will identify stressors inherent in the diagnosis-illness-death period; provide a discussion of coping with the personal, social, and developmental challenges of adolescence as a bereaved sibling, as they search for an identity while simultaneously dealing with the trauma of the bereavement process; explore the awareness that many bereaved adolescents gain that they have grown personally as a result of their suffering; examine their sense of having an ongoing attachment or a continuing bond to their dead sibling; and look at the types of social supports that help to promote their healing.

The final section centers on interventions that help and others that may be barriers to the adaptive recovery of adolescents who grieve the death of a sibling. This chapter is based on stories that children and adolescents have shared with us about their lives as bereaved siblings and the subsequent research we conducted to help better understand sibling grief and what can help or hinder their grieving.

THE DIAGNOSIS AND ILLNESS COURSE

An adolescent's life, and the life of his or her family, changes immediately and immeasurably when a sibling is diagnosed with a life-threatening disease. The parents become preoccupied with providing care and comfort to their ill child, who endures intense medical care that may include radiation, chemotherapy, amputation and other painful treatments that may require repeated hospitalizations (Hogan, Morse, & Tason, 1996; Webster & Skeen, 2012). During this time the parents dedicate their time, energy, and hopes for a cure or at least one more remission as they focus intensely on the care and protection of the ill child (Bank & Kahn, 1982; Hogan, Morse, & Tason, 1996; Packman, Horsley, Davies, & Kramer, 2006). Well children miss their "old family" as they live with the fact that family life as they had known it, with the distinct family rituals, holidays, and familiar routines, are changed or missing (Patistea, Makrodimitri, & Panteli, 2000). The changes in parenting leave the children in the family feeling left out, and sometimes anxious and depressed, even though they know for obvious reasons that the parents must dedicate themselves to the ill child. A review of literature of siblings whose ill sibling was diagnosed with cancer showed that well siblings perceived that there were changes in the family relationships, dynamics, and routines that resulted in multiple losses, such as when parental attention by necessity was centered on the ill child resulting in less time devoted to the well children in the family (Webster & Skeen, 2012). Research indicates that as a result, some well siblings experienced feeling sadness, loneliness, rejection, anxiety, anger, jealousy, guilt, and isolation from peers (Davies, 1999; Hogan & Greenfield, 1991; Martinson & Campos, 1991; Moody, Meyer, Marcuso, Charlson, & Robbins, 2006).

COPING WITH THE CHALLENGES OF ADOLESCENCE

Bereaved adolescents do not have the luxury of delaying the developmental tasks of adolescence while they grieve their siblings' death; instead they must deal simultaneously with the challenges of adolescence while coping with their own grieving within a grieving family. The primary developmental crisis or challenge of adolescence is working through the process of forming an identity. Identity formation is accomplished when adolescents sense that they have a stable sense of themselves and a personal identity that makes them feel unique. Having a firm sense of self is foundational to successfully challenging the next developmental stage in young adulthood, that of forming an intimate relationship with another (Erikson, 1959).

A non-bereaved adolescent's tasks of developing an identity are often fraught with emotional upheaval as the adolescent struggles to figure out who he or she is. The universal questions of identity formation that the adolescent must address are: "Who am I?" "Where am I going?" "How am I going to get there?" and "Who am I taking with me?" This process becomes even more difficult for bereaved siblings who must address the more complicated questions of identity: "Who am I *now*?" "Where am I going *now*?" "How am I going to get there *now*?" and "Who am I taking with me *now*?" Bereaved adolescents must incorporate the fact of their dead sibling into their sense of identity. A preteen sibling, whose only brother died, asked her identity question this way: "Am I still a sister?" (Sims, 1986).

Another key task of adolescence is the teen's need to become progressively more independent from parental oversight. The adolescent seeks the freedom to explore who he or she is separate from the family's identity. To do this, the bereaved sibling must move away from the parents' monitoring and vigilance. For bereaved adolescents, however, their parents have already lost one child, and they may feel the need to be overly protective toward their surviving children.

Developing a sense of self includes developing a sense of belonging to a social group of peers. However, being accepted into a peer group requires fitting in to the peer group and acting like the non-bereaved members. Therefore, to be accepted by the group, the bereaved adolescent must appear "normal," to behave the same as the non-bereaved group members. For bereaved siblings to appear normal when they don't feel normal is quite a feat, but bereaved adolescents often manage it by leading two lives. When they are with friends, teachers, coaches, and other non-bereaved adults they "act normal" for this audience. When they are with their family members, trusted friends, or other bereaved siblings they can let their guard down and assume their identity as a bereaved sibling who, in many ways, is quite different than non-bereaved peers.

ADOLESCENT SIBLING GRIEF

Each bereaved adolescent experiences grief that is unique to his or her personality, worldview, the support available, and gender, although there is little empirical research on gender and grief in adolescence. And while adolescents must do much of their grieving alone, they grieve within the context of their grieving parents and siblings.

Most of the literature and research on the adolescent sibling bereavement process has focused on the negative effects of experiencing a sibling's death, including disrupted patterns of self-esteem; increased likelihood of impulsive behavior; and disrupted peer relationships (Hogan & Greenfield, 1991); anxiety and guilt (Davies, 1999; Fanos, 1991); and symptoms indicative of depression including sleep disturbance, nightmares, poor concentration, feeling powerless or helpless, decreased self-worth, and suicidal ideation (Balk, 1990; Davies, 1999; Hogan & Greenfield, 1991; Martinson, Davies, & McClowry, 1987). As researchers, we were also interested in the normative aspects of grief where we could learn from siblings about the stressors of bereavement and how they coped and adapted to these life crises. Therefore, our adolescent sibling bereavement research is grounded in the stories of bereaved siblings who we have had the privilege to work with in sibling support groups, school-based bereavement support groups, and personal conversations over many years.

The following section identifies the way bereaved siblings make meaning out of becoming a sibling survivor. Tables 1 through 4 display the verbatim or slightly modified phrase that siblings used to describe their grief, personal growth, ongoing attachment, and social support. The initial response of siblings upon learning that their brother or sister has died is shock and numbness that the sibling has really died and that the hope for a cure or another exacerbation is no longer a possibility. This period of shock is soon replaced with hopelessness and despair as they realize that their sibling will permanently be physically absent in their life; life as they had known it before the death will forever be marked by the time reference "before it happened" and "after it happened." The relative control of their emotions that they had been able to manage prior to their sibling's death is replaced with the fear of losing emotional control in the presence of peers. Bereaved teens know that fitting in with their peers requires that they appear "normal;" in part, that means appearing to be preoccupied with the usual teen concerns when, in comparison with what they are going through, the typical trials and tribulations of adolescence now seem trivial. Bereaved siblings come to realize that their priority about what is important in their life has changed.

Their family is different now; it is smaller and there is a pervasive sense of missing and longing for the sibling who died. Some teens may feel guilty that they lived and their sibling died and wonder why they were spared. They may doubt they will ever be happy again, and often begin to reflect on the meaning of life. At home they feel and see the sadness of other family members and wonder if the family will make it intact. It is not uncommon for bereaved adolescents to have difficulty sleeping; when they are quiet and alone, memories may flood their mind, and some adolescents may lose sleep due to nightmares (Hogan & DeSantis, 1996.) With lack of sleep and intrusive thoughts about the death, it is easy to understand why they may have difficulty concentrating in school (Balk, 1990).

Our research with a sample of 157 adolescents between 13 and 18 years old showed that bereaved siblings fit three pathways of grieving and self-image trajectory. One group showed mild intensity of grief correlated with high levels of self-image. A second group showed moderate grief and moderate levels of self-esteem and a third group showed high intensity of grief and significantly lower levels of self-image, particularly in the areas of depression, self-control, and a sense of the lack of mastery in the external world (Hogan & Greenfield, 1991). These findings support studies that most bereaved adolescents grieve the death of their sibling and go on to live lives of meaning and purpose. However, a small percentage of bereaved adolescents become mired in grief and warrant assessment and possibly professional counseling. J. William Worden's book, *Grief Counseling and Grief Therapy: A Handbook for the Mental Health Practitioner,* offers criteria for evaluating complicated grief in adolescents.

Adolescents who successfully work through their grief find no closure to their grief, but in time they realize that their grief softens. They recall that in the beginning of their grief, their life was filled with nearly all-bad days; as time passed, there were a few good days in a row, and finally they were comforted to find that they were having more good days than bad. As time passes they begin to feel more in control of their emotional life; when the bad days come they feel better able to cope with re-grieving episodes that now occur less often, and with less intensity and of less duration. The way siblings describe their grief is displayed in Table 1.

TABLE 1. ITEMS ON THE HOGAN GRIEF REACTION CHECKLIST: GRIEF SUBSCALE

Loss of control
I believe I will lose control when I think about him or her.
I have no control over my sadness.
I believe I have little control over my life.

Sadness
I don't think I will ever be happy again.
I have no control over my sadness.
I feel depressed when I think about him or her.
Family holidays such as Christmas are sad times for my family.

Discomfort when acting normal
I am uncomfortable when I am having fun.
I am uncomfortable when I am feeling happy.

Fears
I believe I am going crazy.
I have panic attacks over nothing.
I am afraid that more people I love will die.
I am afraid to get close to people.
I worry about everything.

Feeling alone
People don't know what I am going through.
I want to die to be with him or her.

Survivor guilt
I should have died and he or she should have lived.

Recognizing the family's incompleteness
My family will always be incomplete.

Hopelessness
I don't care what happens to me.
I do not believe I will ever get over his or her death.

Difficulty concentrating
I have trouble concentrating.

Difficulty sleeping at night
I do not sleep well at night.
I have nightmares about his or her death.

(Hogan, 1990)

Personal Growth

The adolescent sibling bereavement process teaches many harsh, life-changing lessons. Bereaved siblings face the stark reality that death can happen to anyone at any time and they now recognize how fragile life is. As a result, their worldview and priorities change. These teens' sense of their own mortality facilitates their becoming more altruistic at a time when typically adolescents are egocentric and focused primarily on themselves. The survivor siblings gain a sense of other-centeredness by concluding that they think more about others now; they care more deeply for their family and they have become more aware of other people's feelings. They are consciously aware of trying to be kinder and more understanding and compassionate toward others. Because of knowing what it is like to grieve, bereaved siblings often feel competent to reach out to others who are grieving. Because of the strength gained through coping with grief, these teens sense that they have become more tolerant of others and themselves, a value associated with maturity. They compare themselves to their non-bereaved peers and believe that they are more mature than friends; in many ways, they become mature beyond their years (Hogan & DeSantis, 1996). This increased sense of maturity is coupled with a belief that they now have a better outlook on life, and that they can cope better with their problems. A study of 105 bereaved siblings whose brother or sister died due to cancer was compared to a control group of non-bereaved participants on measures of social behavior and peer acceptance. Findings showed teachers reported that bereaved siblings compared to paired non-bereaved siblings were significantly more pro-social and scored higher on leadership and popularity, providing further evidence that increased maturity is a possible outcome for bereaved siblings (Gerhardt et al. 2011). The way siblings describe their personal growth is displayed in Table 2.

TABLE 2. ITEMS ON THE HOGAN GRIEF REACTION CHECKLIST: PERSONAL GROWTH SUBSCALE

Sense of mortality
I have learned that all people die.
I know how fragile life is.
Being grateful
I have changed my priorities.
I don't take people for granted.
Increased sense of maturity
I have grown up faster than my friends.
Increased sense of self
I believe I am a better person.
More altruistic
I care more deeply for my family.
I try to be kinder to other people.
I am a more caring person.
I can give help to others who are grieving.
I am more aware of other's feelings.
I have more compassion for others.
I am more understanding of others.
More tolerant of self and others
I am more tolerant of others.
I am more tolerant of myself.
Increased ability to cope
I have learned to cope better with my problems.
I believe I am stronger because of the grief I have had to cope with.
I have a better outlook on life.
I have learned to cope better with my life.

(Hogan, 1990)

ONGOING ATTACHMENT

In 1982, Bank and Kahn coined the phrase "sibling bond" in their classic book *Sibling Bond*, in which they devoted one chapter to sibling bereavement. This chapter, titled "Siblings as survivors: Bonds beyond the grave," begins with the phrase, "…death ends only a life: it does not end a relationship" (p. 271). However, for nearly 100 years, psychoanalytic theory has been based on the notion that severance of bonds to the deceased is the hallmark of healthy grieving (Freud, 1917). The theory that healthy outcomes include maintaining an ongoing attachment to the dead loved one is conceptually the diametric opposite to the therapeutic goal of severing bonds to the deceased as the desired outcome. In the real world of bereaved children, adolescents, and parents, the belief in a reunion in heaven with siblings and children is common and a basic belief of most world religions (Hogan & DeSantis, 1992). One doesn't sever bonds to someone they plan to see again. The fact that Freud was a proclaimed and devout atheist who did not believe in a reunion in heaven, or in heaven itself, may account for his theory necessitating the separation of bonds to the deceased. It is important when seeking bereavement therapy/counseling to investigate if the practitioner's bereavement care is based on this theory (that one must discontinue bonds with the deceased) or if it is based on the ongoing attachment theory, so the treatment plan matches the bereaved's own belief system.

A common comment heard in years of listening to bereaved children and adolescents is the wish that they could have just one more moment with the deceased loved one. Specifically, the plea was, "If I could just see [name] one more time." To gain an understanding of the meaning behind this supplication, we initiated a nationwide study of bereaved adolescents in which we rephrased the plea to read, "If you could ask or tell your dead sibling something, what would it be?" We analyzed written responses of 157 bereaved siblings that showed that 81% of the responses were reaffirmations of continuing to love and miss their dead sibling. The most common response was, " I miss you and I love you," written in the present tense regardless of the time since death, confirming that surviving siblings in this study had an ongoing attachment to their dead sibling. Having a sense of ongoing attachment with the deceased sibling was described as comforting (Hogan & DeSantis, 1992). The ways siblings describe their sense of their sibling's presence in their lives and their continuing to miss their sibling are displayed in Table 3.

TABLE 3. ITEMS ON THE ONGOING ATTACHMENT INVENTORY: SENSING A CONTINUING PRESENCE AND THE MISSING AND LOVING SUBSCALES

Factor 1: Sensing a continuing presence
Feeling close to my family member helps me feel better.
I feel a continuing bond to him/her.
My family member is a continuing presence in my life.
My family member's presence comforts me.
I believe he or she watches over me.
I feel connected to him or her.
Memories of my family member comfort me.
I feel my family member will always be with me.
My love for him or her is as strong as it was before they died.
I believe I will see my family member in heaven.

Factor 2: Missing and loving
I will always miss my family member.
I continue to miss my family member.
I continue to love my loved one.
I will always love him or her.
My family member continues to be a member of our family.

(Hogan & DeSantis, 1996)

SOCIAL SUPPORT

Many bereaved siblings have found that certain types of social support helped them through their grief. First, they believed that they needed at least one person who would be there for them; often this was a trusted friend. Next, they needed to believe that this support person could be depended upon to be readily available. Third, this trusted person had to take the time to listen while the bereaved adolescents stumbled through trying to make sense of the senselessness of their lives. Fourth, this friend had to be nonjudgmental about how the bereaved adolescents grieved. The bereaved siblings did not want to be judged that they were "doing it wrong" by being told they were grieving too much or too long. When these conditions were met, the bereaved siblings felt that they could express their feelings about their grief openly and honestly, which helped them to feel better (Hogan & DeSantis, 1994). The way siblings describe the characteristics of people needed to provide social support is displayed in Table 4.

TABLE 4. ITEMS ON THE SOCIAL SUPPORT INVENTORY SCALE

> *People take the time to listen to how I feel.*
> *I can express my feelings about my grief openly and honestly.*
> *It helps me to talk with someone who is nonjudgmental about*
>   *how I grieve.*
> *There is at least one person I can talk to about my grief.*
> *I can get help for my grieving when I need it.*

(Hogan & Schmidt, 1991)

SUPPORTS THAT HELP GRIEVING ADOLESCENTS

Webster, a child psychiatrist and pediatrician, and Skeen, a pediatric oncologist, wrote about the psychosocial aspects and clinical interventions in the care of families where a child was diagnosed with a life-threatening disease. The authors stress the importance of communication with seriously ill children and family members about the disease, treatment, and prognosis. Webster and Skeen highlight the "...need for siblings to receive ongoing information about their brothers' or sisters' illness and to have their anxiety and concerns listened to and addressed" (2012). A bereaved sibling in one of our studies stated, "What helped the most was my mother who was totally honest with me from the time Sarah got sick through her death." Another said, "My mom did it for me. She was such a help. I'm not saying she was strong because she wasn't; but she shared her grief so it made it easier for me to feel that all my feelings were normal." A study of bereaved siblings whose sibling had died seven to nine years earlier due to cancer recalled that what helped them were memories of spending time with their sibling during the illness period, having someone to share their grief with, and having family who were supportive of them. Bereaved siblings offered advice to other siblings whose brother or sister was ill: seek information about the sibling's illness to remain informed, spend time with the ill sibling, enjoy the good times together, and stay optimistic (Martinson & Campos, 1991).

Adolescents may be afraid they will break down while in school. If teachers are informed that one of their students has a critically ill sibling, or if they are notified when the ill sibling has died, teachers can be helpful in informing parents about how a child is doing in school. When the sibling dies, the teacher can inform classmates about how to be kind to others who are sad and that crying is a normal part of grieving for children and adults. The teacher can partner with the school nurse or school counselor to support the teen by providing a quiet place where he or she can go to gather his or her emotions or, if they prefer, to talk about their sadness.

After the death of a sibling, survivors need to have open communication with at least one parent who can be there for them. They also need to have the fun and funny things about their dead sibling remembered and enjoyed. One bereaved sibling expressed this by saying, "I would talk to my dad once in a while about the happy memories we all had and stuff my brother did that used to get him in trouble." Other activities that siblings said helped included writing about their feelings, listening to and playing music, or "just screaming, crying, and letting it out." Having friends that could be counted on was very important to the bereaved siblings. Bereaved teens fortunate enough to be in a sibling support group describe how it helped "...to know that there are others who feel just like I do." Peer support groups help by normalizing grief and by providing the newly bereaved adolescents the opportunity to learn from adolescents further along in their grief, seeing that it is possible to get through the hard times and at some point to feel that they have found renewed meaning and purpose in life.

BARRIERS TO HELPING BEREAVED SIBLINGS

Some well-intentioned statements may hinder bereaved adolescents' grief and make it harder to cope, such as being told by others that they are grieving "too much" or "too long," or admonishing the bereaved sibling that "You should be over it by now" and "Just stop thinking and talking about it and you will feel better." These statements make the bereaved adolescent feel like they are doing it wrong and that no one wants to listen to them. And while most young people recover from the death of a brother or sister without needing professional care, a small percentage of bereaved adolescents may need to be seen by a health professional to assess their well-being; signs of concern can include an inability to function in school or work, isolation from friends, self-destructive behaviors, or behavior that is destructive or damaging to others.

It is not uncommon for bereaved adolescents, especially early in their grief, to feel uncomfortable having fun with friends. Bereaved siblings have described having a good time laughing and playing with friends until suddenly remembering their sibling has died and feeling guilty because they may feel they have dishonored their sibling by having fun. Bereaved siblings need to know that laughter feels good and it is okay to have fun. In time, these young people gain a bittersweet new normal in their lives; bittersweet because while they learn to enjoy life again, someone is always missing.

Siblings of a seriously ill child and bereaved siblings need concrete evidence that they are loved. Sometimes parents are just too overwhelmed by their need to constantly care for the ill child, or after the death they may be too distraught in their grieving to perform the tasks of making events special for the surviving sibling. Bereaved siblings need to know they are visible in the family by having their special days celebrated. A family member or friend can fulfill this role and would be honored to be asked to take care of the details of obtaining a birthday cake, inviting guests, buying and wrapping presents, supervising a party, and cleaning up. The memories of having birthday parties helps the young person feel loved and gives them hope that the family is going to make it. In addition, bereaved adolescents feel like they matter when they are invited to create new family rituals that may include the dead sibling. Some bereaved siblings find comfort in hanging a Christmas stocking for their dead sibling, or writing a message to their sibling and then attaching it to a balloon and sending it off to fly into the clouds, planting a tree in his or her name, or donating books to their school library in memory of their dead sibling

It is fitting to end this chapter by thanking the bereaved siblings who have courageously shared their stories about their siblings' death, their grief, and how they, in time, found hope and meaning again. I thank them for sharing about how their dead sibling continued to be an ongoing presence in their lives. It is my hope that I have told their story well so that it may help other bereaved siblings find their way through grief and feel less alone on their journey.

Nancy S. Hogan, PhD, RN, FAAN, is a distinguished professor of nursing at Loyola University in Chicago, IL and a Fellow in the American Academy of Nursing. She teaches research and philosophy courses and has supervised PhD research as well as conducting her own program of research. She recently completed a five-year longitudinal, mixed-method study to investigate the grief response of tissue donor family members to assess the effect of time on their grief reactions, personal growth, and continuing bonds. She has conducted parent-sibling bereavement groups and conducted bereavement research for many years and has published parental and sibling bereavement studies widely in national and international peer-reviewed journals. She has been a board member of the Association for Death Education and Counseling and Fox Valley Hospice and is currently a board member of the International Work Group for Death, Dying, and Bereavement.

REFERENCES

Ångström-Brönnström, C., Norberg, A., Strandberg, G., Söderberg, A. & Dahlquist, V. (2010). Parents' experiences of what comforts them when their child is suffering from Cancer. *Journal of Pediatric Oncology Nursing, 27*, 266-275.

Balk, D. E. (1990). The self-concept of bereaved adolescents: Sibling death and its aftermath. *Journal of Adolescent Research, 5*, 112-131.

Bank, S. P. & Kahn, M. D. (1982). *The sibling bond.* New York, NY: Basic Books.

Davies, B. (1999). *Shadows in the sun: The experiences of sibling bereavement in childhood.* Philadelphia, PA: Brunner/Mazel.

Erikson, E. H. (1959). *Identity and the life cycle.* New York, NY: International Universities Press.

Freud, S. (1917/1967). Mourning and Melancholia. In J. Stachey (Ed.), *The Standard Edition of the Complete Psychological Works of Sigmund Freud.* London, England: Hogarth Press.

Fanos, J. H. & Nickerson, B. G. (1991). Long-term effects of sibling death during adolescence. *Journal of Adolescent Research, 6*, 70-81.

Gerhardt, C., Fairclough, D. L., Grossenbacher, J., Barrera, M., Gilmer, M., Foster, T.,...Vannatta, K. (2011). Peer relationship of bereaved siblings and comparison classmates after a child's death from Cancer. *Journal of Pediatric Psychology, 37*, 209-219.

Hogan, N. S. (1990). Hogan Sibling Inventory of Bereavement (HSIB). In J. Touliatos, B. Perlmutter, & M. Straus, (Eds.), *Handbook of Family Measurement Techniques* (p. 524). Newbury Park, CA: Sage.

Hogan, N. S., & Greenfield, D. B. (1991). Adolescent sibling bereavement symptomatology in a large community sample. *Journal of Adolescent Research*, 6, 97-112.

Hogan, N. S., & DeSantis, L. (1992). Adolescent sibling bereavement: An ongoing attachment. *Qualitative Health Research*, 2, 159-177.

Hogan, N. S., & DeSantis, L. (1994). Things that help and hinder adolescent sibling bereavement. *Western Journal of Nursing Research*, 16, 132-153.

Hogan, N.S., & DeSantis, L. (1996). Adolescent sibling bereavement: Toward a new theory. In C. A. Corr & D. E. Balk, (Eds.), *Handbook of adolescent death and bereavement*. New York, NY: Springer.

Hogan, N. S., Morse, J. & Tason, M. (1996). Toward an experiential theory of bereavement. *Omega: Journal of Death and Dying*, 33, 43-65.

Hogan, N. S., Greenfield, D. A. & Schmidt, L. A. (2001). The development and validation of the Hogan Grief Reaction Checklist, *Death Studies*, 25, 1-32.

Hogan, N. S. & Schmidt, L. A. (2002). Testing grief to personal growth model using structural equation modeling. *Death Studies*, 26, 615-635.

Martinson, I., Davies, B., & McClowry, S. (1987). The long-term effects of sibling death on self-concept. *Death Studies*, 15, 259-267.

Martinson, I. & Campos, R. G. (1991). Adolescent bereavement: Long term responses to a sibling death from cancer. *Journal of Adolescent Research*, 6, 54-69.

Moody, K., Meyer, M., Marcuso, C. A., Charlson, M., & Robbins, L. (2006). Exploring concerns of children with cancer. *Supportive Care in Cancer*, 14, 960-966.

Packman, W., Horsley, H., Davies, B., & Kramer, R. (2006). Sibling bereavement and continuing bonds. *Death Studies*, 30, 817-341.

Patistea, E., Makrodimitri, P., & Panteli, V. (2000). Greek parent's reactions, difficulties and resources in childhood leukemia at the time of diagnosis. *European Journal of Cancer Care*, 9, 86-96.

Sims, A. (1986). *Am I still a sister*. Slidell, LA: Big A & Co.

Webster, M. L., & Skeen, J. E. (2012). Communicating with children: Their understanding, information, needs, and processes. In S. Kreither, M. Ben-Arush, & A. Martin (Eds.), *Pediatric Psychology: Psychosocial Aspects and Clinical Interventions, 2nd ed.* (pp. 72-91). Hoboken, NJ: John Wiley & Sons.

CHAPTER 7

Voices
Giving Back

Alivia Seay

As I have experienced loss, I have also experienced a new beginning that has made me the person I am today. Going through loss for the first time in my life was probably one of the hardest things I had ever dealt with. I was just sixteen and thought that there was no end to the precious thing we call life. My grandma decided after six months of dialysis that the treatments were no longer for her. My mom and I were her primary caregivers, so we called Suncoast Hospice and started preparing for those next few weeks.

Little did I know that nothing I could do would prepare me for that time. I began to talk to the nurses who took care of my grandma and spent countless hours looking up information that Suncoast Hospice offered. Two weeks went by so fast when I look back on it, but it felt like forever. After my grandma passed away I knew I wanted to be a part of Suncoast Hospice. Even if I wasn't a nurse yet I could become a patient and family volunteer and sit with those families: I could let them talk to me like I had just needed someone to do for me. I also knew I was not quite ready to face that experience right away, but continued for the next six months to read about the teen volunteer program.

Finally, I picked up the phone with tears in my eyes and called Suncoast Hospice. When I talked to Jill, the sweetest, kind-hearted angel on earth, I knew that it was my time to be there. No matter what was on my mind about my grandma's death, Jill was there. If I started to talk to anyone and started to tear up, which I did a lot, she would reach out and just give me the biggest hug. Nowhere else would I have been able to get through such a horrible time in my life.

Time passed and things got a little easier as I began to volunteer at Woodside Hospice House, one of Suncoast's inpatient facilities. I began sitting with patients and their families. Being there for people that were in the same situation I had been in just a short time before helped me cope. Having my volunteer coordinator always there just a couple of steps behind me, always there to talk and make sure I was still okay, was the best feeling. Shortly after, my family received a phone call that my aunt was sick and had been admitted into hospice care. I felt, yet again, like my world was turned upside down. I went and talked to Lisa, my volunteer coordinator, and she insisted that I could just let her know if I needed to not volunteer for some time. All I needed, though, was the love and support of those nurses or volunteers. No matter how hard a day was, I knew I would get through it.

One day, I was feeling down and missing my grandma and had just visited my aunt at Woodside. I started to volunteer and as I made my rounds I realized there was a gentleman who I had never talked to before. I knocked on the door and waited for the faint "come in." As soon as I walked in, this gentleman just brightened my whole day. He was eating breakfast, coffee in one hand and fork in the other. I asked if he would like me to leave but he told me no, so I stayed. I then proceeded to ask him how he was feeling that day. Little did I know that what he said next would change my life forever.

He put his coffee down, reached over and grabbed my hand. He looked me in the eyes and told me, "I am feeling wonderful. I woke up with a smile on my face and am just so glad to be here today. I hope you woke up with a smile on your face too, because you should." The next day he passed away. I have never been able to get those words out of my head.

Just a few short months later my aunt passed away. For a long time I could not step back into Woodside, but I have continued volunteering and enjoying every day I have been given. Every experience I have had has changed my life and helped me get through my losses. Volunteering with hospice has opened my eyes to all the wonderful things about life and truly took me out of a dark time. With the help of my wonderful family, friends, and every loving soul who is a part of Suncoast Hospice, I am who I am today and can go on, knowing that I will see my grandma and my aunt again.

Alivia Seay is a nursing major at St. Petersburg College in St. Petersburg, FL. At the age of two she started dance and danced for 13 years until she decided to focus on pursuing her passion for nursing. She is currently working on her Associate in Science degree and will go on to get her Bachelor of Science in Nursing degree along with a Nurse Practitioner degree.

CHAPTER 8

Perinatal Loss in Adolescence: A Double Transition

Carlos Torres, Nicole Alston, and Robert A. Neimeyer

Author's Note: Names have been changed to protect confidentiality.

Sahara was 18 when she lost her baby. The pain she felt while holding her dead child, Iyanna, was unimaginable but not without precedent. Molested by a relative for six years and raped in a classroom by a peer at age 14, she held her pain in silence. Without giving her family any explanation, she dropped out of school and turned to partying, drinking, and smoking. In her family's eyes, she was a burnt-out rebel. But Sahara was just trying her best to cope. She turned to a brother figure, a young man with whom she had been raised and who lived in the house with her family. For several years, he provided her emotional comfort, and their relationship also became a sexual one. She kept that joy in her life a secret as well, knowing her parents would not approve of their relationship. Then Sahara became pregnant. Her family's reaction to the news, given that she was unwilling to disclose any details regarding the baby's father, ranged from disappointment to anger.

> A lot of people were angry at me...I felt so alone. When I first found out that I was pregnant, I expected people in my family to be happy for me, but instead I was getting a whole lot of negative vibes. I guess it's because I'm young. I guess maybe they felt that I wasn't ready. They said that I wasn't going to have any money. They said, it's not going to be easy. They wanted me to get an abortion.

Sahara isolated herself from her family. She no longer wanted to hear their negative comments. However, it was the baby's father's reaction that was the most damaging.

> I was excited, but when I called and told him I was pregnant, his response was, 'That sucks...I'm not ready to be a father, that's gonna be all you, if you go through with this.' He tried to talk me out of having the baby. He tried to convince me to get rid of it...His response opened my eyes and I realized that it was going to be me and my baby, alone, and I was gonna be by myself. Then he disappeared, just like that. Like nothing ever happened between us. So I had my moments when I couldn't wait for her to arrive. Then, other times, I would be depressed and cry. I just stopped talking.

> I just wanted someone who was going to love me forever... and thought the baby would do that. That's the only thing that was going through my head.

Sahara's baby, Iyanna, was born and died the same day.

> At six months, I started to witness a lot of pain in my stomach. Like I said, I would cry day in and day out. I noticed a decrease in movement. And then, when I went to the doctor, her heart rate was getting slower, and slower, and slower. She wasn't growing properly, they told me. The left side of her heart was not fully developed."

> When I went to the hospital, they wanted to give me an emergency C-section, but I was afraid, and I didn't want that. My labor with her...it was hard, but easy at the same time. She came right out. They rushed her to the NICU, so I was trying to cope with that. But something just came to me, I wasn't feeling right. I asked my mom to call the nursery to check on her. Eventually, the docs came and spoke with me. I got to see her...so small with so many tubes. It broke my heart. I just couldn't take it. The doctors told me that she kept having episodes when they tried to feed her. They put her on the breathing machine. It looked like she was improving, but it failed. But I already kinda knew.

> The dad ended up getting someone else pregnant and she was due a couple of months after me.

> We had a funeral and a burial. I didn't make any decisions about the funeral. After I had her, I was quiet for six days. I was quiet and I didn't talk. I wanted nothing to do with the funeral. I didn't think that I'd even make it to the funeral, but I did go. I just didn't stay. I was numb. I couldn't cry.

> A few weeks later, I moved across the country. My first words when I started to open up were that I was moving. I just went to work and came home…all I did was write. I had less of a desire to go to school because of Iyanna's death. I had nothing to show for it. I wanted Iyanna to be proud of me for going back to school. My child wasn't here for me to say, 'Look, Mommy got this,' or, 'Mommy got that.'

After Iyanna's death, Sahara often felt that there was something she could have done to change what happened. Often, she wished she could have switched places with Iyanna.

> I kinda felt like it should have been me that died instead of her. I felt like maybe I shoulda taken better care of myself. I know that I did the best I could at the time, but I tend to beat myself up about stuff that happened.

Eleven months after Iyanna's death, Sahara attended a baby shower. The shower triggered intense emotions.

> I remember that day that I had too much to drink as well…I went to a baby shower with my cousin. At first it didn't bother me, but after I was there, it did. I didn't have the experience of none of it [her own baby shower]. I know that all I was crying for was Iyanna. I let it out so that I was no longer feeling any type of way. Like I said, I was quiet, my body was numb, I couldn't cry, and I finally did cry.

> I was anxious to have another baby…after a while I started to get into relationships not for love, but just for a baby. I didn't know how to cope.

Grief, as it is understood from a meaning reconstruction approach, is most problematic when it shatters our most fundamental worldview assumptions (Neimeyer & Sands, 2011). A loss like Sahara's is likely to shatter the assumptions held by many. For the teenage mother-to-be, whose life may have previously been lived without the weight of such personal loss, assumptions regarding an infinitely possible future are reduced by the reality of miscarriage, stillbirth, or neonatal death. For the mental health professional, whose experiences working with pregnancy loss may not yet have included a client so young, assumptions regarding an "appropriate" age for pregnancy may hinder the helping relationship. But a review of U.S. infant mortality statistics reveals that adolescent pregnancy loss is not so rare. Of the 742,990 pregnant females between the ages of 15 through 19 in 2006, 107,130 miscarried or had a stillbirth (Guttmacher Institute, 2010). Thus, it is an experience many mental health professionals are likely to encounter. Unfortunately, the psychological effects of miscarriage, stillbirth, and neonatal loss on adolescent girls are not well examined.

The psychological sequelae of miscarriage and stillbirth are well documented for adult women, and include protracted grief (Toedter, Lasker, & Janssen, 2001), anxiety (Geller & Klier, 2001), major depressive disorders (Klier, Geller, & Neugebauer, 2000), and post-traumatic stress disorder (PTSD) (Turton, Hughes, Evans, & Fainman, 2000). While this literature may be appropriate for the targeted adult population, there are many important ways that teenagers differ from adults. Thus, what is known about adult perinatal loss may not generalize to adolescents. There is an implicit cultural understanding that teens are just beginning to acquire the life skills that will lead them into adulthood and so their sense of self is just being explored (McLean, 2005). Within that transitional phase into adulthood, adolescent females often lack financial, emotional, and relational stability. Moreover, because it runs contrary to societal norms, teen pregnancy and subsequent loss may be silenced, minimized, or stigmatized, rendering expressing grief and seeking help problematic (Wiemann, Rickert, Berenson, & Volk, 2005).

In working for the first time with adolescent females grieving a perinatal loss, mental health professionals may lean on their understanding of or experience with adult grief or adolescents bereaving other types of losses. Two important questions for mental health professionals working with teens who have experienced a miscarriage, stillbirth, or neonatal loss are: How is a perinatal loss experience different/similar for teens compared to adults? And how is a perinatal loss different for a teenage girl compared to other types of losses?

To answer those questions, we turn to the few studies that have explored perinatal loss among adolescents. Although there may be some overlap between adolescent and adult perinatal loss bereavement, important developmental differences may exist for teens compared to adults with regard to cognitive and emotional processes, as well as important differences in relationships with family, peers, and society. Thus, we examine the effects of miscarriage, stillbirth, and neonatal death experiences on the individual separately from relationships with important others.

GRIEF AFTER A PERINATAL LOSS:
THE INDIVIDUAL EXPERIENCE

Studies have found that, similar to adults, pregnancy loss among adolescents follows a path from shock, to grief, to resolution that is punctuated by the ability to make meaning of the event. Several bereavement models have been found to apply equally well to adolescents and adults. Welch and Bergen (2000), making use of Rando's (1984) 6-R Process Model of grief (recognizing the loss, reacting emotionally, re-experiencing the loss, relinquishing their loss, readjusting, and reinvesting) found that the six Caucasian women they interviewed experienced some form of confusion, disbelief, and feelings of "going crazy." They found this experience to be commensurate with the emotional reaction stage, with difficulty comprehending the loss. Similarly, Sefton (2007) found that the 14 Hispanic adolescents she interviewed initially reacted to their loss with shock, an experience she tracked using Sanders' (1989) Integrated Theory of Bereavement model, which includes shock, awareness of the loss, conservation and withdrawal, healing, and finally renewal. Many of the teens in Sefton's study went on to experience anger, guilt, sadness, and somatic complaints such as headaches in the months following the loss. A study by Wheeler and Austin (2001) found similar results among the adolescents they surveyed. The participants in the Wheeler and Austin study reported that their guilt stemmed from a belief that their body had failed, a belief also held by many adult women who experience a perinatal loss (Frost & Condon, 1996). However, unusual among adult women, Welch and Bergen found that the majority of adolescents in their study had sex as soon as two months after their pregnancy loss, with no feelings of guilt associated with the act.

For some adolescents, sexual intercourse was a conscious attempt to conceive again and fulfill a yearning for motherhood, which some adult women have also reported (Grout, Bronna, & Romanoff, 2000). Some teens in Welch and Bergen's (2000) study expressed their yearning in child-like ways, such as cuddling a teddy bear in baby clothes or purchasing a puppy. However, sex was not always an attempt at conception, and some teens reported engaging in loveless sexual behaviors as an act of avoidance. Along with promiscuity, other teens reported binge drinking and withdrawal from others to avoid or cope with the pain brought on by the loss, as was the case with Sahara. The meaning making that occurred during the re-establishment phase was clearly specific to the adolescent and included beliefs that it was not time to be a mother and a second chance to be a teen was given. Although the majority of Sefton's (2007) participants reported growth from their loss, six reported that their miscarriage continued to affect them in adverse ways. Unfortunately, risk factors for complicated grief among adolescents who experienced a perinatal loss have not been studied, and little is known about what helps or hinders good outcomes from a perinatal loss among adolescents.

GRIEF AFTER A PERINATAL LOSS: RELATIONSHIPS WITH OTHERS

Many teens experiencing a perinatal loss must contend with cultural assumptions that produce problematic responses from others, including negative value judgments against teen pregnancy, minimization of the loss due to the belief that the pregnancy was not wanted by the teen, and a belief that an adolescent is not capable of caring for a child. Indeed, researchers have found that pregnant teens often experience social disdain. Wiemann, Rickert, Berenson, and Volk (2005) found that in a sample of 925 pregnant adolescents, two out of five reported feeling stigmatized. SmithBattle (2009) noted that it's not just peers and family who stigmatize; professionals, such as nurses, meet pregnant teens with bias as well. Thus, family and professionals may meet the teen's loss with unfortunate comments like, "That was God's way of saving you from disgrace" or "You can just have another baby when you're ready."

The social isolation that occurs after a perinatal loss is shared by adults and teens. Hastings' (2000) study with bereaved adult parents may offer a partial explanation. She proposed that identity re-negotiation after parental bereavement is unavoidable and explained that former parental identities can no longer be performed in the same way and thus the death of a child creates a separate cultural identity. Her analysis of ethnographic data found that bereaved parents created specific self-disclosure and identity management rules to avoid imposing on others or to "wear them out." Similarly, one of the participants in Welch and Bergen's (2000) study said, "It's too intense for them…like anyone can understand what it's like to lose your kid" (p. 441). Sahara described several failed attempts at empathy.

> Don't tell me everything is going to be okay…when people say 'I know how you feel'…I hate that! Another is 'let it go.' That bothers me because I had a heartbeat inside of me that was a special bond and that's something I cannot let go.

However, for many teens it appears that distancing others from their loss is not so much an attempt to spare them the seriousness of their loss, but rather is done in order to avoid peers who may not be capable yet of understanding the gravity of the loss. Bereaved teens reported that those peers who did not stay away or ignored them displayed their support by offering to take the grief-stricken teen out to party and forget. Of course, the complexity surrounding the event can affect the adolescent mother-to-be in ways that are too difficult to immediately attend to and thus requires support from others. Welch and Bergen found that several teens in their study deferred medical and funeral decisions to their parents, as did Sahara. Additionally, although a few teen mothers reported receiving adequate and loving support from the child's father, most teens reported that they were not in a sufficiently stable relationship to count on the father's support during their bereavement, a painful reality for Sahara.

ADOLESCENT PERINATAL LOSS: IS IT COMPARABLE TO OTHER TYPES OF ADOLESCENT LOSS?

We have touched briefly on the particular cultural assumptions and the resulting stigma that may accompany adolescent perinatal loss. The minimizing or even silencing of such a loss has been termed *disenfranchised grief.* Grief is disenfranchised when it is "not openly acknowledged, publically mourned or socially supported" (Doka, 1989, p. 4). Explicating the "serious social failure" that occurs when grief is disenfranchised, Attig (2004) described disenfranchised grief as "a political failure involving both abuse of power and serious neglect" (p. 200) as well as "an ethical failure to respect the bereaved both in their suffering and in their efforts to overcome it and live meaningfully again in the aftermath of loss" (p. 201). Among women who've experienced a perinatal loss, that failure appears when interacting with extended family, community, and health professionals (Hazen, 2003; Lang et al., 2011). Adolescent disenfranchised grief is not only limited to perinatal loss, and may occur if the death of a loved one was due to a taboo illness like an AIDS-related complication or a taboo event like suicide or gang-related homicide. However, unlike these other stigmatized death-related losses, perinatal loss may challenge notions of feminine identity, of what it means to be able to embody certain cultural ideals and give birth and become a mother. As such, the idea of a nonfinite loss (Bruce & Schultz, 2001), a loss that is intangible and often ongoing, may apply to adolescents who are struggling to reconstruct a coherent sense of identity amidst the potentially silenced pain of their lost pregnancy.

CLINICAL CONSIDERATIONS

How can a clinician help a bereaved teen honor her child and reconstruct her life? A crucial first step involves understanding the meaning of motherhood, the pregnancy, and the loss held by the adolescent. Here we describe the interplay that development, culture, and family have on the teens' lived experience.

Placing the loss in a developmental context

Substantial empirical evidence shows that a coherent life story and systematic construction of identity begins during adolescence (Meeus, 2011). For example, McLean (2005) found that younger adolescents tended to share memories with parents for the purpose of self-exploration, whereas older adolescents tended to share with peers for the purpose of entertainment. Furthermore, each form of sharing was punctuated with different narrative patterns and meaning making results. Those familiar with Erikson's psychosocial stages of development will notice the similarity with the identity-versus-role-confusion conflict that is present during the adolescence stage, a time when social relationships become increasingly important. Given this, the clinician can explore the impact of pregnancy loss by asking the teen to describe who she was and what she wanted before, during, and after the pregnancy. How did the pregnancy fulfill or frustrate her emerging life goals? In our case study, Sahara shared that she "just wanted someone who was going to love me forever," a response that, given her sexual abuse history and belief that "no one cared…no one wanted me to be happy," is consistent with a self seen as unlovable. How has the loss impacted (or possibly confused) the teen's sense of self? Sahara provided one concrete example of how Iyanna's death affected her sense of self when she explained that she had lost desire to continue her studies because she no longer had a loving child who would "be proud of me for going back to school." However, loss often impacts us in ways that are more abstract than concrete. For example, one of the authors of this chapter (Torres) worked with a client who explained that she thought of her body as "broken" after having a miscarriage, a personal belief that was informed by broader culture-specific beliefs, which will be explained in more detail in the next section.

Situating the loss in cultural terms

As briefly noted in the last section, personal beliefs are produced, shaped, and managed by broader cultural and community beliefs. Our culture provides templates to produce individualized selves. As such, notions of pregnancy, motherhood, and loss are significantly affected by the teen's historical and geographical context. For the client described above, the belief that her miscarriage revealed a "broken" body stemmed from her understanding that the woman's role was to provide children for her husband, a belief that was explicitly and implicitly taught to her by the small rural Mexican community where she grew up. The pain of her loss turned to a shame that was guided by her community's prevailing belief systems. In her case, teen pregnancy was not regarded as taboo in her community, but the miscarriage was quickly silenced by her family because of its cultural implication.

However, for teens growing up elsewhere, negative reactions from others may start with the pregnancy itself. Of course, those examples dwell on the negative; certainly, it is possible that a community may support a teen through her pregnancy as well as through her grief. The clinician is advised to ask the teen not only how she saw herself before, during, and after her pregnancy, but where she learned to hold those views. Culture also affects how grief is experienced and expressed. Thus, beyond response to the pregnancy, culture considerations should also examine loss-related concerns, including death-related rituals and ceremonies. For example, a teen raised with traditional Mexican customs, like the one described above, may find comfort in giving voice to her grief by creating an altar for her unborn child during the *Dia de los Muertos* (Day of the Dead). The clinician may benefit from addressing spiritual and religious upbringing and beliefs as well, as they significantly impact grief and meaning making. Notions of sin, redemption, afterlife, and continuing bonds may be particularly salient for a teen raised in a religious environment who is mourning a pregnancy loss.

Evaluating the family context

Culture provides teens with raw materials from which to carve out identity, including general norms to follow and values to hold. The family system provides the teen with specific guidelines and instructions, including communication styles and relational approaches. How the teen approaches her pregnancy loss, including whom she talks to and what coping strategies she takes on, will be largely influenced by her exposure to the rules and values held by her family. In Sahara's case, her pregnancy was met with castigation, which led her to isolate herself. Moreover, the complexity sharply increases if conflict and mixed messages regarding pregnancy, loss, or expression of emotion are found among the family. Understanding the teen's responses to her pregnancy loss is crucial for knowing how the family has supported or castigated the teen during her pregnancy as well as how the family has responded to or ignored her loss. The clinician can further understand the teen's familial context by asking to whom in her family she feels safe talking. For many teenagers the family will comprise not just parents and siblings, but extended family as well, which sometimes includes individuals not related to the teenager, such as godparents or close family friends.

INTERVENTION RECOMMENDATIONS

We end our chapter with intervention suggestions suited for teens bereaved by a perinatal loss. Our attempt here is to weave together the aforementioned research findings and clinical considerations into practical and potent principles of practice.

Assess current coping strategies

As was true for Sahara and many other teens who participated in the aforementioned research studies, negative coping, including substance abuse and risky sexual behaviors, is a major concern. Thus, it is important for the clinician to assess the teen's coping behaviors and directly ask about substance use, self-harm, and risky sexual behaviors. Given that the teen is a minor and in a vulnerable situation, and may have entered the therapeutic relationship for reasons as diverse as personal choice, family request, or mandate by another, there may be resistance to share. Thus, the clinician must first establish a trusting relationship before asking direct questions. This is especially true if the teen previously felt judged by medical professionals during her pregnancy. To that end, accompanying the teen in her story with a supporting, listening presence, being there to "feel and deal" with her, can "help undo the client's aloneness" (Fosha, 2009, p.45).

Establish a support system

Many of the teens in research studies also reported that their substance use was encouraged by well-meaning friends and peers who wanted to help. Other teens reported talking very little about their loss with peers, and they refused any help from others. Sahara, who attempted to isolate herself by moving away from her family, explained that she eventually "couldn't take the pain anymore...I was tired of feeling alone," and that she decided to seek professional help because she was "ready to open up." However, most teens reported that they had not sought out mental health professionals, something Sahara acknowledged: "No, they are not going to come forward easily. Some teens who have been through what I've been through are just going to try to block the memory out and try not to think about it." It is important for the clinician working with the bereaved teen to acknowledge her courage for seeking help. Additionally, the clinician should assess whether the teen needs help establishing other supportive contacts in her community. Having evaluated the family system and the teen's community network, the clinician can begin to work with the teen to determine who might be a safe family member or relative to lean on for support, whether it be financial or emotional. The clinician should determine whether the baby's father (and, possibly, his family) is a source of support. Close friends may become distant, and the clinician should take time to help the teen decide which friends have remained helpful. If the teen is religious, she may feel comfortable turning to supportive figures in her spiritual community. With the possibility of a silenced and stigmatized loss, the clinician may need to remind the teen that her grief is justified and that her loss should be honored. The clinician may need to play coach as well to equip the teen with the communication skills necessary to ask for support as well as refuse comments she finds disparaging.

Pursue artful means to therapeutic ends

Though a teen might be willing to share her story with the clinician, she may find it difficult to express herself in concrete terms. Any loss that shakes the very foundations of our sense of self produces an ephemeral catalogue of emotions that may sting sharply but remain elusive nonetheless. Expressing loss and change through creative endeavors occurs in all cultures and is often highly engaging for adolescents. In her isolation, Sahara turned to writing as a means of making sense of her loss. Similarly, one of the authors of this chapter (Torres) has had much success with teens who struggled to narrate stories of loss and transition with words but found that they could chart their complex inner world by cutting and pasting collages and drawing pictures. Research supporting the use of arts-based grief interventions is scant, but growing (Torres, Neff, & Neimeyer, 2014). However, a simple invitation to explore her loss artfully can easily accompany a clinician's more traditional approach. Many excellent resources are at the clinician's disposal offering ready-made templates ready to be combined with other therapeutic techniques. The Pongo Teen Writing website (www.pongoteenwriting.org), for example, offers a large selection of writing activities geared toward teens, several of which are geared specifically toward loss. Teens might come to the clinician with journals or artwork they've already created. Inviting teens to share their poetry, drawings, paintings, music and other creative expressions can encourage intimate explorations of loss and foster restorative pursuits. Eliciting stories associated with memorial tattoos, memorial jewelry, or other keepsakes can acknowledge and strengthen naturally occurring continuing bond practices between teen and child.

Respect talking and not talking

As important as it is for a teen to tell her story, it is just as important for the clinician to respect her silence. The clinician should not assume that silence means avoidance. To the contrary, silence is often an important component of successful coping and emotion regulation during bereavement (Hooghe, Neimeyer, & Rober, 2012). The teen's silence may also be infused with cultural meaning that is meant to show respect for authority (where silence pertains to the clinician-client relationship) or exemplifies a stance toward discussing loss (where silence pertains to communicating loss-specific details).

CONCLUSION

In this chapter, we considered how adolescent perinatal loss is similar to and different from adult perinatal loss, which has received greater attention in the bereavement literature. Reviewing the brief literature on adolescent perinatal loss, we noted that while bereavement trajectories are similar between teens and adults, coping and meaning making endeavors differ due to developmental and cultural differences. Expanding on those differences, we provided clinicians with recommendations that focused on intra- and inter-personal considerations that impact teens particularly. We paid attention to the impact social and familial stigma may have on the teen's loss and on her particular identity-forming needs. We then offered practical interventions that assessed the teen's coping style, evaluated and explored her support system, made use of developmentally appropriate artistic modalities, and respected the teen's story-telling and silence.

Conception and loss in adolescence confronts teens with a complex double transition at a vulnerable stage in the development of their sense of self and intimate relationships. A teenager may initially be reluctant to share her loss with the clinician, an "authoritative adult." However, just like any other bereaved individual, she will yearn to express her story because doing so keeps the memory of her child alive, even if she never had the chance to hold her baby. The clinician's empathic, patient, and supportive presence may be the first safe space that has been offered to her. We hope that our attempt to explore the meaning of such transitions in light of the current literature makes the voices of teens who have suffered this experience more audible, and provides clinicians with some principles that can contribute to more empathic practice as their clients negotiate the twin challenges of anticipated motherhood and subsequent bereavement.

Carlos Torres is currently a clinical psychology PhD candidate at the University of Memphis. His research interests include bereavement experience and expression in culture and identity transformation after traumatic loss. He has particular interests investigating deaths that are stigmatized and silenced. He champions the use of arts-based research methods and enjoys engaging clients with creative and self-exploratory therapeutic techniques.

Nicole Alston is the founder and executive director of the Skye Foundation, a nonprofit foundation established in memory of her stillborn daughter Skye. Drawing on experiential knowledge, she has spoken to audiences internationally about providing comprehensive psychosocial support for families who are grieving the death of a baby. She is also a contributing author for the Open to Hope Foundation and has written a number of other publications. Since 2012, Alston has been the bereavement coordinator for the Circle of Life Children's Center in Newark, NJ, a wide-ranging program that provides support and psycho-education to families, as well as palliative and end-of-life care for children with life-limiting illness.

Robert A. Neimeyer, PhD, is a professor in the Psychotherapy Research Area of the Department of Psychology, University of Memphis, where he also maintains an active clinical practice. Neimeyer has published 25 books, including Techniques of Grief Therapy: Creative Practices for Counseling the Bereaved; Grief and Bereavement in Contemporary Society: Bridging Research and Practice, *and* The Art of Longing, *a book of contemporary poetry. The author of nearly 400 articles and book chapters, he is currently working to advance a more adequate theory of grieving as a meaning-making process, both in his published work and through his frequent professional workshops for national and international audiences.*

References

Attig, T. (2004). Disenfranchised grief revisited: Discounting hope and love. *Omega: Journal of Death and Dying, 49*(3), 197-215.

Bruce, E. & Schultz, C. (2001). *Nonfinite loss and grief: A psychoeducational approach.* Baltimore, MD: Brookes Publishing.

Doka, K. J. (1989). *Disenfranchised grief: Recognizing hidden sorrow.* Lexington, MA: Lexington Books.

Fosha, D. (2009). Healing attachment trauma with attachment (and then some). In M. Kerman, *Clinical pearls of wisdom: 21 leading therapists offer their key insights* (pp. 43-56). New York, NY: Norton

Frost, M., & Condon, J. T. (1996). The psychological sequelae of miscarriage: A critical review of the literature. *Australasian Psychiatry, 30*(1), 54-62.

Geller, P. A., Klier, C. M., & Neugebauer, R. (2001). Anxiety disorders following miscarriage. *Journal of Clinical Psychiatry.* 62(6), 432-438.

Grout, A., Bronna, D., & Romanoff, L. (2000). The myth of the replacement child: parents' stories and practices after perinatal death. *Death Studies, 24*(2), 93-113.

Guttmacher Institute. (2010). U.S. Teenage Pregnancies, Births and Abortions: National and State Trends and Trends by Race and Ethnicity [data file]. Retrieved from: http://www.guttmacher.org/pubs/USTPtrends.pdf

Hastings, S. O. (2000). Self-disclosure and identity management by bereaved parents. *Communication Studies, 51*(4), 352-371.

Hazen, M. A. (2003). Societal and workplace responses to perinatal loss: Disenfranchised grief or healing connection. *Human Relations, 56*(2), 147-166.

Hooghe, A., Neimeyer, R. A., & Rober, P. (2012). "Cycling Around an Emotional Core of Sadness:" Emotion Regulation in a Couple after the Loss of a Child. *Qualitative Health Research, 22*(9), 1220-1231.

Klier, C. M., Geller, P. A., & Neugebauer, R. (2000). Minor depressive disorder in the context of miscarriage. *Journal of Affective Disorders, 59*(1), 13-21.

Lang, A., Fleiszer, A. R., Duhamel, F., Sword, W., Gilbert, K. R., & Corsini-Munt, S. (2011). Perinatal loss and parental grief: The challenge of ambiguity and disenfranchised grief. *Omega: Journal of Death and Dying, 63*(2), 183-196.

McLean, K. C. (2005). Late adolescent identity development: narrative meaning making and memory telling. *Developmental Psychology, 41*(4), 683-691.

Meeus, W. (2011). The study of adolescent identity formation 2000–2010: A review of longitudinal research. *Journal of Research on Adolescence, 21*(1), 75-94.

Neimeyer, R. A., & Sands, D. C. (2011). Meaning reconstruction in bereavement: From principles to practice. In R. A. Neimeyer, H. Winokuer, D. Harris, & G. Thornton (Eds.), *Grief and bereavement in contemporary society: Bridging research and practice* (pp. 9-22). New York, NY: Routledge.

Rando, T. (1984). *Grief, death and dying: Clinical interventions for caregivers.* Champaign, IL: Research Press Company.

Sanders, C. (1989). *Grief: The mourning after.* New York, NY: Wiley.

Sefton, M. (2007). Grief analysis of adolescents experiencing an early miscarriage. *Hispanic Health Care International, 5*(1), 13-20.

SmithBattle, L. (2009). Pregnant with possibilities: Drawing on hermeneutic thought to reframe home-visiting programs for young mothers. *Nursing Inquiry, 16*(3), 191-200.

Toedter, L., Lasker, J., & Janssen, H. (2001). International comparison of studies using the perinatal grief scale: A decade of research on pregnancy loss. *Death Studies, 25*(3), 205-228.

Torres, C., Neff, M., & Neimeyer, R. A. (2014). The expressive arts in grief therapy: An empirical perspective. In Thompson, B. E., & Neimeyer, R. A. (Eds.), *Grief and the expressive arts: Practices for creating meaning.* New York, NY: Routledge.

Turton, P., Hughes, P., Evans, C. D. H., & Fainman, D. (2001). Incidence, correlates and predictors of post-traumatic stress disorder in the pregnancy after stillbirth. *The British Journal of Psychiatry, 178*(6), 556-560.

Welch, K. J. & Bergen, M. B. (2000). Adolescent parent mourning reactions associated with stillbirth or neonatal death. *Omega: Journal of Death and Dying, 40*(3), 435-452.

Wheeler, S. R. & Austin, J. K. (2001). The impact of early pregnancy loss on adolescents. *MCN: The American Journal of Maternal/Child Nursing, 26*(3), 154-159.

Wiemann, C. M., Rickert, V. I., Berenson, A. B., & Volk, R. J. (2005). Are pregnant adolescents stigmatized by pregnancy? *Journal of Adolescent Health, 36*(4), 352.

CHAPTER 9

Accidents and Traumatic Loss: The Adolescent Experience

Illene Noppe Cupit and Karissa J. Meyer

C onrad Jarrett is a teenage boy living in an affluent suburb of Chicago. His brother, Buck, the "perfect" older brother, died in a sailing accident 18 months ago. Conrad attempted suicide after this traumatic loss, and is home after spending four months in a psychiatric hospital. Thus begins a riveting film drama, *Ordinary People,* based on the book written by Judith Guest (1976), which won five Academy Awards in 1980. While coping with post-traumatic stress disorder and survivor guilt, the family dynamics are played out by Conrad's rejecting mother who attempts to recreate their impeccable home where death is not acknowledged, and Conrad's father, who awkwardly tries to mediate between his surviving troubled son and his wife.

The many layers of this story speak to the complexity of adolescent bereavement due to accidental death. In addition to learning about the sensitive thoughtful nature of Conrad, we find that he and his older brother, both on the swim team, were a close sibling pair. Confident in their swimming abilities, they did not heed the storm warnings that ultimately caused the boating accident. The death also deeply affects Conrad's parents, and certainly their ways of handling the death contribute to the difficulties Conrad experiences. However, in this family, the financial resources are in place for psychotherapeutic help, which sadly are not available to many grieving adolescents. And unlike many others in similar circumstances, Conrad ultimately is able to reintegrate within his peer group.

Why did this film rivet moviegoers so, and why does the story still have contemporary appeal? In both reality and drama, adolescent death and its aftermath on family members and extended family is still not given adequate serious attention. In 1976, when the book was first published, the consequences of death were poorly understood, and adolescents certainly were marginalized in their grief (Raphael, 1983). The novel's story illustrates that such deaths have ripple effects that magnify existing family dynamics and fare best under carefully considered intervention. In addition, there is a social and cultural context that provides a specific lens for which the narratives of adolescence and death due to accidents are filtered. Finally, the story reflects the truths that most adolescent deaths are due to accidents; that adolescent grievers are profoundly affected by such deaths; and that despite their mature understanding of death, the emotional needs and developmental tasks of adolescence create "the perfect storm" of a difficult grief experience in a context of misunderstanding or benevolent negligence from the adolescent's social environment. Drawing upon the themes of this fictional story, the purpose of this chapter is to broaden knowledge about adolescent traumatic loss due to accidents. Adolescents lose their lives in accidents and are grievers from such deaths, which include not only the deaths of their peers, but family members, teachers, and celebrities. There are two contextual themes that wrap around each discussion. The first is that adolescent death, grief, and responses to intervention are affected by the social, cognitive, physical, and interpersonal developmental tasks that often are tension-ridden by their own dialectical drama. The second is that adolescent death and adolescent grief do not occur in a vacuum. Rather, the experience is rooted in a wider social, cultural, and historical context which is addressed by ecological systems theory (Bronfenbrenner, 1994).

ADOLESCENT ACCIDENTAL DEATH AS A FUNCTION OF DEVELOPMENTAL PROCESSES

It is assumed that adolescents have mastered a mature concept of death, i.e., the universality, nonfunctionality, and irreversibility of death (Noppe & Noppe, 1991). Though they may hold the textbook "mature conception" about death, their position in the life cycle leaves many questions about death unanswered, and these can affect the way in which an adolescent responds to the accidental death of a parent, sibling, or friend. Despite their age and understanding, adolescents do experience a number of losses: their childhood, their innocence, belongings they have outgrown, and relationships they have outgrown. Such nondeath losses, nevertheless, frequently trigger grief responses (Harris, 2011). As Noppe and Noppe (1991) describe, the ambiguous relationship with death that develops during adolescence can be characterized by four dialectic themes: the biological dialectic, the cognitive dialectic, the social dialectic, and the affective dialectic. Noppe and Noppe (1991) consider such themes to be dialectical as encounters with death bring to the forefront the tensions between the life-affirming growth orientation of this age period and the inevitable losses of developmental transitions. Such tensions may explain why adolescents are particularly at risk for accidents and why their reactions to such deaths are intense and tangled.

The biological dialectic refers to adolescents' understanding that physical maturation of the body ultimately ends in the cessation of bodily functions. By the time children reach adolescence, they typically have a good understanding of the fact that everyone ages and eventually must die. However, teens seem to feel so physically alive that it occasionally borders on invincibility. Despite this feeling of "it won't happen to me," they know, to an extent, that eventually they too will come to an end. This conflict may channel itself in various kinds of risk-taking behavior. Death-defying behavior can present itself in the forms of reckless driving, drug and alcohol abuse, or sexual promiscuity (Noppe and Noppe, 1991). Every day, adolescents die from activities such as texting and driving, driving under the influence of alcohol or drugs, speeding, and accidental overdoses on drugs and alcohol. Such fatalities often are perceived as being potentially preventable and are just another example of adolescents' grasp of their physical peak falling short. Based on what we know about adolescents' sensation of invincibility, many of these fatal accidents could have resulted after the victim assumed that he or she is far too healthy, fast, and can beat the odds. Regardless of disconfirming evidence, death only happens to "the other guy" and to the old.

The second theme described by Noppe and Noppe (1991) is the cognitive dialectic. As a result of formal thought, adolescents have a greater ability to understand all of the possibilities of life, hold a sophisticated reasoning power that allows them to think about both life and death, and question childhood ideas regarding religion, spirituality, ethics, and the meaning of life (Noppe and Noppe, 1991). Because they now have the ability to plan ahead, set goals, and work out long-term strategies, they must ultimately accept death as the conclusion to life. This is no easy feat and can potentially be even more difficult if the adolescent has mixed feelings about the afterlife or if he or she has already had a first death experience through the death of a peer, family member, or pet. Hypothetical thought enables adolescents to plan for a future that will bring them happiness whether it be in the form of success, a family, traveling the world, or money. The plan that is often constructed depends heavily on the fact that each person lives a long and healthy life. Such a life plan may be threatened by the actual or envisioned accidental death of the self or a loved one.

Formal thought is also the reason for the egocentricity behind their belief in being immune to destruction. As Noppe and Noppe (1991) describe, they "fail to recognize how ordinary and human they are" (p. 34). Until an adolescent is personally affected by the death of someone significant, it remains mostly an abstract thought (Balk, 2008). Cognitions certainly change when there is an unexpected death. Brent, Melhem, Donohoe and Walker (2009) found that many cognitive changes take place in adolescents after a death of a parent due to a sudden and unexpected accident.

The third dialectic described by Noppe and Noppe (1991) involves the social context of development. It is expected that during adolescence the loss of one's childhood buddies are replaced by an ever-widening circle of new friends. However, adolescents experiencing the accidental loss of a parent, peer, or sibling may feel marginalized from their peers who do not realize the impact the death has on their friend. The sudden shock of an accidental death may heighten the inherent tension between the need to affiliate and the desperate realization of one's existential aloneness.

Finally, Noppe and Noppe (1991) consider the affective dialectic to include an emerging sense of identity and a need for independence while still being emotionally and physically dependent upon parents. Mastery and control become important themes when one feels so out of control of one's body, cognitions, and feelings. A sudden and unanticipated death challenges all of these: identity ("Who am I without you?" and "How will I be remembered?"); independence ("I now am afraid to be alone or on my own."); and control and mastery ("Why did I not prevent the death and can death happen to me at any instant?"). Ambivalent, insecure attachments with a significant other who dies in an accident can set the adolescent up for complications in grief (Noppe, 2000).

THE ECOLOGICAL CONTEXT AND ADOLESCENTS WHO DIE FROM ACCIDENTS

Adolescence is a loosely defined stage of life that is more of a Western social construction than a physical reality. The "stage" emerges out of a developing economic and political landscape that necessitates extended time in education, dependence upon immediate family, extensive socialization within a peer group, and self-identification as a "teen." There are varying accounts of what ages constitute adolescence, with many researchers and writers extending the upper limit as far as age 24. A more useful approach is to look at the developmental tasks of this period, which involve emotional separation from one's parents, achieving a sense of personal autonomy, and developing intimacy and commitment with others (Balk, in press). These characteristics uniquely position adolescents in terms of their own mortality as well as how they respond to the death of others.

There are many physical changes that occur during this period, but it also is one of the healthiest periods of the lifespan. In the US, where the number one cause of death for the overall population is cardiovascular disease, during adolescence it is death due to accidents, and mostly vehicular accidents (Centers for Disease Control and Prevention, http://www.cdc.gov/nchs/data/nvsr).

TABLE 1

NUMBER OF DEATHS BY AGE: UNITED STATES 2010

Cause of Death	All Ages	Under 1	Ages 1 to 4	Ages 5 to 14	Ages 15-24	Ages 25-34
Motor Vehicle Accidents	35,332	79	449	890	7,250	5,746
Other land transport accidents	1,029	2	17	30	154	134
Water, air, and other transport accidents	1,600	–	3	36	145	210
Falls	26,009	10	24	28	211	299
Accidental discharge of firearms	606	–	25	37	145	107
Accidental drowning	3,782	39	436	251	656	476
Accidental exposure to flames, smoke, & fire	2,782	21	147	135	127	155
Accidental poisoning	33,041	6	34	54	3,183	6,767
Other and unspecified accidents	16,678	953	259	182	470	679
All Accidents/ Unintentional Injuries	120,859	1,110	1,394	1,643	12,341	14,573

Source: CDC National Vital Statistics Report (2013)

In 2010, the death rate for adolescents age 15 to 19 was 49.4 per 100,000 (Child Health USA, 2012) with 63.8% of these due to motor vehicle accidents. For this age group, the adolescent mortality rate for males is more than twice that of females (69.6 per 100,000 for males; 28.1 per 100,000 for females) and is chiefly due to unintentional injuries, homicide, and suicide. For all racial/ethnic groups and males and females, unintentional injury was the number one cause of death. Furthermore, the Insurance Institute for Highway Safety (2013) reports that in 2011, 59% of the deaths of teenage passengers in motor vehicles occurred when the vehicle was driven by another teenager. Alcohol may play a significant role in such deaths. The Youth Risk Behavior Surveillance System (U.S. Department of Health and Human Services, 2011) reports that 24.1% of adolescents indicated that in the 30 days prior to taking the survey they had ridden one or more times in a car with someone who had been drinking alcohol. Furthermore,

8.2% of students had actually driven a vehicle one or more times after having consumed alcohol. Of relatively recent concern is accidents due to the distractions of texting or e-mailing. In 2011, 32.8% of students surveyed by the Youth Risk Behavior Surveillance System indicated that they had engaged in such activities while driving.

During this age period, death due to accidents is also caused by firearms. In 2009, 114 children and adolescents younger than age 20 died as a result of firearm accidents (Council on Injury, Violence and Poison Prevention Executive Committee, 2012). The Centers for Disease Control and Prevention (CDC) reports smaller numbers of U.S. deaths due to unintentional injuries for 2010 for children age 5 to 14 and 15 to 24 (see Table 1). In addition to the causes cited above, these include deaths due to falls, drowning, drug-induced deaths, and poisoning. These findings are similar to global trends, which suggest that most deaths of youth around the world, many due to traffic accidents, were preventable (World Health Organization, 2013).

These untimely deaths have a ripple effect throughout an entire community, reflect social trends in a culture at a particular point in history, and mirror prevailing attitudes about youth and death. The ecological systems theory of Bronfenbrenner (1994) offers a good contextual framework for understanding how the effects of adolescent death due to accidents extend beyond the individual who has died. At the first level of analysis, the *Microsystem* centers on the individual and his or her relationship to peers, family, school, health services, and any institution or group that has a direct immediate impact on the adolescent. For example, with increasing age, adolescents move away from the watchful eyes of their home base. Those who have access to cars, cell phones, and drugs, who have free time, disposable income, and a penchant for risk-taking, may be more prone to accidental death. In all countries, males are more prone to die this way than females. An inability to accurately assess the consequences of one's actions, as well as bowing under peer pressure, which are functions of an immature neurological system, comes into play as well (Noppe & Noppe, 2009). At the next level are the *Mesosystems,* created by linking together two or more microsystems. These involve the linkages between teachers, families, peers, and the adolescent. Effective intervention strategies may capitalize on the relationships of these groups because open communication from so many sources may ultimately reduce risk-taking behavior. It is also at this level that adolescents may be responsive to bereavement support. Conversely, youth who live in areas where they may have easy access to drugs and firearms are at greater risk for death due to an unintentional injury. What these youth might not have available to them are mental health facilities that can provide educational and psychological support to help them with effective decision making and their grief when a family member or friend dies (Walker, 2009).

The *Exosystem* is identified as links between various social networks in which the adolescent is not directly involved. Communities which do not recognize the seriousness of the consequences of adolescent accidents may not target their resources toward pre- or postvention.

According to Bronfenbrenner (1994), the macrosystem describes the overall culture of a society, with its implicit belief systems, values, and identity. In many cultures, males are given more latitude to explore and "be wild," accounting in part for the large disparity in accidental deaths between the two genders. And according to a report from the Centers for Disease Control and Prevention (Gilchrist & Ballesteros, 2012), the U.S. rate for unintentional injuries for persons age birth to 19 is worse than in other developed nations, which may be due to the fact that at present the US lacks a national, action plan to prevent such unintentional injury deaths. From 2000 to 2009, the death rate in the US due to poisoning almost doubled, primarily because of drug overdoses from prescription drugs. Fatalities due to texting and driving also are on the rise, a function of the greater usage and ownership of mobile devices.

Overlaying these four systems is the *Chronosystem* which in part represents social historical change. For example, deaths due to car accidents are more prevalent today than 100 years ago, when farm accidents and other work-related injuries led to death (Noppe and Noppe, 2009). In the past, close-knit families and communities, prior exposure to death, and adult-like responsibilities may have buffered the adolescent's suffering. Today, the social world of adolescents is vastly different. What may have replaced some of the community and family connections of the past is the Internet, which teens frequently turn to for connection and solace from their peers.

Understanding Adolescent Bereavement as a Result of Death Due to Accidents

Adolescent grievers have lots of company, despite the fact that most are not aware of their compatriots in this sad journey. Many adolescents are grieving the loss of their parents, co-workers, family members who are not teenagers, and even celebrities due to accidental deaths. Because so much of the research lumps deaths due to accidents together with death of a peer from suicide and homicide, it is difficult to determine if an accidental death is particularly troublesome for adolescent mental health.

The Centers for Disease Control reports that for all ages during 2010, the number of deaths in the US due to accidents was 120,859 (Murphy, Xu, & Kochanek, 2013) with the majority of these occurring in people age 35 to 64. This age range is where the parents and other adults who are involved in the lives of teenagers are found. As in adolescent accidental death, such deaths are unanticipated, traumatic, and may involve body mutilation. Additionally, many adolescents experience the death of a peer. Compounding the problem is the perception that the death may have been preventable. Noppe and Noppe (2009) point out that such deaths may involve putting the accident victim on life support, which frequently places the family and peers into conflict about medical ethical dilemmas. This may especially be the case for youth because they are much less likely to have an advance directive than individuals older than age 65 (Jones, Moss & Harris-Kojetin, 2011). As Raphael (1983, p. 28) noted:

> There has been no opportunity for anticipation, for preparation beforehand. The death brings an extra effect of shock over and above the normal. It is at the same time a most potent reminder of human mortality and human impotence, since one cannot know or control the time of the death. The bereaved is confronted by the power of death to kill and deprive and human helplessness in the face of it.

According to a number of theories of bereavement and grief, the myriad of responses that people experience are normative, culturally defined, and usually adaptive (Corr & Corr, 2013). It is also generally believed that with time the intensity of the emotional responses wanes and is replaced by coping responses that focus on reintegrating one's life (Stroebe & Schut, 1999). Finally, contemporary approaches to the grief response refer to meaning making in a person's narrative about the death, or an attempt to make sense out of what has happened so that it forms a coherent narrative (Neimeyer, 2001).

How do these assumptions play out for the adolescent griever, especially in the case of accidental death? First, consider who dies. The unanticipated death of a parent typically throws a family into emotional, financial, and functional crises. Excepting the case of suicide, where adolescents are targeted as needing special attention, many adults do not recognize that adolescents require emotional support and understanding that is tailored to their developmental needs. The accidental death of a parent throws into conflict the adolescent's need for separation from one's parents, as they may become vigilant and protective of the surviving parent. The adolescent's sense of mastery may be compromised by cognitions that he or she did nothing to prevent the death, and the need for intimacy may butt up against the sad reality that peers are not very tolerant of prolonged sadness. Some adolescents feel abandoned by their parents (Walker, 2009). Although they are cognitively mature enough to understand the random nature of an accident, unanswered questions may result in irrational feelings that their deceased parent abandoned them, which is damaging to the adolescent's self-esteem. Many adolescents feel that something is wrong with them because they want to maintain a connection between their deceased parent and can't seem to "get over it." Contemporary grief theory acknowledges the griever's need to maintain a connection with the deceased (Klass, Silverman, & Nickman, 1996) but how many people who are not bereavement specialists have heard of "continuing bonds" theory? Some professionals may still adhere to older theories that propose a specific endpoint to the bereavement experience, which is generally not an easily achievable standard for adolescents. Adolescents may also feel that they need to step into the role of their deceased parent, bearing some of the financial and parenting responsibilities of younger siblings. They may avoid socializing with their peers. Gender may also come into play as stereotypes are intensified for this age group, and males in particular hesitate to seek out help and confide about their grief.

Brent, Melheim, Donohoe, and Walker (2009) looked at the effects of loss of a parent due to suicide, accident or sudden natural death on children ages 7 to 25. The researchers found that nearly two years past the death, the children of parents who had died from either suicide or accident manifested higher rates of depression and alcohol or substance abuse as well as higher levels of anxiety. This proved to be particularly the case when it was the mother who had died.

Losing one's sibling from an accident presents another array of complicating factors. Such losses are not unusual. Data from the National Longitudinal Study of Adolescent Health and the Wisconsin Longitudinal Study suggest a prevalence rate of sibling death that ranges between 5% and 8% (Fletcher, Mailick, Song, & Wolfe, 2012). The surviving siblings find themselves coping with both their own responses as well as their bereaved parents, with negative effects particularly apparent when the death is traumatic and unanticipated (e.g., accident, suicide and homicide). The evidence also suggests that adolescents who experience such a death within the context of a more integrated and communicative family tend to do better over time than those who come from more emotionally distant families (Balk, 2009). Fletcher et al. (2012) report that experiencing a sibling death prior to age 25 is harder for sisters than brothers, and results in fewer years of schooling, lowered test scores, and effects on labor market earnings. Sisters appear to be impacted more by sibling death due to illness, but sibling death due to accidents or suicide had a greater impact on brothers. Unfortunately, no breakdown by age is given, so the assumption that the age of the bereaved sibling may make a difference in the grief response is unknown. Fletcher et al. (2012) suggest that surviving siblings may respond to the death of their sibling by questioning the meaning of life, experiencing fear that they too may die, and losing their religious beliefs. These outcomes appear to be more typical of an adolescent response than that of a younger child. What is apparent from this study, however, is how the death's impact upon family dynamics (the mesosystem) may have long-term consequences for the surviving sibling.

According to Servaty-Seib (2009), adolescents who experience the unintentional death of a peer may experience grief reactions that are similar to those of when a family member dies. This finding should not be surprising because adolescent friendships often serve as the replacements for the family relationships of childhood. The quality of the peer relationship and the degree to which the adolescent felt that she or he was "close" to the deceased peer affects the intensity and duration of the grief experience. Adolescents claim that such deaths are life-altering events that offer opportunities for positive growth (e.g., a greater appreciation of life) as well as negative outcomes.

FACTORS AFFECTING ADOLESCENT RESPONSES TO ACCIDENTAL DEATH

The role of the Internet

Today, social media is central to the way in which adolescents learn about death and cope with death. The Internet comes into play at all systemic levels of developmental ecology. Adolescents are exposed to a plethora of information and misinformation regarding death on a daily basis (Sofka, 1999; Sofka, Cupit & Gilbert, 2013) and they use social media sites to post information about the death of their friends and to memorialize the deceased. Sadly, some adolescents first learn about the accidental death of a friend through social media sites such as Facebook (Sofka, 2013). but the consequences of being informed this way are unknown. However, research is accruing that suggests that the Internet can also serve as a place where adolescents have the opportunity and freedom to feel safe about processing the death with their friends, communicate with the deceased, and express their confusion and intense feelings (Williams & Merten, 2009).

There are multiple ways in which adolescents who have experienced a loss due to accident use online communications to cope with their grief. Online memorial sites for celebrities, many who die in accidents (e.g., Princess Diana—car accident; Michael Jackson—accidental drug poisoning) may be a haven for adolescents who experience strong mourning responses to their deaths (Sanderson & Cheong, 2010). Spontaneity, seen in the many roadside memorials that often commemorate accidents, seems to be a key factor in adolescent expression of grief (Walter, Hourizi, Moncur & Pitsillides, 2011-2012). One might find a digitized RIP or other iconic signs suggesting one is in mourning.

Disenfranchised grief and the Internet

Without using the term "disenfranchised grief," Raphael (1983) described teenagers who were forgotten mourners when a friend or romantic partner died. Partly this was a function of the dominating needs of the bereaved family. Social groups tend to marginalize certain people who are mourning a loss by failing to acknowledge the significance of the death to that mourner. According to Doka (1989), disenfranchised grief refers to a death that is not socially supported. For example, there are few "grieving rules" or social norms established for the adolescent whose friend has died (Servaty-Seib, 2009). As Corr (2002) states, such disenfranchisement reflects "an active process of disavowal, renunciation, and rejection" (p. 40). Adolescents are particularly prone to disenfranchisement, hiding their grief as they fear social disapproval for mourning beyond the funeral, shame if they somehow were involved in the accident, and neglect because they are viewed as adults and thus should have developed adequate coping strategies to handle their grief (Rowling, 2002). This is especially true for adolescent males, who need a modality for expressing their grief in ways that are in keeping with their developing identity as young men (Rowling, 2002). And although there are a number of studies that have examined the grief responses of lesbian, gay, bisexual, transgender, and queer/questioning (LGBTQ) youth as a function of loss of friends and family from AIDS, currently there is no research that examines their mourning the accidental loss of a friend or romantic partner.

The Internet may provide an arena where adolescent grief "enfranchisement" may occur. Through blogs, social network sites, and gaming, adolescents find a venue for accepted expression of grief and a community of support. Perhaps the fact that it is spontaneous, peer driven, and perceived to be uniquely associated with youth, makes seeking solace via online communications particularly appealing to adolescents (Walter et al., 2011-2012). Another factor that is especially potent in the face of accidental death is the immediacy of the Internet. A sudden death jolts an adolescent peer group, rendering rapid communication with peers an appealing digitized option. Except for the occasional "Like" on Facebook, there are minimal expectations of returned messages. Thus, once the reality of the accidental death has sunk in, this form of communication promotes a continued relationship with the deceased and yet another venue for the expression of grief. Such communications have also been found to be helpful in making sense of the death (DeGroot, 2012). Adolescents, who are so self-conscious, are afforded the option to both hide their grief and be completely open about it at the same time.

Meaning making and styles of coping

When a death occurs, it may challenge the bereaved's ability to integrate his or her past, present, and future into a coherent story line. Since the construction of such a narrative is a major task of adolescence, an unanticipated death due to an unintentional injury may be particularly problematic. Making sense of death when there is a fatal accident is a difficult challenge for most bereaved (Currier, Holland & Neimeyer, 2007), but the conflict between identity construction, especially if there is a strong identification with the deceased, may render meaning making especially hard for the adolescent (Balk, in press). Given that their life cycle "roadmap" is under construction, the unpredictability of the death event could reinforce the capricious nature of the future, its pointlessness, and the lack of control over the forthcoming life cycle.

According to the dual process model of coping with bereavement (Stroebe & Schut, 2010), grief involves an oscillation between confronting the loss emotionally (loss orientation) and focusing on how to manage the tasks of life in the face of the loss (restoration orientation). Adolescents who have the skills (and support) to frame an accidental death within a meaningful coherent context that promotes a sense of self-efficacy may fare better in the face of accidental death. Using technology (but not exclusively) may be one avenue that may lead to a more positive outcome (James, Oltjenbruns, & Whiting, 2008). However, adolescents who perceive the death as traumatic may have difficulty oscillating between these two forms of coping skills, as their attempt at coping may be to avoid thinking about the death altogether (Walker, 2009).

Adolescent grief due to accidental death: Complicated grief

Complicated grief as a psychotherapeutic construct has undergone a number of transformations in recent years. At its basic level, clinicians regard a grief response that leads to prolonged dysfunctional behavior, primarily in terms of long-term depression and/or anxiety, as complicated (Stroebe, Schut, & VanDenBout, 2013). The ensuing distress frequently is intense and negatively affects the bereaved's social and psychological functioning. There are a number of risk factors of complicated grief that have been identified, but those that may be particularly significant for understanding adolescent grief due to an accidental death include being young, having difficulty finding meaning in the death, and difficulty integrating the death in one's sense of identity, life or future (Stroebe et al., 2013). Low levels of social support also may contribute to complicated grief, as do poor coping skills, a sense of vulnerability, and a belief that one has little control over life events. On all systemic levels of the developmental ecosystem, the adolescent may fail to find the social and psychological resources that are helpful in coping with the accidental death, particularly if it is a parent who has died. Peer groups are especially important for teens in coping with their losses, and their support (both in person and online) typically is harnessed in the case of the death of a peer. The death of a parent or a sibling, on the other hand, may be threatening or misunderstood in terms of its impact and it is here that an adolescent may be isolated in his or her grief.

One final factor to consider in regard to grief complications from accidental loss are those sad situations when there are multiple deaths. National and local databases do not keep records on unintentional fatalities for more than one person in the same accident. These may be accessed via police reports and newspaper stories. It is not hard to imagine, however, that a number of bereft adolescents are suffering from the simultaneous loss of family members or friends because of a plane crash, storm, vehicle accident, or fire. For example, in the village of Pulaski, WI on an October evening in 1988, five seventh-grade girls were walking on a sidewalk and were instantly killed by a car that careened into them. The driver was a 17-year-old male who lost control of the car due to a seizure. As recently reported in the October 12, 2013 *Milwaukee-Journal Sentinel*, a best friend of two of the girls who organized a memorial tribute 25 years later described her life-long effort to cope with the deaths. She spent a number of years abusing drugs, dropped out of school, and ran away from home. Ultimately, she herself became a funeral arrangements counselor, perhaps her way to make meaning out of the deaths. Sadly, the article reports that few have forgiven the driver of the car, and "...can't imagine how much he has been tormented over the years knowing he caused five deaths."

Therapeutic implications

Clinicians and researchers attest to the power of the peer group in helping adolescents cope with loss due to accidents. Peers can provide social support at a time when adolescents are trying to separate from their families. Peers also can help the adolescent work through the meaning making process by offering their interpretations of the loss (Walker, 2009). At the college level, National Students of AMF (http://www.studentsofamf.org) has helped to organize student-led grief support groups and promote community service projects to commemorate loved ones who have died. Currently, there are more than 40 college chapters nationwide responding to a need as evidence suggests that one in three college students experiences the death of a close family member or peer each year (Balk, Walker, & Baker, 2010). In a study of two college campuses, researchers found that over 20% of the deaths experienced by their grieving students (who made up over 45% of the student body within the past 24 months) were due to accidents (Cupit, Servaty-Seib, Parikh, Walker, & Martin, in preparation).

Physical and virtual contact with peers can help to affirm a bereft adolescent's self-identity, sense of autonomy from parents, and a belief in the continuity of relationships. It can also help to normalize the "crazy" way bereft adolescents feel who have had little education or preparation for handling an unexpected death. Seeking comfort, information, and expression online should not be discouraged, as forbidding or restricting the use of technology will alienate the adolescent from his or her parents (Sofka, 1999). Sofka recommends that adults actually encourage adolescents to share how they are using the Internet to cope with their grief. This can open up avenues of communication wherein the adult can offer guidance as to how to keep a grieving teenager from being victimized by predatory and malicious users of social media sites.

Psychotherapeutic intervention can also capitalize on the adolescents' natural tendency to engage in restorative coping strategies. These can involve engaging in physical activities that provide a new way to attain a sense of mastery and control (e.g., training for a half marathon); creating or participating in memorial activities; or developing organizations or participating in drives that work towards preventing future accidental deaths (e.g., advocating for laws against texting and driving, promoting workplace safety, or participating in a student group against drunk driving).

Schools have become more open to holding special programs and activities when there is an accidental death of a student, although many teachers still lack training and education in how to deal with student grief (Servaty-Seib, 1999). Bringing in outside teams of "grief counselors" with whom teens have had little prior contact does not seem to be effective. High school students do seem to appreciate when schools hold commemorative and symbolic events and offer the services of teachers and guidance counselors who had established a positive rapport with the students prior to the death.

Finally, attending a camp for grieving adolescents may be a very potent form of psychotherapeutic intervention. The bereavement experiences of the camp attendees typically are varied, from losses ranging from illness to suicide and accidental death. It is in the context of such intense short-term group experiences that adolescents find peers with similar experiences, and learn effective coping strategies and insights from trained personnel. The effects can be life transforming and long-term, although currently the data that attests to such positive results are mostly anecdotal (Cupit, 2013).

CONCLUSION

Death due to accidents represents a unique constellation of challenges for adolescents. Adolescents are at greater risk for dying from such deaths, as well as becoming the grieving survivor. There is an ongoing need to further assess the efficacy of prevention programs to reduce the risk of death due to unintentional injuries, the impact of social media on coping with loss due to accidents, and how coping strategies can help or hinder the bereaved. Research has yet to explore the effects such deaths have on those adolescents who already feel alienated from mainstream society. Across the globe, teenagers are experiencing death in dangerous working conditions, mass transit accidents, and the debris left in war-torn areas. These teens are suffering from multiple accidental deaths in communities plagued by chaos and disruption, and yet we do not know how they are faring in the face of such losses. Clearly there is much to learn.

In sum, adolescence represents a span of the life cycle where biological, cognitive, social and affective tensions exist that are personally affirming of life and sensitizing of death. These "dialectical dilemmas" appear within a biosocial context that includes the immediate social circles of teenagers within the prevailing cultural and historical environment. The confluence of all of these ultimately result in making sense out of death within the context of development.

Figure 1

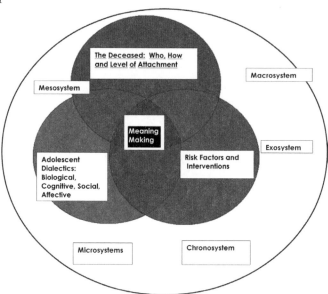

Factors Affecting Adolescent Meaning Making as a Consequence of Accidental Death

Death due to accidents certainly presents challenges for the adolescent, but we would be remiss not to also acknowledge the power of adolescent resiliency in the face of death due to accidents. As Balk (in press) notes, adolescents who maintain their sense of optimism, develop effective problem-solving skills, and have strong attachments with parents and adults can find a positive pathway toward growth enhancement in the face of loss—and many are able to do so.

Illene Noppe Cupit, PhD*, a graduate of Temple University, is professor of human development at the University of Wisconsin-Green Bay. She developed the Dying, Death & Loss course on her campus over twenty years ago. Dr. Cupit's research focuses on college student bereavement, adolescent grief, death education and developmental issues. Dr. Cupit recently co-edited a book with Carla Sofka and Kathy Gilbert entitled* Dying, Death and Grief in an Online Universe *(Springer Publishers, 2012). She also founded Camp Lloyd, a day camp for grieving children. She was the president of the Association for Death Education and Counseling (ADEC) for 2012-2013.*

Karissa J. Meyer is majoring in human development and psychology at the University of Wisconsin-Green Bay. She plans to go to graduate school for a doctorate in clinical psychology.

REFERENCES

Balk, D. E. (in press). *Dealing with dying, death, and grief during adolescence.* New York, NY: Routledge.

Balk, D. E. (2009). Adolescent development: The backstory to adolescent encounters with death and bereavement. In D.E. Balk & C.A. Corr (Eds.), *Adolescent encounters with death, bereavement, and coping* (pp. 3-20). New York, NY: Springer.

Balk, D. E., Walker, A. C., & Baker, A. (2010). Prevalence and severity of college student bereavement. *Death Studies, 34,* 459-468.

Balk, D. E. (2008). The adolescent's encounter with death. In Doka, K. J. & Tucci, A. S. (Eds.), *Living with grief: Children and adolescents* (pp. 25-42). Washington, DC: Hospice Foundation of America.

Brent, D., Melhem, N., Donohoe, M. B., & Walker, M. (2009). The incidence and course of depression in bereaved youth 21 months after the loss of a parent to suicide, accident, or sudden natural death. *American Journal of Psychiatry, 166(7),* 786-794.

Bronfenbrenner, U. (1994) Ecological models of human development. *International Encyclopedia of Education* (2nd ed., Vol. 3, pp. 1643-1647). Oxford, UK: Pergamon.

Corr, C. A. (2002). Revisiting the concept of disenfranchised grief. In K. J. Doka (Ed.), *Disenfranchised grief: New directions, challenges, and strategies for practice* (pp. 39-60). Champaign, IL: Research Press.

Corr, C. A. & Corr, D. M. (2013). *Death and dying, life and living* (seventh ed.). Belmont, CA: Wadsworth.

Council on Injury, Violence, and Poison Prevention Executive Committee. (2012). Firearm-related injuries affecting the pediatric population. *Pediatrics, 130*(5), doi: 10.1524/peds.2012-2481.

Cupit, I. N. (2013). *A university-based camp for grieving children.* Paper presented to the National Bereavement Camp Conference, Philadelphia, PA. October 10, 2013.

Cupit, I. Noppe, Servaty-Seib, H. L., Parikh, S.T., Walker, A. & Martin, R. (in preparation) *Forging a pathway through college during bereavement and grief: Findings of the National College Student Grief Study.*

Currier, J. M., Holland, J. M., & Neimeyer, R. A. (2007). The effectiveness of bereavement interventions with children: A meta-analytic review of controlled outcome research. *Journal of Clinical Child & Adolescent Psychology, 36,* 253-259.

DeGroot, J. M. (2012). Maintaining relationship continuity with the deceased on Facebook. *Omega, 65,* 195-212.

Doka, K. J. (1989). *Disenfranchised grief.* Lexington, MA: Lexington Books.

Fletcher, J., Mailick, M., Song, J., & Wolfe, B. (2012). A sibling death in the family: Common and consequential. *Demography, 50,* 803-826.

Gilchrist, J. & Ballesteros, M. F. (2012). Vital signs: Unintentional injury among persons aged 0–19 years—United States, 2000-2009. *Centers for Disease Control and Prevention Morbidity and Mortality Weekly Report.* Retrieved from http://www.cdc.gov/mmwr/ preview'mmwrhtml/mm6115a5.htm

Guest, J. (1976). *Ordinary people.* New York, NY: Penguin.

Harris, D. L. (Ed., 2011). *Counting our losses: Reflecting on change, loss, and transition in everyday life.* New York, NY: Taylor & Francis.

James, L., Oltjenbruns, K. A. & Whiting, P. (2008). Grieving adolescents: The paradox of using technology for support. In K. J. Doka and A. S. Tucci (Eds.), *Living with grief: Children and adolescents* (pp. 299-315). Washington, DC: Hospice Foundation of America.

Insurance Institute for Highway Safety. (2011). *Teenagers: Driving carries extra risk; Teenagers: 2011.* Retrieved from http://www.iihs. org/iihs/topics/t/teenagers/fatalityfacts/teenagers

Jones, A. L., Moss, A. J., & Harris-Kojetin, L. D. (2011). Use of advance directives in long-term care populations. *NCHS Data Brief, 54,* 1-8. Retrieved from http://www.ageiowa.org/files/public/advance_ directives.pdf

Klass, D., Silverman, P. R., & Nickman, S. L. (Eds.). (1996). *Continuing bonds: New understandings of grief.* Washington, DC: Taylor and Francis.

Kübler-Ross, E. (1969). *On death and dying.* New York, NY: Macmillan.

Murphy, S. L., Xu, J., & Kochanek, K. D. (2013). Deaths: Final data for 2010. *National Vital Statistics Reports, 61*(4), 1-17. Retrieved from http://www.cdc.gov/nchs/data/nvsr/nvsr61/nvsr61_04.pdf

Neimeyer, R. A. (Ed.). (2001). *Meaning reconstruction and the experience of loss.* Washington, DC: American Psychological Association.

Noppe, I. C., & Noppe, L. D. (2009). Adolescents, accidents, and homicides. In D. E. Balk & C. A. Corr (Eds.), *Adolescent encounters with death, bereavement, and coping* (pp. 61-79). New York, NY: Springer.

Noppe, L. D., & Noppe, I. C. (1991). Dialectical themes in adolescent conceptions of death. *Journal of Adolescent Research, 6,* 28-42. In K. J. Doka (Ed.), *Disenfranchised grief: New directions, challenges, and strategies for practice* (pp. 275-292). Champaign, IL: Research Press.

Raphael, B. (1983). *The anatomy of bereavement.* New York, NY: Basic Books.

Rowling, L. (2002). Youth and disenfranchised grief. In K. J. Doka (Ed.), *Disenfranchised grief: New directions, challenges and strategies for practice* (pp. 275-292). Champaign, IL: Research Press.

Sanderson, J. & Cheong, P. H. (2010). Tweeting prayers and communicating grief over Michael Jackson online. *Bulletin of Science Technology Society, 30,* 328-340.

Servaty-Seib, H. L. (2009). Death of a friend during adolescence. In D. E. Balk & C. A. Corr (Eds.), *Adolescent encounters with death, bereavement, and coping* (pp. 61-79). New York, NY: Springer.

Sofka, C. J. (2009). Adolescents, technology, and the Internet: Coping with loss in the digital world. In D. E. Balk & C. A. Corr (Eds.), *Adolescent encounters with death, bereavement, and coping* (pp. 155-173). New York, NY: Springer.

Sofka, C. J. (2013). The net generation: The special case of youth. In C. J. Sofka, I. N. Cupit, & K. R. Gilbert (Eds.), *Dying, death, and grief in an online universe* (pp. 47-60). New York: Springer.

Sofka, C. J., Cupit, I. N., & Gilbert, K. R. (Eds.). (2013). *Dying, death, and grief in an online universe.* New York, NY: Springer.

Stroebe, M. & Schut, H. (1999). The dual process model of coping with bereavement: Rationale and description. *Death Studies, 23,* 197-224.

Stroebe, M., Schut, H., & VanDenBout, J. (Eds.). (2013). *Complicated grief: Scientific foundations for health care professionals.* New York, NY: Routledge.

U.S. Department of Health and Human Services, Health Resources and Services Administration, Maternal and Child Health Bureau. *Child Health USA 2012.* Rockville, MD: U.S. Department of Health and Human Services, 2013.

United States, Department of Health and Human Services, National Center for Health Statistics, Centers for Disease Control and Prevention. (2013). FastStats: Leading causes of death. Retrieved from http://www.cdc.gov/nchs/fastats/lcod.htm

Walker, A. C. (2009). Adolescent bereavement and traumatic deaths. In D. E. Balk & C. A. Corr (Eds.), *Adolescent encounters with death, bereavement, and coping* (pp. 253-270.). New York, NY: Springer.

Walter, T., Hourizi, R., Moncur, W., & Pitsillides, S. (2011-2012). Does the Internet change how we die and mourn? Overview and analysis. *Omega, 64*(4), 275-302.

Williams, A. L., & Merten, M. J. (2009). Adolescents' online social networking following the death of a peer. *Journal of Adolescent Research, 24,* 67-90.

United States, Department of Health and Human Services, National Center for Health Statistics, Centers for Disease Control and Prevention. (2011). Youth risk behavior surveillance system: 2011 national overview. Retrieved from http://www.cdc.gov/healthyyouth/yrbs/pdf/us_overview_yrbs.pdf

CHAPTER 10

Adolescent Suicide

Lillian Range

S uicide is a critical problem for people of all ages, but is the third leading cause of death for adolescents. In a 2011 survey, 16% of students reported seriously considering suicide, 13% reported creating a plan, and 8% reported trying to take their own life in the previous 12 months (Centers for Disease Control, 2013). This chapter covers suicide prevention (school or community programs to reduce the suicide rate); suicide intervention (therapy with specific individuals to prevent them from committing suicide); and suicide postvention (counseling designed to help suicidally bereaved individuals, or protocols for schools or other agencies to enact that would discourage others from copying the suicidal act).

PREVENTION

Prevention can include resiliency training, gatekeeper training, screening, education, crisis hotlines, and means restriction. Many programs combine some or all of these components.

Resiliency training ranges from brief one-hour programs to multiple week units with lectures and experiential exercises to increase students' knowledge about suicide. In-school programs might be three to five days of in-class instruction using educational videos, presentations, and discussions. Videos might depict young people experiencing suicidal and/or depressed feelings; discussion groups might cover ways to deal with someone who is depressed or suicidal, and the link between suicide and mental disorders. Some programs include both teaching and screening (Robinson et al., 2013).

Example

The Penn Resiliency Program for adolescents (PRP-A) is designed for adolescents who reported high anxiety or high depression (Gillham et al., 2012). PRP-A has two components: cognitive-behavioral treatment that teaches connections between interpretations and feelings, and how to challenge unrealistic pessimistic beliefs; and interpersonal problem-solving. Adolescents meet in teacher-led groups for 90 minutes for ten to twelve months, and then participate in six group booster sessions five months later. In a randomized controlled trial, PRP-A reduced hopelessness and depressive symptoms at post-test, but not 6-month follow-up, and tended to reduce anxiety symptoms, particularly for students who reported high hopelessness initially (Gillham et al., 2012). Though designed for depression rather than specifically for suicide, this prevention approach seems promising, and suggests that teachers and counselors can deliver these programs.

Gatekeeper training for teachers, counselors, coaches, youth workers, and afterschool program leaders can improve early identification of students at high risk for suicide, facilitate timely mental health referrals, heighten intent to offer help, and increase commitment to suicide awareness and prevention. Gatekeeper training typically includes strategies for questioning students about suicide and increasing awareness of referral protocols for suicidal students. Gatekeeper training can increase knowledge and self-efficacy.

Example

Question, Persuade, and Refer (QPR), a 90-minute program taught by certified instructors, includes rates of youth suicide; warning signs and risk factors; procedures for asking a student about suicide, persuading a student to get help, and referring a student for help; local rates of student suicidal behavior; and the district protocol for responding to suicidal students (Reis & Cornell, 2008). In two studies, QPR increased self-reported knowledge and appraisals of efficacy (Tompkins, Witt, & Abraibesh, 2009; Wyman et al., 2008), especially for younger teachers not previously trained and unfamiliar with suicidal youth (Wyman et al., 2008). Also, trainees responded positively, with most rating the program as good to excellent, and reporting that they would recommend it to others (Tompkins et al., 2009).

Example

Another gatekeeper training, Sources of Strength (SOS) (Wyman et al., 2008), includes a video (with a discussion guide) that has dramatizations of suicidal and depressed people, recommended ways to react to someone who is depressed and suicidal, and interviews with real people whose lives have been touched by suicide (Aseltine, James, Schilling, & Glanovsky, 2007). SOS also includes a screening instrument completed anonymously and scored by students themselves. Compared to untreated control youths, those involved in SOS had more knowledge, more adaptive attitudes about depression and suicide, and significantly fewer suicide attempts three months later (Aseltine et al., 2007). SOS includes both gatekeeper training and screening components.

Suicide screening questionnaires are available. Targeted to college students, the Suicidal Ideation Scale (Rudd, 1989) lists 10 suicide ideas statements (e.g., "I have been thinking of ways to kill myself.") depending on how respondents felt or behaved during the *past year*. In versions for high school students (30 items) or junior high students (15 items), the Suicidal Ideation Questionnaire (Reynolds, 1987) is thoughts about suicide in the *past month* (e.g., "I thought it would be better if I were not alive."). Not designed for adolescents but completed on a computer or with paper and pencil, the Self-Rated Scale for Suicide Ideation (Beck, Steer, & Ranieri, 1988) is 19 prompts (e.g., "Wish to live"), with an unspecified timeline. Only four easy-to-complete questions, the Suicide Behaviors Questionnaire (Cole, 1988) is quite straightforward (e.g., "Have you ever thought about or attempted to kill yourself?"), and comes in a slightly simplified version with a third-grade reading level (Cotton & Range, 1993). These screening tools are publicly available, easily scored, and user friendly, so would be a useful first step in identifying adolescents at risk. They are available in languages other than English as well. In addition to questionnaires, screening programs exist.

Example

The College Screening Project (American Foundation for Suicide Prevention) is an interactive, web-based method to identify students at risk, support them in getting help, and determine the proportion who actually enter treatment. An assessment project sent students an e-mail invitation from a campus official that described the project and provided a link to a secure website that had screening questions on depression, past suicide attempts, anxiety, panic, rage, desperation, loss of control, and alcohol/drug use (Haas et al., 2008). After completing the questions, students were told to expect a personal assessment from a counselor, which came within the day for high-risk students. The counselor's e-mail encouraged them to ask questions or elaborate on a particular problem or situation, urged all at-risk students to call or e-mail the counselor to schedule an in-person evaluation, and gave the option of participating in an online anonymous dialogue with the counselor. Among high-risk students, 91% viewed the counselor's personalized assessment, 34% emailed the counselor, 20% came for an in-person evaluation, and 15% entered treatment; a few others sought treatment outside the project. Counselors considered these students unlikely to have come in without the screening procedure. The dialogue feature of the website was particularly important in resolving concerns, removing perceived treatment barriers, and forming a therapeutic relationship with the counselor. Screening can identify adolescents not otherwise known as being at risk.

Education about suicide in adolescence can include classroom curriculum-based modules for students, in-service training modules for gatekeepers such as teachers or health professionals, or public education campaigns. Education improves knowledge and attitudes, and may or may not impact behavior.

There are several curriculum-based suicide prevention classroom modules.

Example

A 50- to 75-minute program called Raising Awareness of Personal Power educated students about depression, bipolar disorder, and suicide warning signs, taught a three-step process (Listen, Ask, Take Action) of how to respond, and described local resources. Taught by trained peer counselors and adult volunteers, this program included lectures, interactive games, role plays, and analysis of several stories. This program improved students' knowledge, attitudes, and efficacy in responding to a suicidal peer (Cigularov, Chen, Thurber, & Stallones, 2008).

Example

Another program of four 50-minute sessions involved reading, role play, and class discussion on suicide facts, stress coping strategies, and recognizing and responding to depression. Targeted to high school students, this program diminished suicide ideas, plans and attempts, and improved self-efficacy and intent to get help from pre- to three-month follow-up (King, Strunk, & Sorter, 2011). Though potentially effective, suicide education modules often miss the most at-risk students, who are more likely to miss the training in the first place and be unresponsive to intervention attempts in the second place (Westefeld et al., 2000).

Suicide prevention education is a part of in-service training and/or continuing education requirements for many professionals.

Example

A primarily didactic workshop for social workers working with mentally ill homeless and previously homeless adults assisted staff members in recognizing indicators of suicide risk, obtaining and coordinating care for suicidal clients, documenting this work appropriately, and communicating effectively with coworkers and external service providers. This workshop was effective in increasing the suicidality-related knowledge of both professional and paraprofessional staff both at post-test and 21-month follow-up (Levitt, Lorenzo, Yu, Wean, & Miller-Solarino, 2011).

Example

A three-hour educational workshop for a multidisciplinary sample of clinicians with clinical responsibilities in acute and outpatient care was designed as a practical and authentic skill-building experience. It began with a clinical vignette about an at-risk patient, followed by six minutes to document suicide risk, and also included lecture and case-based discussions. Participants' knowledge, confidence, and documentation skills improved significantly from pre- to posttraining (Pisani, Cross, Watts, & Conner, 2012). Other successful in-service training modules have been reported. For example, a 4-hour program for Chinese second-year student nurses reduced judgmental attitudes and improved attitudes toward suicide attempters (Sun, Long, Huang, & Chiang, 2011). A 90-minute program for practicing nurses in Taiwan enhanced suicide awareness and willingness to refer patients to counseling (Tsai, Lin, Chang, Yu, & Chou, 2011). Gatekeepers who interact with adolescents are responsive to suicide in-service training.

Public education campaigns typically are often initiated with the goal of reducing suicide risk. In Austria, a local multimedia awareness campaign, *Reasons to love life*, aimed to draw public attention to suicide prevention and crisis intervention and increase help-seeking behavior in suicidal individuals (Till, Sonneck, Baldauf, Steiner, & Niederkrotenthaler, 2013). It included an initial press conference, billboards, electronic infoscreens in railways and on traffic junctions, and small placards sent to community centers and psychosocial institutes. However, this campaign had no effect on calls to a telephone crisis line or area suicide rates (Till et al., 2013). In northern California, a suicide-prevention project included developing a Teen Resource Card and a community resource brochure targeted at teens, and offering education for the public and school officials to raise awareness about suicide (Pirruccello, 2010). The suicide rate dropped in this community from four in the previous year to zero in the year after this program, but without a control group it is impossible to know if this drop was due to the program.

For students, suicide education programs can improve knowledge, attitudes, help-seeking and self-reported likelihood of suicide ideas and attempts (Robinson et al., 2013). For gatekeepers, educational programs increase knowledge, improve attitudes, and further confidence, and sometimes lead to self-reported improvements in practice (Robinson et al., 2013). Reviews of classroom programs for students and in-service trainings for gatekeepers are typically positive, but evaluating public education campaigns is quite difficult.

Crisis centers and suicide hotlines typically use a combination of trained volunteers and paid staff to provide telephone counseling to individuals in crisis. The centers may also be linked to mental health services and other associated social welfare agencies. In the United States, a national network of suicide prevention crisis lines, the National Suicide Prevention Lifeline (http://www.suicidepreventionlifeline. org) is a key component of many suicide prevention programs and prominent in public awareness messages and websites (Gould, Munfakh, Kleinman, & Lake, 2012). In 2008, Lifeline received over 500,000 calls (Gould et al., 2012). Much of the Lifeline research focuses on adults. In Australia, a similar program, Kids Help Line, is designed for callers under age 18. Available 24/7, it requires no identifying information or parental involvement; it aims to empower callers rather than refer them to adults (King, Nurcombe, Bickman, Hides, & Reid, 2003). In an evaluation of over 100 calls involving suicidality lasting on average 40 minutes, urgency reduced considerably from beginning to end of the call (King et al., 2003). Thus, a telephone hotline for suicidal adolescents seemed to help, and would likely be a good resource for bereaved teens grieving a death by suicide.

A follow-up evaluation of almost 400 adult crisis calls (Gould, Kalafat, HarrisMunfakh, & Kleinman, 2007) found that more than 50% of callers (more women than men) had current plans to harm themselves when they called, nearly 10% had acted to hurt or kill themselves immediately prior to their call, and almost 60% previously attempted suicide. These adult callers reported significant decreases in suicidality over the course of the telephone session, with continuing decreases in hopelessness and psychological pain in the following weeks. In a U.S. survey of 500+ high school students, only seven had used a hotline. Reasons for non-use included shame, wanting to be self-reliant, and having no time or knowledge. Further, those most hopeless or impaired had the most negative attitudes (Gould, Greenberg, Munfakh, Kleinman, & Lubell, 2006). Suicide hotlines, although widely available, free, accessible, anonymous, and in sync with the pervasiveness of phones in adolescent lives, may or may not be used.

Finally, *means restriction* is another aspect of suicide prevention. The data is clear: there is an association between firearms in the home and completed suicide, with higher risks (four to five times higher compared to homes with no firearm) associated with loaded guns and handguns in the home (Brent & Bridge, 2003). Also, there is a relationship between greater restrictiveness of gun control laws and lower overall and firearm suicide rates, although some studies fail to show an effect or show method substitution. In a prospective study, handgun purchasers had an elevated risk for suicide for up to 6 years after the purchase (Brent & Bridge, 2003).

In a review, Brent and Bridge (2003) concluded that the risk conveyed by gun availability may be particularly high among adolescents and young adults, and an increase in suicide by firearms primarily accounts for the dramatic increase in the American youth suicide rate since 1960. Means restriction, either individually or via population methods, may substantially reduce suicide rate, particularly in the US, where guns are the most common suicide method for both men and women. Given their impulsiveness, restricting adolescents' access to guns is imperative.

Prevention efforts such as resiliency training, screening, education, crisis hotlines, and means restriction aim to reduce the likelihood that adolescents will resort to suicide. Gatekeeper training aims to help people know how to respond promptly and helpfully if they do.

INTERVENTION

Intervention in a suicidal crisis can entail crisis intervention, brief or longer term therapy, medication, and/or hospitalization. Many treatment programs include several of these aspects.

Crisis intervention begins with an assessment of risk. The clinician obtains specific information about the adolescent's suicide ideas, plan, and intent. Regardless of whether the adolescent brings up any information about suicide, the therapist should ask directly about ideas, plan, and intent (Miller & Emanuele, 2009). An example of a question would be, "Are you feeling like you might hurt or kill yourself?" Commonly, the clinician interviews both adolescent and parent/guardian separately, and, when possible, teachers as well. If the adolescent is acutely suicidal, the therapist may need to violate confidentiality. Crisis intervention is typically short- term and designed to help the adolescent get past the crisis.

Example

Family-based crisis intervention (FBCI) is a single-session emergency room (ER) treatment for adolescent suicide attempters. Based on cognitive-behavioral and family systems theory, it involves nonjudgmental collaboration between social worker, adolescent, and family. First, the social worker holds separate meetings with the adolescent and family members to assess the sequence of events and differing perceptions leading to the suicidal problem. During these meetings, the social worker helps each party tell his or her story, exploring what each person thinks would be necessary for the adolescent to return home safely. Next, the social worker meets with the whole family together, attempting to construct a single, unified perception of the problem and improve communication among family members. Compared to a matched group who came to the ER during the previous 18 months, suicidal adolescents and families who received FBCI were significantly less likely to be admitted to an inpatient psychiatry unit, and significantly more likely to be referred to an intensive outpatient service (Wharff, Ginnis, & Ross, 2012). The ER is a good place for crisis intervention for suicidal adolescents.

Therapy is typically longer-term than crisis intervention and has the goal of changing behavior that may lead to crisis. Components of therapy for suicidal adolescents include helping them delay impulses toward self-harm, restoring hope, solving the current problem, reducing high risk behaviors, committing to a safety-maintaining plan of action, and anticipating recurrence of suicide ideas (Miller & Emanuele, 2009). The therapist stays available to be contacted, typically by pager or cell phone. One strategy is to give all suicidal patients an emergency card that contains important telephone and pager numbers (Miller & Emanuele, 2009).

One possible component of therapy for suicidal persons is a *no-suicide contract*. Typically, the no-suicide contract includes a specific time component, such as a week, a day, or until the next appointment; and it includes a plan if the client realizes that he or she is unable to keep the contract or the appointment. No-suicide contracts can be verbal or written. If written, they are typically signed and kept by both parties. One recommendation is to have the suicidal person write the contract. Given the possibility that adolescents can be rebellious, an alternative recommended by some experts is a *commitment-to-treatment statement*, a written agreement between patient and clinician that articulates what it means to be invested in treatment. It includes frequency of sessions, level of involvement, agreement to complete homework, willingness to experiment with new behaviors, and a crisis response plan (Rudd, Joiner, Trotter, Williams, & Cordero, 2009). No-suicide contracts or commitments-to-treatment are no guarantee against suicidal behavior; they can help if they foster the alliance between suicidal adolescent and therapist, they can hurt if they hinder this alliance.

Some therapy interventions are designed specifically for suicide. Cognitive approaches to suicide focus on the automatic thoughts that influence emotions and behaviors. The fundamental idea is that people absorb information filtered through belief systems that trigger thoughts about the meaning of the situation or event (Miller & Barber, 2002). The therapist challenges the behaviors and automatic thoughts of suicidal clients, and trains them to question the evidence for negative automatic thoughts when they arise. Clients learn to examine logically their beliefs and adjust those beliefs when they are unsupportable. Clients practice self-instruction to stop or reduce ruminating about failures and increase more positive automatic thoughts. Interpersonal psychotherapy for suicide focuses on problems in suicidal clients' interpersonal relationships; 12-week treatments that include frequent telephone contacts have been successful (Shaffer et al.,

2001). An adaptation for adolescents addresses common adolescent developmental issues, such as separating from parents, exploring authority in relationship to parents, developing dyadic interpersonal relationships, facing the loss of a relative or friend, and dealing with peer pressure.

Example

Dialectical Behavior Therapy (DBT) has four aspects: individual therapy using a cognitive behavioral approach, group skills training, telephone-based skills coaching between sessions, and a weekly consultation team meeting with therapists (Linehan & Kehrer, 1993). In DBT, the therapist conducts a detailed behavioral analysis of each self-injury episode to determine coping strategies, triggers, and reinforcements, being careful to avoid inadvertently reinforcing the suicidal actions; the therapist also works with family members to ensure that they are not reinforcing the adolescent's problem behaviors but are rewarding positive behaviors (Miller, Rathus, & Linehan, 2007). Didactic, multifamily group sessions teach a new skill each week and include homework on that skill. Skills include mindfulness (attentiveness to emotions without evaluating them or acting on them), interpersonal effectiveness (adaptive ways to communicate needs to others and cope with interpersonal problems that lead to strong negative emotions), distress tolerance (distraction and self-soothing), and emotional regulation (labeling and identifying emotions, reducing vulnerabilities, increasing behaviors that lead to positive emotions, and decreasing negative emotions). DBT would probably work best for multi-problem adolescents, because adolescents who attempt suicide frequently have co-morbid psychiatric diagnoses and life stressors such as loss, as well as characteristics of borderline personality disorder (Neece, Berk, & Combs-Ronto, 2013).

For therapy to work, therapist and client must establish an alliance. Treatment compliance may be improved by offering definite, closely spaced follow-up appointments, being flexible with appointments if a crisis should arise, and reminding the client of the next appointment by phone or e-mail (Shaffer et al., 2001). Although they are typically a multi-problem group, thus especially difficult to treat, suicidal adolescents can get help from therapy.

Medicine may help reduce suicide risk for adolescents. Three classes of psychotropic drugs relevant to suicide are antidepressants, antipsychotics, and antimania drugs.

Antidepressants can reduce depression, which is strongly associated with suicide. Reviews of treatments for adolescents indicate that certain antidepressants and time-limited cognitive-behavior therapy work better than no-treatment control interventions to decrease depression, but relapse is high when the treatment is discontinued, and research on depression often excludes suicidal adolescents (Miller & Glinski, 2000). Tragically, overdosing on antidepressants is one method used to commit suicide. Because medicine could be a potential self-harm agent, experts recommend close monitoring of anyone receiving antidepressants.

For people with schizophrenia and schizoaffective disorders, clozapine therapy reduces suicide risk (Mamo, 2007). Marketed under the brand names Clozaril and FazaClo, clozapine can cause numerous side effects so should be monitored closely. Clozapine is sometimes given for bipolar disorder as well as schizophrenia. For adolescents, some experts recommend a similar drug, olanzapine. De Giacomo, Lozito, and Portoghese (2008), following 12 adolescents for an average of one year, had good medicine compliance and suicidality reduction using a daily dose of olanzapine plus psychological support.

Lithium, sometimes classified as an antimania drug, reduces recurrence of suicide attempts in adults with bipolar disorder, or other major affective disorders (Shaffer et al., 2001). In a meta-analysis of 31 studies (typically of adults), the overall risk of suicides and attempts was five times less among lithium-treated than non-lithium treated people (Baldessarini et al., 2006). However, adolescents may not respond the same as adults.

Research on psychotropic drugs is often riddled with problems, such as being non-controlled, retrospective, and potentially biased in those selected for treatment, and whether clients use other drugs, take their medicine as instructed, or discontinue it (Ernst & Goldberg, 2004). Nevertheless, extensive literature reports reductions in suicidal behavior with antidepressants for depression, clozapine for schizophrenia, and lithium for bipolar disorders, although research is much less common for adolescents than for adults. Anyone being treated with medicine needs close monitoring, and the therapist and prescribing physician need a collaborative relationship (Westefeld et al., 2000). Medication for suicidality may co-occur with outpatient therapy or inpatient hospitalization.

Hospitalization may be necessary for adolescents who are suicidal. Clinicians should be prepared to admit as inpatients suicide attempters who express a persistent wish to die and/or have a concrete plan. Reasons for hospitalization include psychosis or hallucinations telling the person to kill self or someone else; history of overdose on psychotropic medication; having a severely strained relationship with the therapist; being unresponsive to outpatient therapy; escalating suicide threats; severely abusing alcohol or drugs; refusing to remove lethal items from home or use an emergency card; feeling profoundly hopeless and unable to identify reasons for living; and inability to identify social supports (Miller & Emanuele, 2009). Hospitalization should continue until the adolescent's mental state or level of suicidality has stabilized and a responsible third-party is able to provide adequate supervision and support (Shaffer et al., 2001). Hospitalization is not always necessary, however, and is only a short-term treatment.

Intervention is often necessary when adolescents suffer loss or other important life stressors. Either alone or in combination, crisis intervention, brief or longer term therapy, medication, and/or hospitalization can help.

POSTVENTION

Suicide postvention programs aim to minimize distress, inhibit the development of psychiatric disorders, and reduce the chance of a suicide cluster occurring. Postvention can take various forms, depending on the context in which the suicide or suicide attempt takes place, but typically can include individual or group counseling for those affected by the suicide, and protocols for schools or other agency officials to follow to discourage contagion.

Individual or group therapy may be needed after a suicidal death, and is not always available. In a study of 166 relatives and friends bereaved by suicide in Australia, 94% indicated a need for help to manage their grief, but only 44% received help. Further, only 40% of those who received professional support felt satisfied with it (Wilson & Marshall, 2010). These people who lost a loved one by suicide believed that they needed mental health help. Little has been written about individual counseling specifically for suicidally bereaved individuals, but a few descriptions exist of group therapy.

One group therapy postvention is an eight-week bereavement support group designed for children who lost a parent or other family member through suicide (Mitchell et al., 2007). Facilitated by an advanced practice registered nurse, it typically consists of six to eight children (age 7 to 13) whose parent died two to six months ago. The facilitator uses activities such as drawing pictures and playing games to encourage the children to talk about their feelings and counseling adolescents who have experienced the suicide of someone such as a parent, sibling, or friend. Mitchell et al. (2007) reported favorable responses to this group, but no research analysis has been conducted of this postvention effort.

Another group therapy treatment after a loved one's suicide is a hospital-based ten-session, flexibly manualized, and culturally relevant psychoeducational group (Kaslow, Ivey, Berry-Mitchell, Franklin, & Bethea, 2009). Each two-hour session includes a supportive discussion, problem-focused psychoeducation and skill building, and an activity, and most also include handouts and homework. Designed for family members of all ages, this group contains separate child components for youth age 6 to18 (Kaslow et al., 2009). This group is most applicable to families who are open to talking about the suicide with one another, whose religious convictions do not hinder them from receiving support, and whose grief is unresolved. Though promising, no research analysis has been conducted of this postvention effort either.

School-based suicide postvention *protocols* may involve psychological debriefings for students, staff and parents; individual and group counseling; focus groups; consultation with immediate family of the deceased student; a community response plan; screening high-risk individuals; and media liaison (Robinson et al., 2013). A published toolkit for schools is available (American Foundation for Suicide Prevention and Suicide Prevention Resource Center, 2011). For schools, physical memorials on school grounds may mystify or glamorize the suicide. Most experts recommend some other type of memorial activity such as a fund drive for a worthy cause (Lamb & Dunne-Maxim, 1987). For news outlets, simplistic, repetitive, sensationalistic news coverage or how-to descriptions may encourage copycat behavior, so experts recommend that the media liaison provide journalists with information about mental health resources to accompany news stories, and that the media liaison distinguishes between the talented person and the drug abuser who ultimately killed himself (Jobes, Berman, O'Carroll, Eastgard, & Knickmeyer, 1996).

Example

Responding to Loss (RTL), a crisis response program, provides strategies to help high school crisis teams in their structured response following the suicide of a student or staff member (Underwood, Dunne-Maxim, & Ahrens, 1995). RTL has three components: Preparing for Crisis Training, Peer Witness Intervention, and Crisis Consultation.

Example

Another systematic postvention effort, Local Outreach to Suicide Survivors Program (LOSS), includes a first-response team comprised of crisis center staff members and paraprofessional survivor volunteers, all trained in responding to suicide scenes, including crime scene procedures, precautions for exposure to pathogens, and supportive counseling training (Campbell, Cataldie, McIntosh, & Millet, 2004). At the suicide scene, LOSS team members comfort survivors, answer questions, and provide referrals. LOSS relies heavily on the bond between the newly-bereaved person and the paraprofessional survivor, and works closely with other first responders to offer the newly-bereaved persons choices that might not be available otherwise. For an example of a well-coordinated postvention effort following the death of celebrity rock musician Kurt Cobain, see Jobes et al. (1996).

Suicide is very upsetting, and can catch individuals, schools and agencies off guard. So it is very important for schools and other agencies to have plans in place for offering individual or group counseling to those affected, and protocols in place to discourage contagion.

Prevention, intervention, and postvention efforts may at times overlap. For example, a prevention screening might identify at-risk adolescents (prevention), and also offer them counseling (intervention). Or, a gatekeeper training program might teach how to respond to a suicidal student (prevention), as well as how to respond after a suicidal death (postvention). All programs are aimed to help those touched by suicide deal with their grief, shock, anger, relief, or other emotions, and to encourage all to work together to prevent other suicidal deaths.

Lillian Range, PhD, is professor of psychology at Our Lady of Holy Cross College and professor emerita at The University of Southern Mississippi. An associate editor of Death Studies, *she is a member of the editorial board of* Suicide and Life-Threatening Behavior, Journal of Loss and Trauma, *and* Journal of Personality Assessment; *her research focus has included suicide, suicide prevention, bereavement, and health promotion. A licensed clinical psychologist in the states of Louisiana and Mississippi, she has served on the psychology licensing board in Mississippi. Range is a fellow of the American Psychological Association through Divisions 12 (Clinical) and 35 (Women), she is Secretary-Treasurer of Clinical Emergencies and Crises (Section VII of Division 12 of APA), and a past president of Southeastern Psychological Association.*

REFERENCES

American Foundation for Suicide Prevention and Suicide Prevention Resource Center. (2011). After a suicide: A toolkit for schools. Newton, MA: Education Development Center. Retrieved from http://www.sprc.org/library/AfteraSuicide-ToolkitforSchools.pdf

Aseltine, R. H., James, A., Schilling, E. A., & Glanovsky, J. (2007). Evaluating the SOS suicide prevention program: A replication and extension. *BMC Public Health, 7,* 161-168.

Baldessarini, R. J., Tondo, L., Davis, P., Pompili, M., Goodwin, F. K., & Hennen, J. (2006). Decreased risk of suicides and attempts during long-term lithium treatment: A meta-analytic review. *Bipolar Disorders, 8*(5 pt 2), 625-639.

Beck, A., Steer, R., & Ranieri, W. (1988). Scale for Suicide Ideation: Psychometric properties of a self-report version. *Journal of Clinical Psychology, 44,* 499-505.

Brent, D. A., & Bridge, J. (2003). Firearms availability and suicide: Evidence, interventions, and future directions. *American Behavioral Scientist, 46,* 1192-1210.

Campbell, F. R., Cataldie, L., McIntosh, J., & Millet, K. (2004). An active postvention program. *Crisis: The Journal of Crisis Intervention and Suicide Prevention, 25*(1), 30-32.

Centers for Disease Control and Prevention. (2013). Youth suicide. Retrieved from http://www.cdc.gov/mmwr/

Cigularov, K., Chen, P., Thurber, B., & Stallones, L. (2008). Investigation of the effectiveness of a school-based suicide education program using three methodological approaches. *Psychological Services, 5*(3), 262-274.

Cole, D. A. (1988). Hopelessness, social desirability, depression, and parasuicide in two college student samples. *Journal of Consulting and Clinical Psychology, 56,* 131-136.

Cotton, C., & Range, L. (1993). Suicidality, hopelessness and attitudes toward life and death in children. *Death Studies, 17,* 185-191.

De Giacomo, A., Lozito, V., & Portoghese, C. (2008). Olanzapine in adolescents with schizophrenia who manifest suicidal behaviour. *Early Intervention in Psychiatry, 2*(2), 114-115.

Ernst, C. L., & Goldberg, J. F. (2004). Antisuicide properties of psychotropic drugs: A critical review. *Harvard Review of Psychiatry, 12,* 14-41.

Gillham, J. E., Reivich, K. J., Brunwasser, S. M., Freres, D. R., Chajon, N. D., Kash-MacDonald, V. M., ...Seligman, M. E. P. (2012). Evaluation of a group cognitive-behavioral depression prevention program for young adolescents: A randomized effectiveness trial. *Journal of Clinical Child and Adolescent Psychology, 41*(5), 621-639.

Gould, M. S., Greenberg, T., Munfakh, J. L., Kleinman, M., & Lubell, K. (2006). Teenagers' attitudes about seeking help from telephone crisis services (hotlines). *Suicide and Life-Threatening Behavior, 36*(6), 601-613.

Gould, M. S., Kalafat, J., HarrisMunfakh, J. L., & Kleinman, M. (2007). An evaluation of crisis hotline outcomes: Part 2: Suicidal callers. *Suicide and Life-Threatening Behavior, 37*(3), 338-352.

Gould, M. S., Munfakh, J. L. H., Kleinman, M., & Lake, A M. (2012). National Suicide Prevention Lifeline: Enhancing mental health care for suicidal individuals and other people in crisis. *Suicide and Life-Threatening Behavior, 42*(1), 22-35.

Haas, A., Koestner, B., Rosenberg, J., Moore, D., Garlow, S. J., Sedway, J., Nicholas, L., ...Nemeroff, C. B. (2008). An interactive web-based method of outreach to college students at risk for suicide. *Journal of American College Health, 57,* 15-22.

Jobes, D. A., Berman, A. L., O'Carroll, P. W., Eastgard, S., & Knickmeyer, S. (1996). The Kurt Cobain suicide crisis: Perspectives from research, public health, and the news media. *Suicide and Life-Threatening Behavior, 26,* 260-271.

Kaslow, N. J., Ivey, A. Z., Berry-Mitchell, F., Franklin, K., & Bethea, K. (2009). Postvention for African American families following a loved one's suicide. *Professional Psychology: Research and Practice, 40*(2), 165-171.

King, R., Nurcombe, B., Bickman, L., Hides, L., & Reid, W. (2003). Telephone counselling for adolescent suicide prevention: Changes in suicidality and mental state from beginning to end of a counselling session. *Suicide and Life-Threatening Behavior, 33*(4), 400-411.

King, K. A., Strunk, C. M., & Sorter, M. T. (2011). Preliminary effectiveness of Surviving the Teens® Suicide Prevention and Depression Awareness Program on adolescents' suicidality and self-efficacy in performing help-seeking behaviors. *Journal of School Health, 81*, 581-590.

Lamb, F., & Dunne-Maxim, K. (1987). Postvention in schools: Policy and process. In E. Dunne, J. McIntosh, & K. Dunne-Maxim (Eds.), *Suicide and its aftermath: Understanding and counseling survivors* (pp. 245-262). New York, NY: Norton.

Levitt, A. J., Lorenzo, J., Yu, V., Wean, C., & Miller-Solarino, S. (2011). Teaching note from suicide awareness and prevention workshop for social workers and paraprofessionals. *Journal of Social Work Education, 47*, 607-613.

Linehan, M. M. & Kehrer, C. A. (1993). Borderline personality disorder. In D. Barlow (Ed.), *Clinical handbook of psychological disorders: A step-by-step treatment manual* (2nd ed.) (p. 396-441). New York, NY: Guilford.

Mamo, D. C. (2007). Managing suicidality in schizophrenia. *Canadian Journal of Psychiatry, 52*, 59S-70S.

Miller, A. L., & Emanuele, J. M. (2009). Children and adolescents at risk of suicide. In P. Kleespies (Ed.), *Behavioral emergencies: An evidence-based resource for evaluating and managing risk of suicide, violence, and victimization* (pp. 79-101). Washington, DC: American Psychological Association.

Miller, A. L., & Glinski, J. (2000). Youth suicidal behavior: Assessment and intervention. *Journal of Clinical Psychology, 56*(9), 1131-1152.

Miller, A. L., Rathus, J. H., & Linehan, M. M. (2007). *Dialectical behavior therapy with suicidal adolescents.* New York, NY: Guilford.

Miller, K. & Barber, J. G. (2002). Brief intervention strategies for the prevention of youth suicide. *Brief Treatment and Crisis Intervention, 2*(3), 217-231.

Mitchell, A. M., Wesner, S., Garand, L., Gale, D. D., Havill, A., & Brownson, L. (2007). A support group intervention for children bereaved by parental suicide. *Journal of Child and Adolescent Psychiatric Nursing, 20*(1), 3-13.

Neece, C. L., Berk, M. S., & Combs-Ronto, L. A. (2013). Dialectical Behavior Therapy and suicidal behavior in adolescence: Linking developmental theory and practice. *Professional Psychology: Research and Practice, 44,* 257-265.

Pirruccello, L. M. (2010). Preventing adolescent suicide: A community takes action. *Journal of Psychosocial Nursing and Mental Health Services, 48*(5), 34-41.

Pisani, A. R., Cross, W. F., Watts, A., & Conner, K. (2012). Evaluation of the Commitment to Living (CTL) curriculum: A 3-hour training for mental health professionals to address suicide risk. *Crisis: The Journal of Crisis Intervention and Suicide Prevention, 33*(1), 30-38.

Reis, C., & Cornell, D. (2008). An evaluation of suicide gatekeeper training for school counselors and teachers. *Professional School Counseling, 11*(6), 386-394.

Reynolds, W. M. (1987). *Suicide Ideation Questionnaire: Professional manual.* Odessa, FL: Psychological Assessment Resources.

Robinson, J., Cox, G., Malone, A., Williamson, M., Baldwin, G., Fletcher, K., & O'Brien, M. (2013). A systematic review of school-based interventions aimed at preventing, treating, and responding to suicide-related behavior in young people. *Crisis: The Journal of Crisis Intervention and Suicide Prevention, 34*(3), 164-182.

Rudd, M. D. (1989). The prevalence of suicidal ideation among college students. *Suicide and Life-Threatening Behavior, 19,* 173-183.

Rudd, M. D., Joiner, T. E., Trotter, D., Williams, B., & Cordero, L. (2009). The psychosocial treatment of suicidal behavior: A critique of what we know (and don't know). In P. Kleespies (Ed.), *Behavioral emergencies: An evidence-based resource for evaluating and managing risk of suicide, violence, and victimization* (pp. 339-350). Washington, DC: American Psychological Association.

Shaffer, D., Pfeffer, C. R., Bernet, W., Arnold, V., Beitchman, J., Scott Benson, R., Buksbein, O., ... & Kroeger, K. (2001). Practice parameter for the assessment and treatment of children and adolescents with suicidal behavior. *Journal of the American Academy of Child and Adolescent Psychiatry, 40*, 24S-51S.

Sun, F., Long, A., Huang, X., & Chiang, C. (2011). A quasi-experimental investigation into the efficacy of a suicide education programme for second-year student nurses in Taiwan. *Journal of Clinical Nursing, 20*(5-6), 837-846.

Till, B., Sonneck, G., Baldauf, G., Steiner, E., & Niederkrotenthaler, T. (2013). Reasons to Love Life: Effects of a suicide-awareness campaign on the utilization of a telephone emergency line in Austria. *Crisis: The Journal of Crisis Intervention and Suicide Prevention.* doi: 10.1027/0227-5910/a000212

Tompkins, T. L., Witt, J., & Abraibesh, N. (2009). Does a gatekeeper suicide-prevention program work in a school setting? Evaluating training outcome and moderators of effectiveness. *Suicide and Life-Threatening Behavior, 39*, 671–681. Doi 10.1521/suli.2009.39.6.671

Tsai, W., Lin, L., Chang, H., Yu, L., & Chou, M. (2011). The effects of the Gatekeeper Suicide-Awareness Program for nursing personnel. *Perspectives in Psychiatric Care, 47*, 117-125. Doi 10.1111/j.1744-6163.2010.00278.x

Underwood, M. M., Dunne-Maxim, K., & Ahrens, R. (1995). Managing sudden violent loss in the schools. *Social Work in Education, 17*, 125-128.

Westefeld, J. S., Range, L. M., Rogers, J. R., Maples, M. R., Bromley, J. L., & Alcorn, J. (2000). Suicide: An overview. *The Counseling Psychologist, 28*(4), 445-510.

Wharff, E. A., Ginnis, K. M., & Ross, A. M. (2012). Family-based crisis intervention with suicidal adolescents in the emergency room: A pilot study. *Social Work, 57*, 133-143.

Wilson, A., & Marshall, A. (2010). The support needs and experiences of suicidally bereaved family and friends. *Death Studies, 34*, 625-640. Doi 10.1080/07481181003761567

Wyman, P. A., Brown, C. H., Inman, J., Cross, W., Schmeelk-Cone, K., Guo, J., & Pena, J. B. (2008). Randomized trial of a gatekeeper program for suicide prevention: 1-year impact on secondary school staff. *Journal of Consulting and Clinical Psychology, 76*(1), 104–115.

CHAPTER 11

Voices
Zach's Suicide

Dylan Rieger

When my friend Zachary killed himself there were a lot of warning signs, for many years, leading up to the moment. He'd always been a fiery personality who had the respect of many people. But a lot of the respect came from his impulsiveness and ability to do things most people are too afraid to do. He would often race his car at breakneck speeds and at one time could have five girlfriends. There were times in school he could become so upset he could be in tears, but twenty minutes later you wouldn't think anything at all happened to him. He lived for the moments and adrenaline rushes. Even in middle school, Zach, big and strong for his age, would challenge two people at a time in wrestling matches and pretty easily pin both. His motto in high school was, "If I get a thought, I have to go through with it" and "If I make it to 21, I'll be happy." At the time, all those things seemed cool but he never seemed to grow out of it.

As we got older, he became more and more depressed about life and the future. A few months before he hung himself, he told me that he was afraid of the future and he could not stop thinking about it. When another friend died eight months before his own death, Zach told me the person "got the easy way out" because he died in a car accident and didn't have to grow old. About a month before he hung himself, his girlfriend of a couple years broke up with him and he went off the deep end. He began posting stuff on Facebook that hinted at suicide. He began to stalk his ex-girlfriend. A few days before he hung himself, he even slashed her tires. Yet, while this sounds like highly erratic behavior, it was typical of Zach. This is how he handled everything. He would do something over the top then come back to earth.

When I finally got the call that Zach had killed himself I was very upset. I remember I cried pretty much the whole night. In the months following his death, I began just thinking of all the warning signs and how I could have helped and maybe prevented his death. I beat myself up for not being there for him and just not giving him a call to check in the days preceding his death

But as more time goes by, the more and more I realize it was a decision he made on his own. When you remember the things he lived by—"If I get a thought I have to go through with it" or "If I make it to 21 I'll be happy"—you can see why he didn't see any quality of life. He was always looking for temporary thrills to satisfy himself and never anything long-term. He feared the future so much because it would mean growing up and not having the excuse of being young to cover up how he lived and what he did. I still miss him and I'll probably never meet another person like him again. I'll remember the day I got the call about his death for the rest of my life. But I can look back and be satisfied with the type of friend I was to him and the times we did have. Zach was fun to be around.

I realize now that Zach's death wasn't my fault, or anyone else's. It was a lot of factors coming together. The only person who truly could have prevented Zach's suicide was Zach himself.

Dylan Rieger is 23 and graduated from a small high school in Pawling, NY. His passion has always been sports and he was athlete of the year in high school. He is currently studying marketing at Siena College and will graduate in 2015.

CHAPTER 12

Adolescents and Homicide

Tashel C. Bordere

IMPACT OF HOMICIDE LOSS ON ADOLESCENT GRIEF

A growing number of youth must find their way as they cope with deaths of cared-about persons through homicide loss. In 2010, the homicide rate reached a record low among youth ages 10 to 24 across all racial and ethnic groups (Centers for Disease Control and Prevention, [CDC] 2012b). Despite the hopeful decline, the rate remains a public health concern as the third leading cause of death among youth ages 10 to 24, showing an increase in later adolescence as the second leading cause of death among youth ages 15 to19. Firearms were used in 85% of teen homicides.

Homicides occurring in school settings receive a great deal of media attention. However, a small percent (1%) of homicides actually occur on school grounds (Robers, Kemp, & Truman, 2013). Similarly, mass shootings attract large amounts of media coverage, but single victim homicides are much more common (95%) (Bureau of Justice Statistics, 2013).

Victims and perpetrators tend to be geographically similar to each other (e.g., similar age, race, gender) with violent death rates differentially impacting youth populations. Males ages 15 to 19 are eight times more likely than females to die as a result of gun violence and are six times more likely than females to be victims of homicide (CDC, 2012b). Firearm deaths are highest among African American teens with homicide being the leading cause of death for African American male youth (51.7 per 100,000). Hispanic adolescent males and American Indian male youth have the second (17.9 per 100,000) and third highest (11.9 per 100,000) homicide rates.

A preponderance of literature exists as it relates to violence (e.g., Apel, Dugan, & Powers, 2011; Buckner & Bordere, 2012; DuRant, Cadenhead, Pendergrast, Slavens, & Linder, 1994; Howard, Kaljee, & Jackson, 2002; McMahon, 2009; Voisin, Bird, Hardesty, & Shiu, 2011) with limited but increasing attention to the death, loss, and grief experiences of adolescents that result from violence (e.g., Barrett, 1996; Bordere, 2008-09c; Currier, Holland, Coleman, & Neimeyer, 2006; Johnson, 2010; Vigil & Clements, 2003; Salloum, Avery, & McClain, 2001). The scarcity of literature connecting grief to violence and violent death contributes to perceptions of male youth, African American male youth in particular, as desensitized or devoid of feelings, yielding apathy and service delivery that may neglect to take into account affective reactions and grief support in the development of programs and interventions.

WAYS THAT HOMICIDE MAY COMPLICATE GRIEF

Grief is rarely uncomplicated. However, youth coping with deaths due to homicide face unique challenges in traveling along what might already be experienced as an arduous journey through grief. Several factors may intersect to complicate the grief process.

Relationship to the deceased

The high rate of homicide among youth ages 10 to 24 means that many adolescents are experiencing grief around the loss of significant persons in their lives including friends, peers, significant others, or siblings to violence. This may be especially so for African American youth who may be experiencing multiple peer losses resulting from violence. Friendship losses are significant as peers serve an increasingly vital role during adolescence as sources of support as youth develop their identities and greater independence from parents (Erikson, 1968). Due to the high levels of intimacy and trust that characterize adolescent friendships, teens may feel closer to peers than actual family members or may even view close friends as "fictive kin," the family we choose (Chatters, Taylor, & Jayakody, 1994). Emotional closeness has been related to grief response in adolescence (Servaty-Seib & Pistole, 2006-07), with friendship loss impacting the grief responses of youth in ways similar to that of family member loss (Dyregrov, Gjestad, Wikander, & Vigerust, 1999). Thus, youth may be responding intensely to the deaths of peers with whom they maintained a strong or close relationship in a culture that disenfranchises or neglects to recognize adolescent bereavement, particularly that of male youth (Doka, 1989). Youth may be further disenfranchised by the generalized lack of recognition of friendship losses within the larger culture.

The lack of acknowledgment from others combined with the "personal fable," or exaggerated thinking about their uniqueness (i.e., "No one understands me or my pain over this loss.") (Elkind, 1978) during adolescence may leave youth isolated in processing these losses. Adolescents are at a stage of development in which they are able to think abstractly, or hypothesize and speculate, about their perceptions, feelings, and experiences (Piaget, 1972). Thus, they may be thinking deeply and frequently about the death (e.g., Will my friend go to heaven? Should I make someone else feel how I feel through retaliation?) and about their grief experience (e.g., Why can't I stop crying? Why don't I feel anything?) but may be hesitant to discuss their thoughts with others due to the personal fable.

Suddenness of the loss

Deaths due to homicide may be complicated by their sudden and largely unanticipated nature. Due to the suddenness, it is unlikely that surviving youth were present at the time of death to say goodbye. Those present at the death scene may be barred from approaching their cared-about person by individuals investigating what is now a crime scene. This may be especially the case with adolescent friendship loss as youth and friends have even fewer rights than family members, who often surreptitiously or forcefully bypass the infamous yellow tape surrounding their loved one's body. In this way, youth are unable to have a role, for example, as caregiver or protector, in their cared-about person's "dying story" (Rynearson, 2001). Additionally, adolescent survivors frequently have little or no information about the death and are left to craft a "dying story" based on police records, media accounts, and/or peer and neighborhood speculations. This is to be distinguished from deaths due to natural or health-related causes where bereaved teens have factual or clear-cut health related labels to account for the death (e.g., My friend died of sickle cell anemia.) that can also be used to convey the cause of death to others, such as teachers. According to Rynearson (2001), in the absence of information, homicide survivors may have reoccurring "reenactment fantasies" about the person's last moments, fantasies about what the person may have been thinking and feeling in the moments before death. Teens may be struggling with repetitive thoughts about their cared-about person's last moments. However, they may be less likely than adults to share these troubling reenactment fantasies with others due to the "personal fable" or an exaggerated sense of their uniqueness, characteristic of normal adolescent development, and the accompanying belief that others will not understand.

Mode of death

The mode of death may further complicate the grief process for adolescents. Death by homicide is considered a non-natural or non-normative form of death as compared to deaths due to aging or deteriorating health. In general, such deaths are not socially supported or sanctioned and are thus stigmatized or considered disenfranchising deaths (Attig, 2004; Doka, 1989, 2002) contributing to *secondary victimization* (Rynearson, 1994). Homicidal deaths may garner less support than deaths due to natural causes as they are deemed preventable. It follows that if the death is preventable someone must have caused it. In cases of violent death, causation may be assigned to the homicide victim, such as through negative perceptions of the deceased as a participant in criminal activities. Further, the character of peers associated with the deceased may be questioned; bereaved friends may be criminalized due to guilt by association. This sentiment has been apparent in my research with teen survivors of violent death losses. I have met many parents who have not believed that their adolescents qualified for study participation; reflecting stereotypical perceptions of the deceased, I am frequently met with responses such as "My son doesn't know anybody like *that*." In the school system, families may not disclose the homicidal nature of the death to teachers due to fear of being stigmatized or worry that their child may be stereotyped (Bordere, 2009b).

Legal aspects

In deaths due to natural or normative causes, youth are typically able to participate in funeral rituals and move forward in processing their grief. Homicide survivors may have special difficulty with their grief process as they must wait for the state to try the case and reach a verdict (Peach & Klass, 1987). The legal process can be quite lengthy, lingering on for months or even years. Emotional stress may be exacerbated through legal proceedings where many people experience a sense of "revictimization" (Herman, 2003); this may be particularly so if the verdict reached is experienced as unjust. Fairness and justice are hallmarks of the adolescent period of development. Thus, the suddenness of the death through violence combined with a perception of the verdict as unjust may shake the teens' assumptions of the world and how it should work (Janoff-Bulman, 1992; Kauffman, 2002). Teens invalidated in their experiences with violent death losses and bereavement have been referred to as "the walking wounded" (e.g., Webb, 2010) and may become self-protective or self-destructive (Balk, 2011). Some youth may have thoughts of revenge or seek justice and control through the perpetration of violence. Gender socialization practices that promote the "Boy Code," or the expectation for males to be tough, aggressive, unemotional and strong even when feeling fearful (Terr, 1990), may contribute to such behaviors.

Salloum (2012) emphasized the need for breaks from feeling unsafe and from reminders of trauma experiences for youth bereaved by homicide loss. The court system is the antithesis of this in forcing homicide survivors to face alleged perpetrators and listen to vivid details about the violent death of their cared-about person that may both add to their trauma and to their fears of personal safety.

It can be difficult to conceptualize the reactions that adolescents may have to losses related to gun violence and the complications that may come with serving as a teen witness on trial in such a case. The highly publicized and public trial investigating the shooting death of Trayvon Martin, an unarmed, adolescent, African American male, gives us a glimpse into another adolescent's experience: Rachel Jeantel, his friend who served as a star witness in the case.

During the trial, Rachel Jeantel, now an adolescent homicide survivor, was forced to recount details chronicling the final moments that she shared with her best friend Trayvon in their cell phone conversations and events leading up to his violent death. In the trial, Rachel, who testified that she had elected *not* to attend her friend's funeral ("I didn't wanna be there, Sir.") had to explain her otherwise private reasoning for not attending the services to the public.

Lawyer: Why didn't you go to the wake or to the funeral?

Rachel: (sits in silence, shaking her head and struggling to get out words as she mumbles) I didn't want to see the body.

Lawyer: I'm sorry, what?

Rachel: I didn't wanna see the body (louder and clearer voice).

Lawyer: You didn't wanna see the body?

Rachel: No. (reaches for tissue).

She further had to describe details given to her about the funeral that confirmed the finality of his death.

Rachel: My friend went to the wake.

Lawyer: A friend of yours went to the wake?

Rachel: Yea, like some of my friends went to the wake....and they had said, his body...was there, that his body...he dead. He dead.

Despite Rachel's desire to not see her friend's lifeless body, unsightly images of her deceased friend were displayed during the course of the trial as a part of normal processes in legal proceedings (i.e., "State Shows Graphic Images of Slain Trayvon Martin," CNN) and in the media.

Homicides are often public deaths and hence may receive significant media attention and focus across social networks. This creates a lack of privacy at a period of development when adolescents are increasingly self-conscious, often possessing an "imaginary audience" or exaggerated sense of being assessed or scrutinized by others (Elkind, 1967). A glaring example could be observed in the attitudes and behaviors of Rachel, who directly and indirectly communicated that she did not desire to be in the public eye following her friend's death. For example, when an attorney offered a break that would prolong her trial participation until the next day ("Maybe we can break until the morning."), Rachel interrupted, expressing her desire not to do so. She exclaimed, "No! I'm being done today! I'm leaving today!" (WESH 2 News, 2013). Although teens often have a false or exaggerated sense of being watched and criticized by others, in this case, criticism from others was very real and came at a most vulnerable time for Rachel as she grieved her best friend's death. She received high scrutiny and degradation across media networks and social media for her demeanor and resistance to testifying; some sample headlines read, "Does Rachel Jeantel's Body Language Speak Volumes?" (CNN, 2013) and "The Social Media Stoning of Rachel Jeantel" (Backbone Women, 2013).

Court systems do have the potential to foster healing (Herman, 2003) among otherwise disenfranchised adolescent homicide survivors by providing public acknowledgment of their losses. However, one goal in court proceedings is to question the credibility of a witness, which may, in turn, overshadow opportunities for acknowledgment of grief. This was the case for Rachel, who instead of receiving external recognition and support surrounding *her sense of hurt* (as a survivor), had attention paid to whether *she hurt* his credibility through her testimony (e.g., "Rachel Jeantel: Did She Hurt Trayvon Martin's Case", Rickey Smiley Morning Show, 2013). This shift from survivor to actor in court proceedings may lend itself to feelings of guilt among vulnerable teens such as Rachel, who as a part of normal adolescent development are already "egocentric" (Elkind, 1967) in assuming fault or connection to things in which they are not to blame. For example, after learning of her friend's death, Rachel described looking at her phone to see if it occurred near the time that she had last spoken to him. She explained, "Yea, my friend had sent a text, a [sic] article saying Trayvon's name… that he died. And I asked her what time he died. And I had looked at my phone. My phone said 7:16 that the phone hung up."

Additionally, as the last person in contact with her deceased friend, Rachel's grief could be further complicated by feelings of guilt about what, if anything, she could have done to prevent his death. During the trial, Rachel expressed such feelings of guilt. Shaking her head, she said in a low tone, "I felt guilty." When asked by the attorney her reasoning for feeling guilty, Rachel explained,

> By them [Trayvon Martin's parents] finding out I was the last person, that I was the last person who he talked…..who talked to his [Trayvon Martin's father] son (voice lowered)…. That I was the last person that talked to they [sic] son.

Rynearson (2001) highlights that one aspect of the healing process is being able to tell the story of your loss experience in a coherent way in your own time. The court system, on the contrary, may subpoena or force bereaved youth to participate in court proceedings based on scheduled trial dates, possibly hastening the timing in which they share about their losses. According to Herman (2003), the court frequently demands survivors to respond to "yes or no questions" that dismantle their attempts to share a meaningful story. One major strength of the court proceedings in the trial involving Trayvon Martin was that of the judge's reassurance to Rachel that she would be heard. For example, after being asked a question and not immediately responding, the judge reassured Rachel, "We will listen to your answer, you may answer."

Further, the perpetrator and victim are frequently known to each other. They may have been childhood friends, attended the same school, or lived in the same community. In cases where there is insufficient evidence for a trial, homicide victims may feel a sense of disenfranchisement as they continue to see the alleged perpetrator in their local community. Regional and economic circumstances, conjoined with fears of personal safety and inequalities regarding legal actions and protections, can further disenfranchise and complicate the grief process.

When there is sufficient evidence for a trial, homicide survivors must face the alleged perpetrator in court. Again, this may be particularly challenging if the perpetrator is known to the victim and survivors as it may be experienced as a double loss; the loss of the loved one to violence and loss or severing of relationships with the perpetrator's family, all while frequently continuing to see each other and reside in the same neighborhood.

In highly publicized and televised trials such as the Trayvon Martin case, there is the chance to build or restore trust. Apart from the trial's legal implications, the verdict in the case had looming implications in diminishing trust in societal institutions to protect and in communicating and reinforcing to African American male youth that their lives and personal safety are not valued, what Holloway (2003) has termed the "color-coded death" (p. 57).

BRIDGING THE GAP BETWEEN KNOWLEDGE AND PRACTICE

The high violent death rate that pervades many communities is, no doubt, a public health concern (e.g., Barrett, 1993; Hammond & Yung, 1993). We know much about the clinical implications of homicide loss as associated with complicated grief, post-traumatic stress disorder, depression, and problems with substance abuse (e.g., Burke, Neimeyer, & McDevitt-Murphy, 2010; Hibberd, Elwood, & Galovski, 2010; Miller,

2009; Nader & Salloum, 2011; Overstreet & Braun, 2000; Rheingold, Zinzow, Hawkins, Saunders, & Kilpatrick, 2012). Yet, little is actually being done from a practical standpoint to meet the needs of some of the most marginalized groups of youth impacted by such losses, African American teens. Thus, the larger question remains. Why do such disparities exist in grief support for underserved youth bereaved by homicide loss and, more importantly, how will we overcome them so that our youth are able to benefit from this much-needed support?

The simple truth is that it can be difficult at best to focus on math and science when your best friend was shot in the head just two doors down from your home ten minutes after parting the prior evening, and neither recognition nor support of the loss is offered in the home or upon the return to school. We cannot expect youth to regulate emotions that were not validated in the first place or even at midstream and then penalize them when their grief expressions are manifested in less recognizable or socially acceptable ways. Molaison, Bordere, and Fowler (2011) found that anxieties, fears, and grief around violence were "masked" in angry displays. Behavioral difficulties or academic struggles may lead to mislabeling otherwise bereaved youth as behavior disordered. Once labeled, these youth are put on a trajectory in which future behaviors that may actually be related to unrecognized or unsupported grief reactions to multiple ongoing losses are also assigned to this potentially misconstrued early diagnosis, as opposed to early bereavement intervention. This may be particularly so for African American youth who are disproportionately represented in special education classes for the behavior disordered (Anderson, 1992; Chinn & Hughes, 1987; Ogbu, 1990). Another example may be charging an adolescent a fine or criticizing the teen for the creation of an urban street memorial at the location of the violent death. In doing so, we contribute to the suffocated grief of youth, where penalties surrounding their grief expressions serve to further stifle their bereavement process and contribute to increased externalizing behaviors. In a sample of bereaved adolescent youth, Boelen and Spuij (2008) found that complicated grief and depression were significantly correlated with negative cognitions about the appropriateness of their grief reactions.

There are, no doubt, other factors (e.g., self-esteem, opportunity structure, violence at home) that contribute to externalizing behaviors among youth. My hope is just to highlight grief as "the elephant in the room," requiring greater attention in understanding reactions around homicide loss and rates of youth violence among marginalized groups. Salloum, Avery, and McClain (2001) are notable exceptions in putting research into practice through the use of a grief and trauma intervention (GTI) with a nonclinical sample of underserved adolescent homicide loss survivors. The intervention was effective in reducing trauma symptoms and in facilitating communication about their grief experiences that included living memories of their cared-about person.

CULTURALLY APPROPRIATE PRACTICE WITH ADOLESCENT HOMICIDE SURVIVORS

Enfranchising grief

The good news is that we can do much in the way of enfranchising the grief experiences of youth. This may be achieved in several ways, including what I propose as a *cultural iconic approach* or recognition and acknowledgment of cultural symbols as expressions of loss. This approach could include acknowledging memorial t-shirts as "walking monuments" of the deceased (Bordere, 2008-2009c); memorial tattoos (Martin, 2000, 2010); music (e.g., rap and hip hop); and urban street memorials and murals (Barrett, 2009) as valuable tools for coping and maintaining connections with the deceased among youth populations. In the case of urban street memorials and murals, providing an established place such as a community center for such gestures may help circumvent the creation of memorials in less feasible locations, like on private property.

Creative interventions are needed to reach youth less likely to enter clinical settings and more likely to rely on informal community networks of support. In addition to direct services for bereaved adolescents, training opportunities such as death education courses and educational resources must be provided to individuals in most contact with youth including educators, parents, religious leaders and groups, health professionals, coaches, directors of recreational centers, and youth as peer supports in adolescent bereavement.

Be aware of the medicalization (e.g., complicated grief, traumatic grief, post-traumatic grief) of reactions and processing regarding violent death losses. Although homicide survivors are at risk for adverse outcomes, not every adolescent impacted by homicide loss shows psychiatric symptoms. Some youth simply experience the loss with sadness or other normal reactions to a death loss and are able to move forward and adjust to the loss. Further, youth are most effected by deaths that matter to them. Meanings constructed around loss can impact bereavement (Armour, 2003; Currier, Holland, & Neimeyer, 2006). In cases of multiple violent death losses, what may appear to be desensitization may actually be attempts on the part of youth to decide how they will allocate their ever-diminishing emotional resources. Servaty-Seib and Pistole (2006-07) suggest assessing the bereaved adolescent's level of closeness to the deceased in counseling youth.

While violent death is thought to complicate grief due to its sudden and unexpected nature, it is noteworthy that for some youth, a homicidal death may be viewed as sudden but not necessarily unexpected. For example, the teen may not find the death surprising if he or she believes the deceased engaged in risky behaviors that precipitated the death. This underscores the importance of assessing beliefs about the timing of the death and its significance to the teen.

In the literature, there is a wide focus on homicide bereavement as complicated by a loss of the assumptive world. Because perceptions of loss and experiences with grief vary across cultures (e.g., geographic region, developmental stage, race and ethnicity, gender, spirituality) (Bordere, 2009a; Corr, Corr, & Bordere, 2013; Lopez, 2011; McGoldrick, Schlesinger, Lee, Hines, Chan, Almeida, et al., 2004; Rosenblatt, 1993), it is important to confirm with youth their personal thoughts about the world. From a cultural standpoint, views of the assumptive world among minority youth may differ from that of youth from majority or privileged cultures who may experience the world as more just. More specifically, differences in views about the assumptive world may contribute to grief reactions of underrepresented youth due to different expectations for outcomes that might be just in homicide loss. As part of racial and ethnic socialization processes, many underrepresented youth have been reared to understand that life may not be fair (as in Langston Hughes' poem *Mother to Son*: "Life for me ain't been no crystal stair," 1922) and to remain steadfast through prayer and education amid unjust circumstances (Halgunseth, Cushinberry, & Bordere, 2003). In a sample of African American families, Rosenblatt and Wallace (2005) found that steadfastness or "being strong" in grief may in part be related to feeling alone or lacking support from accessible or culturally appropriate mental health services.

Many youth remain functional due to support derived from family, peers, religious/spiritual beliefs, or intricate community networks. I remember vividly the notification I received that my young research participant had been shot multiple times. In earnest, as a researcher, first human, I struggled with the violations that had occurred to my long-time participant. I found it astounding, yet consistent with research on African American populations, that this youth and his family remained resilient despite this and other significant violent death losses. I have witnessed the sadness and anger expressed by this youth over the murder of his older brother in interviews and the tears of his mother at his bedside following his shooting and subsequent firearm injuries. Yet, seemingly, the biggest stressor for this youth and his family in this ordeal (once it was clear that he had survived) was how they would have the home reconstructed to accommodate his new needs. Moving forward or "going on" once past the initial pain of the loss (Rosenblatt & Wallace, 2005) does not diminish its impact. It may simply be reminiscent of a culture's adaptation to multiple losses and intention to survive life amid otherwise unfathomable circumstances.

The homicide happens, the funeral passes, but the lack of safety remains for many adolescents residing in high crime areas. Thus, youth may experience and need support with thoughts about surviving death coupled with thoughts about surviving *life*. It is important to remember that despite the facts and negative stereotypes often maintained in the larger society about homicide victims, these young men and women occupied significant roles in the lives of surviving youth, often as protectors, confidants, and providers. Teens may be struggling both with the death of their loved one as well as with the life that they will now lead or survival in the absence of the deceased. Thus, it is important to explore secondary losses, such as protection or income, associated with the death. For example, in cases where adolescents believe they have lost a peer who served a major protective role (e.g., "He told me to go inside when it got dark."), it may be important to assist the teen in finding other healthy ways to maintain a sense of safety outside of weapon carrying in the absence of their loved one. In a national survey of high school students, 16.6% reported carrying a weapon (e.g., gun, knife) on at least one day during the 30 days prior to completing the survey with rates highest among males – white males (27.2%), black males (21%), and Hispanic males (24.5%) (Centers for Disease Control and Prevention, 2012a). Barrett (1996) recommends survival education.

Youth need to see more examples of social justice so they can feel reassured that external sources such as police, teachers, or those in the court system can, in fact, be relied on for help and protection, for their physical safety and emotional safety. In a study of African American youth in the justice system, participants expressed little trust in the criminal justice system for help and instead took action themselves or sought out other youth for support (Wilson, 2006). Further, teens generally feel that they are unheard or too unique to be understood (i.e., personal fable), and that their thoughts are minimized by adults. Court systems, by nature of normal legal processes, may unintentionally reinforce these beliefs and serve to further disenfranchise and suffocate the grief of youth. To help overcome this challenge, more accountability is needed and alliances built between entities such as criminal justice workers, therapists, churches, schools, and youth and families. In fairness, it is not the job of the court to be a forum for grief support. However, recognizing that youth bereaved by homicide loss may experience legal proceedings as adversive (e.g., story dismantled) or unjust, collaboration is needed between juvenile justice workers and youth specialists so that preparation may be given to adolescents about the culture of court proceedings. Adolescents could be made aware that that their thoughts and experiences may be questioned, coupled with debriefing and reinforcement that their perceptions and experiences surrounding their loss are still valuable. Resources should also be provided (e.g., a listing of community support services or helpful literature, such as *The Bill of Rights of Grieving Teens*—The Dougy Center, www.dougy.org) on coping with grief and loss following trial participation. Grief support might also be offered in juvenile justice facilities and diversion programs.

There are opportunities for growth through tragedy and trauma (Tedeschi & Calhoun, 1995, 2004). African American youth and families are no strangers to injustices that accompany death through violence. They share a history rooted in the sudden violent deaths of loved ones through slavery and have adapted a repertoire of mechanisms in coping with such losses. In outreach and counseling with bereaved youth, it is important to explore both negative reactions as well as what Park, Cohen, and Murch (1996) describe as "stress-related growth." In a study exploring posttraumatic growth among participants who had experienced major life events, Milam, Ritt-Olson, and Unger (2004) found that religious participants showed posttraumatic growth. In a separate study of African American adolescent girls, a focus on academic success allowed the teens to demonstrate resilience in moving forward with their lives following homicide loss (Johnson, 2010).

Because violent deaths can be disenfranchising, rituals may also serve an important role in the healing process for youth, serving as opportunities to say goodbye and promote the maintenance of continuing bonds with the deceased (Klass, Silverman, & Nickman, 1996; Stroebe, Schut, & Boerner, 2010). The New Orleans second-line funeral ritual has been found to give adolescents another way to look at death (Bordere, 2008-09). Compared to more conventional funerals in a church or funeral home, where the overarching emotion observed was sadness, second-lines communicated an understanding of death as a cause for celebration, remembrance, and unity. The second-line funeral procession typically consists of a small brass band, memorial t-shirts, and dancing or "hopping" and "jumping" as participants travel in a parade-like fashion past the favorite places (e.g., school, park), and sometimes the death scene, of the deceased.

> *Mostly all the family members had on a shirt with a picture of him. And they went to the spot where he got killed at…. staying right there….and it was raining that day…and they started standing right there and they started dancing and stuff and they…some of them was crying. I was watching 'em. I was watching them dance in the mud. They were dancing where he got killed at…under that tree.*

Although all forms of grief are welcome and expressed, second-lines promote a positive outlook on death through joyful "send-offs" and allow for more *instrumental styles* of grief (Martin & Doka, 2000) in encouraging movement or dancing. This ritual may be particularly useful for male youth reared with the "Boy Code" or female youth possessing more of an action-oriented style of grief in giving them an outlet for expressions suited to their personalities.

The second-line ritual also functions as a reminder of the life led by the deceased as youth work to construct a meaningful narrative (living and dying story) that takes into account their memories with the deceased. New Orleans second-lines serve to enfranchise the otherwise unacknowledged grief of youth. They demonstrate in a public way to teens that their feelings surrounding the homicidal death of their loved one matters and that the life of the deceased had value.

Tashel C. Bordere, PhD, CT, is an associate professor of child and family development at the University of Central Missouri where she has developed and taught courses related to death, dying, bereavement, and adolescent development. She is currently editor of The Forum, *the quarterly publication of the Association for Death Education and Counseling (ADEC). She is a past board member of ADEC, past chair of ADEC's People of Color/Multicultural Committee, and member of the National Council on Family Relations. Bordere has written works relating to diversity and resilience through grief, her most recent being* The remedy is NOT working: Seeking socially just and culturally conscientious practices in bereavement, *a co-authored work, in* Grief and Bereavement in Contemporary Society. *She is a Certified Thanatologist. Her research focuses on homicidal violent death and grief among African American youth, cultural death customs, parenting approaches within context, and culturally sensitive practices in research and work with youth and families.*

References

Anderson, M. G. (1992). The use of selected theatre rehearsal technique activities with African-American adolescents labeled "behavior disordered." *Exceptional Children, 59*(2), 132-140.

Apel, R., Dugan, L, & Powers, R. (2011). Gender and injury risk in incidents of assaultive violence. *Justice Quarterly.* DOI: 10.1080/07418825.2011.619558

Armour, M. (2003). Meaning making in the aftermath of homicide. *Death Studies, 27*(6), 519-540.

Attig, T. (2004). Disenfranchised grief revisited: Discounting hope and love. *Omega, 49*(3), 197-215.

Backbone Women. (2013, June 27). The social media stoning of Rachel Jeantel. Retrieved from http://www.backbonewomenonline.com/2013/06/the-social-media-stoning-of-rachel.html

Balk, D. (2011). Adolescent development and bereavement: An introduction. *The Prevention Researcher, 18*(3), 3-9.

Barrett, R. K. (1993). Urban adolescent homicidal violence: An emerging public health concern. *Urban League Review, 16*(2), 67-75.

Barrett, R. K. (1996). Adolescents, homicidal violence & death. In C. Corr & E. Balk (Eds.), *Handbook of adolescent death and bereavement.* New York, NY: Springer.

Barrett, R. K. (2009). Emerging and universal trends in urban memorials. *The Forum, 35*(4), 17-18.

Boelen, P. A., & Spuij, M. (2008). Negative cognitions in loss related emotional distress in adolescent girls: A preliminary study. *Journal of Loss & Trauma, 13,* 441-449.

Bordere, T. (2009a). Culturally conscientious thanatology. *The Forum, 35*(2), 1-4.

Bordere, T. (2009b). Culturally sensitive approaches to support grief in the classroom. Retrieved from http://www.education.com/reference/article/cultural-approaches-support-grief/

Bordere, T. (2008-2009c). 'To look at death another way': Black teenage males' perspectives on second-lines and regular funerals in New Orleans. *Omega, 58*(3), 213-232.

Buckner, P., & Bordere, T. (2012). African American female youth violence: Making sense of the senseless. *The Forum, 38*(2), 15.

Burke, L. A., Neimeyer, R. A., & McDevitt-Murphy, M. E. (2010). African American homicide bereavement: Aspects of social support that predict complicated grief, PTSD, and depression. *Omega, 61*(1), 1-24.

Centers for Disease Control and Prevention. (2011). Youth Risk Behavior Surveillance. MMWR 2012; 61(No. SS-4).

Centers for Disease Control and Prevention. *Web-based Injury Statistics Query and Reporting System (WISQARS) (Online).* (2012b). National Center for Injury Prevention and Control, Centers for Disease Control and Prevention (producer).

Chatters, L., Taylor, R. J., & Jayakody, R. (1994). Fictive kinship relations in Black extended families. *Journal of Comparative Family Studies, 25*(3), 297-312.

Chinn, P., & Hughes, S. (1987). Representation of minority students in special education classes. *Remedial and Special Education, 8*(4), 41-46.

CNN. (Producer). (2013, June 27). Does Rachel Jeantel's body language speak volumes? [Video file] Retrieved from https://www.youtube.com/watch?v=SrYAF9rrHJU

Corr, C., Corr, D., & Bordere, T. (2013). Cultural patterns and death. In C. A. Corr & D. M. Corr (Eds.), *Death and dying, life and living* (7th ed.). Belmont, CA: Wadsworth.

Currier, J., Holland, J., Coleman, R., & Neimeyer, R. A. (2006). Bereavement following violent death: An assault on life and meaning. In R. Stevenson & G. Cox (Eds.), *Perspectives on violence and violent death.* Amityville, NY: Baywood.

Currier, J. M., Holland, J. M., & Neimeyer, R. A. (2006). Sense-making, grief, and the experience of violent loss: Toward a mediational model. *Death Studies, 30,* 403-428.

Currier, J. M., Holland, J. M., & Neimeyer, R. A. (2007). The effectiveness of bereavement interventions with children: A meta-analytic review of controlled outcome research. *Journal of Clinical Child and Adolescent Psychology, 36*(2), 253-259.

Doka, K. J. (1989). *Disenfranchised grief: Recognizing hidden sorrow.* Lexington, MA: Lexington Books.

Doka, K. J. (2002). *Disenfranchised grief: New directions, challenges, and strategies for practice.* Champaign, IL: Research Press.

DuRant, R. H., Cadenhead, C., Pendergrast, R. A., Slavens, G., & Linder, C. W. (1994). Factors associated with the use of violence among urban Black adolescents. *American Journal of Public Health, 84*(4), 612-617.

Dyregrov, A., Gjestad, R., Wikander, A. M. B., & Vigerust, S. (1999). Reactions following the sudden death of a classmate. *Scandinavian Journal of Psychology, 40,* 167-176.

Elkind, D. (1967). Egocentrism in adolescence. *Child Development, 38*(4), 1025-1034.

Elkind, D. (1978). Understanding the young adolescent. *Adolescence, 13*(49), 127-134.

Erikson, E. (1968). *Identity: Youth and crisis.* New York, NY: Norton.

Halgunseth, L., Cushinberry, C., & Bordere, T. C. (2003). Race, ethnicity, and parenting styles. In M. Coleman & L. Ganong (Eds.), *Controversial relationship and family issues in the 21ˢᵗ century.* Los Angeles, CA: Roxbury.

Hammond, W. R., & Yung, B. (1993). Psychology's role in the public health response to assaultive violence among young African-American men. *American Psychologist, 48*(2), 142-154.

Herman, J. L. (2003). The mental health of crime victims: Impact of legal intervention. *Journal of Trauma Stress, 16*(2), 159-166.

Hibberd, R., Elwood, L. S., & Galovski, T. E. (2010). Risk and protective factors for posttraumatic stress disorder, prolonged grief, and depression in survivors of the violent death of a loved one. *Journal of Loss & Trauma, 15,* 426-447.

Holloway, K. (2003). *Passed on: African American mourning stories: A memorial.* Durham, NC: Duke University Press.

Howard, D. E., Kaljee, L., & Jackson, L. (2002). Urban African American adolescents' perceptions of community violence. *American Journal of Health Behavior, 26*(1), 56-67.

Janoff-Bulman, R. (1992). *Shattered assumptions: Towards a new psychology of trauma.* New York, NY: Free Press.

Johnson, C. (2010). African American teen girls grieve the loss of friends to homicide: Meaning making and resilience. *Omega, 61*(2), 121-143.

Kauffman, J. K. (2002). Safety and the assumptive world. In J. Kauffman (Ed.), *Loss of the assumptive world: A theory of traumatic loss* (pp. 205-212). New York, NY: Routledge.

Klass, D., Silverman, P. R., & Nickman, S. L. (1996). *Continuing bonds: New understandings of grief.* Philadelphia, PA: Taylor & Francis.

Lopez, S. A. (2011). Culture as an influencing factor in adolescent grief and bereavement. *The Prevention Researcher, 18*(3), 10-13.

McGoldrick, M., Schlesinger, J. M., Lee, E., Hines, P. M., Chan, J., Almeida, R., et al. (2004). Mourning in different cultures. In F. Walsh & M. McGoldrick (Eds.), *Living beyond loss: Death in the family* (2nd ed.) (pp. 119-160). New York, NY: W.W. Norton & Company.

McMahon, S. (2009). Community violence exposure and aggression among urban adolescents: Testing a cognitive mediator. *Journal of Community Psychology, 37*(7), 895-910.

Martin, A. (2000). On teenagers and tattoos. *Reclaiming Children and Youth, 9*(3), 143-144 & 150.

Martin, A. (2010). *Rhetorical analysis on teenagers and tattoos.* Researchomatic. Retrieved from http://www.researchomatic.com/essay/Rhetorical-Analysis-On-Teenagers-And-Tattoos-49594.aspx

Martin, T. L., & Doka, K. J. (2000). *Men don't cry...women do.* Philadelphia, PA: Brunner/Mazel.

Miller, L. (2009). Family survivors of homicide: I. Symptoms, syndromes, and reaction patterns. *The American Journal of Family Therapy, 37*(1), 67-79.

Milam, J., Ritt-Olson, A., & Unger, J. B. (2004). Posttraumatic growth among adolescents. *Journal of Adolescent Research, 19*(2), 192-204.

Molaison, V., Bordere, T., & Fowler, K. (2011). "The remedy is NOT working": Seeking socially just and culturally conscientious practices in bereavement. In R. Neimeyer, H. Winokuer, D. Harris, & G. Thornton (Eds.), *Grief and bereavement in contemporary society: Bridging research and practice.* New York, NY: Routledge.

Nader, K., & Salloum, A. (2011). Complicated grief reactions in children and adolescents. *Journal of Child and Adolescent Trauma, 4*(3), 233-257.

Ogbu, J. (1990). Minority education in comparative perspective. *Journal of Negro Education, 59*(1), 45-57.

Overstreet, S., & Braun, S. (2000). Exposure to community violence and post-traumatic stress symptoms: Mediating factors. *American Journal of Orthopsychiatry, 70*(2), 263-271.

Park, C. L., Cohen, L. H., & Murch, R. L. (1996). Assessment and prediction of stress-related growth. *Journal of Personality, 64*(1), 72-105.

Peach, M. R., & Klass, D. (1987). Special issues in the grief of parents of murdered children. *Death Studies, 11,* 81-88.

Piaget, J. (1972). Intellectual evolution from adolescence to adulthood. *Human Development, 15,* 1-12.

Rheingold, A. A., Zinzow, H., Hawkins, A., Saunders, B. E., & Kilpatrick, D. G. (2012). Prevalence and mental health outcomes of homicide survivors in a representative US sample of adolescents: Data from the 2005 national survey of adolescents. *Journal of Child Psychology and Psychiatry, 53*(6), 687-694.

Rickey Smiley Morning Show. (2013, June 28). Rachel Jeantel: Did she hurt Trayvon Martin's case. [Audio file] Retrieved from http://rickeysmileymorningshow.com/1204491/rachel-jeantel-trayvon-martin-testimony/

Robers, S., Kemp, J., & Truman, J. (2013). *Indicators of School Crime and Safety: 2012* (NCES 2013-036/NCJ 241446). National Center for Education Statistics, U.S. Department of Education, and Bureau of Justice Statistics, Office of Justice Programs, U.S. Department of Justice. Washington, DC.

Rosenblatt, P. C. (1993). Cross-cultural variation in the experience, expression, and understanding of grief. In D. P. Irish, K. F. Lundquist, & V. J. Nelsen (Eds.), *Ethnic variations in dying, death and grief: Diversity in universality* (pp. 13-19). Philadelphia, PA: Taylor & Francis Publishers.

Rosenblatt, P. & Wallace, B. (2005). *American-American grief.* New York, NY: Routledge.

Rynearson, E. K. (1994). Psychotherapy of bereavement after homicide. *Journal of Psychotherapy Practice and Research, 3,* 341-347.

Rynearson, E. K. (2001). *Retelling violent death.* New York, NY: Taylor & Francis.

Salloum, A. (2012). *Grief and trauma intervention for children.* Invited Featured Speaker Presentation at the Annual Conference of the Association for Death Education and Counseling, Atlanta, GA.

Salloum, A., Avery, L., & McClain, R. P. (2001). Group psychotherapy for adolescent survivors of homicide victims: A pilot study. *American Academy of Child and Adolescent Psychiatry, 40*(11), 1261-1267.

Servaty-Seib, H. L., & Pistole, M. C. (2006-2007). Adolescent grief: Relationship category and emotional closeness. *Omega, 54*(2), 147-167.

Stroebe, M., Schut, H., & Boerner, K. (2010). Continuing bonds in adaptation to bereavement: Toward theoretical integration. *Clinical Psychology Review, 30*(8), 259-268.

Tedeschi, R. G., & Calhoun, L. G. (1995). *Trauma & transformation: Growing in the aftermath of suffering.* Thousand Oaks, CA: Sage.

Tedeschi, R. G., & Calhoun, L. G. (2004). Posttraumatic growth: Conceptual foundations and empirical evidence. *Psychological Inquiry, 15*(1), 1-18.

Terr, L. (1990). *Too scared to cry.* New York, NY: Harper & Row.

U.S. Department of Justice, Bureau of Justice Statistics (2013). *Homicide in the U.S. known to Law Enforcement, 2011* (NCJ 243035). Washington, DC. Retrieved from http://www.bjs.gov/index.cfm?ty=pbdetail&iid=4863

Vigil, G., & Clements, P. T. (2003). Child and adolescent homicide survivors. *Journal of Psychosocial Nursing & Mental Health Services, 41*(1), 30-39.

Voisin, D. R., Bird, J. D., Hardesty, M., & Shiu, C. S. (2011). African American adolescents living and coping with community violence on Chicago's southside. *Journal of Interpersonal Violence, 26*(12), 2483-2498.

Webb, N. B. (2010). Mental health approaches to the treatment of traumatized children. *The Forum, 36*(4), 22-23.

WESH 2 News. (Producer). (2013, June 26). Trayvon Martin's friend testifying: I'm leaving today. Retrieved from https://www.youtube.com/watch?v=sY3XPf912-k

CHAPTER 13

Adolescent Grief: The Death of a U.S. Service Member

Heather R. Campagna, Tina Saari, and
Jill Harrington-LaMorie

The death of a parent or sibling is a stressful life event for children and their families. Since 2001, there have been approximately 16,000 men and women who have died serving on active-duty in all components (Active, Guard, and Reserve) and branches (Army, Navy, Air Force, Marines, and Coast Guard) of the United States (U.S.) Armed Services (Defense Manpower Data Center (DMDC), 2013).

Whether by suicide, accident, combat-related death or illness, the vast majority of service members die between the ages of 18 to 40 by sudden and/or violent circumstances of death. Given the young age of service members at the time of their death, many have surviving family members that are adolescent children or siblings. The impact to these adolescent survivors can be profound, long-lasting, and disenfranchising. While few researchers have studied adolescent grief in military families, the common observation is that the death of a U.S. service member presents unique factors that can contribute to risk or resilience in bereaved families. Studies of school-age children and teens with deployed parents have found increased risk for problems with peer relationships, physiological signs of stress, emotional and behavioral problems, depression, increased use of alcohol or drugs, suicidal thoughts, and use of mental health services (Lester & Flake, 2013). While the literature grows on the impact of military service in the past decade on military children and their families, there is scant information on the impact of a service member's death on the family. The need for research in the surviving adolescent population is critical to help those that may be at-risk and support all those who cope and adapt to the death of their family service member.

A factor that may contribute to risk or difficulty for adolescent survivors can be that they represent an extremely small and distinctive population in American society. Lack of a peer group and feeling disenfranchised or poorly understood could be effects of the growing disconnection between military personnel and their families with the broader U.S. civilian population. Unlike countries such as Israel, where all adults serve in the armed forces, children and siblings of active-duty service members represent families of less than one percent of the American population. Of this one percent, approximately one percent of those have died in uniform since 2001. Disconnection from the military and lack of understanding from the community can contribute to increased vulnerability and feelings of social isolation in these young people and families.

Given the lack of research and the unique factors that may complicate grief and other potential challenges posed to bereaved adolescents, education is essential to both the military and civilian community to better understand and support this distinctive population. Since adolescence is one of the most vulnerable times in human development for formation of identity and crises that challenge it, the experience of a sudden and/or violent military family member death can add great distress to children and teens who are now faced with a task out of sync with a "normative" expected family lifecycle.

This chapter will explore adolescent grief in the context of the death of a family member on active-duty and reserve U.S. military service. For the purpose of our discussion, we will focus on the military and influences to the family since the inception of the Global War on Terrorism on September 11, 2001, and will encompass all deaths that occur while serving, to include killed-in-action, natural causes, accidents, and suicide. The goal of this chapter is to provide clinicians and caregivers an overview of (a) demographics of the deceased and the survivors, (b) the influence of development on bereavement in adolescents, (c) core aspects of military death and issues affecting surviving adolescent siblings and children, (d) considerations for clinicians and educators, (e) normative grief compared to traumatic grief, and (f) issues specific to siblings and dependent children.

DEMOGRAPHIC INFORMATION

Military personnel on active duty

Since 9/11/2001, more than 16,000 uniformed service members have died on active-duty (DMDC, 2013). As stated earlier, the majority of service members die between the ages of 18 to 40 years old by sudden and/or violent circumstances of death. Approximately one-third of these deaths are combat-related deaths, occurring in Iraq and Afghanistan. Approximately 97% of all who have died are male; enlisted personnel have the highest occurrence of death across all service branches (DMDC, 2013). Circumstances of death include: mass-casualties, accidents, homicides, suicides, killed-in-action, terrorist attacks, and sudden illness. Since 2001, there has been a significant rise in suicide rates in military personnel across all branches of service; nearly one in every five suicides nationally is a U.S. veteran.

Surviving families

Today's military service members are young and likely to be married although, according to the Department of Defense (DOD), the majority of service members who die are actually single. In addition, each year, there are 90,000 children born to active-duty service members. Those who die on active-duty are also young (18 to 40). Therefore, they typically are survived by young family members, who may include young parents, young siblings, a young spouse or adult partner, infant to adolescent children (some unborn), and generally a younger group of extended family members and friends (Harrington-LaMorie, 2011).

Military families do not exist in isolation; they live in civilian communities, on military installations, and overseas. Family survivors, whether by origin (parents and siblings) or procreation (spouses and children), reside in all fifty states and outside the continental US. Adolescent siblings will more than likely be living with one or both of the service member's surviving parents at the time of their sibling's death and adolescent children with the surviving spouse, ex-spouse, adult partner, or guardian. National Guard and reserve families tend to live in their "home communities," while active-duty children and spouses live on or near installations and make frequent moves after a death. Nearly 80% of all children of uniformed military personnel attend a civilian school. Surviving children are less likely to continue their education for more than one year at a Department of Defense School, mainly due to policies that transition families off installation housing.

Since 9/11/2001, over 10,000 grieving children and adolescents have lost their special person through a military death. Approximately 4,900 of those were dependent children who have been left behind after the death of a parent serving in the military, while around 5,500 siblings have lost their brother or sister in service to our country (Tragedy Assistance Program for Survivors, 2013).

ADOLESCENT DEVELOPMENT AND BEREAVEMENT

There is conflicting discussion in the literature as to when adolescence begins and ends. For the purposes of this article, we will refer to adolescence as the part of the lifespan between ages 13 to 19. Despite the widespread belief that adolescence is a developmental period of stress and confusion, the majority of adolescents weather this time fairly well. Nevertheless, adolescence is a period in which the most difficulty with development is likely to arise. For the adolescent, there are numerous transitions occurring bio-psychosocially, such as cognitive changes, biological changes (growth and hormonal), psychological changes, and social changes, most notably in the areas of identity and peer relationships.

These changes occur across a broad range of micro and macro systems to include peers, family, school, community, and larger society. Changes within these systems have a significant impact on the development of each individual adolescent. When an adolescent experiences a sudden death of a relative or peer, this event can inflict major stress during an already vulnerable period of their human development. The family composition is abruptly altered and this unexpected major life shift brings intense grief reactions and magnified difficulties with tasks associated with this developmental period.

Violent deaths experienced by teens can be the most difficult circumstances of death for them to understand and present a serious challenge to bereavement and adaptation to loss. However, Balk and Corr (2009) have observed that research on adolescent bereavement has been limited in its existence, and the empirical literature on its effects on bereavement during adolescent development is limited. Nonetheless, what is commonly observed is that the death of a significant person during adolescence may cause difficulty with achieving autonomy, mastery, competency, control, and intimacy, all of which are important developmental tasks of this period.

Adolescents, more than school-age children, often deal with self-esteem and identity issues. A major task of this life stage is differentiation. A normative task for teens is the desire to differentiate themselves from their parents. An adolescent who experiences a sudden, unexpected death may experience an interruption of age-appropriate activities for a life event in which they are not developmentally prepared. The change in family dynamics or shift in focus on the grieving parent or parents may further isolate them from peers and complicate their emerging internal drive to differentiate and individuate. Evidence suggests that when a child loses a parent, the surviving parent's response to death is related to how children respond (Holmes, Rauch, & Cozza, 2013). Children who may be at risk in their bereavement and may have later difficulties are those that experience inadequate parental functioning, poor environmental support and lack of a supportive relationship with their surviving parent or guardian (Holmes, Rauch, & Cozza, 2013). When a surviving parent has previously struggled with depression, anxiety, sleep or health problems prior to the death, children and teens are less likely to adjust well and are at risk for the development of childhood traumatic grief (CTG) (Holmes, Rauch, & Cozza, 2013). Adolescents often express their grief and loss issues through their body language and acting out behavior. In addition, adolescents might be internally preoccupied with death, which might be manifested through poor school performance.

One of the most important developmental challenges for adolescents is the need to fit in with their peers, considering that the social landscape and peer support is such an important part of adolescence. If the adolescent feels different from his or her peers, this can disenfranchise grief and he or she may be more hesitant to express grief reactions. However, support from peers during this time can provide an important element of comfort during their grieving process and allow for a supported environment for expression of grief. The literature suggests that peer support is one of the main sources of help for a bereaved adolescent.

MILITARY FACTORS IN ADOLESCENT GRIEF

Many unique aspects are present for a young person who has experienced the death of a parent or sibling in the military. These factors can affect adolescent survivors not only short term but throughout their lives. Given that a military death impacts such a small population of American society, adolescents may struggle first with peers supporting them in their experience and second with connecting with other adolescent peers who have experienced a similar loss.

Deployment

Deployment times can range anywhere from 3 months to 15 months, and most service members have done multiple deployments in a combat zone in another country, spending that time away from home. When a service member dies while deployed, the family often feels as though the service member is still deployed and not dead, as they are accustomed to long-term separations (Beard, Mathewson, Saari, & Campagna, 2008). This can lead to delays in grief reactions as survivors employ coping mechanisms to imagine their service member is "deployed," delaying the finality of accepting the death. This is known in the field as deployment-delayed grief (Harrington-LaMorie, 2011).

Notification of death

A key component for military children experiencing the death of a service member starts with the notification of death. The military protocol for death notifications consists of two uniformed military personnel going to the home to inform the family of their special person's death. Young people who are raised in a military household are often aware of what this means when they see uniformed personnel show up on their doorsteps, so this event can be extremely upsetting and possibly traumatic. In addition, observing the parent's reaction to the notification of this news can be devastating as well, for both the child of the service member as well as a sibling.

Military burial

Military burial can be another complicated factor for military children. The memorial and burial process may be lengthy compared to the same rituals on the civilian side. When a death happens overseas, it may take up to a week for the body to return stateside. For combat-related deaths, there are dignified transfer ceremonies for the deceased returning through Dover Air Force Base that the family can choose to attend. There are times when there are no identifiable remains to be viewed; in this case, a young person may have a hard time conceptualizing the death of their service member and believe he or she will be returning home. In some cases when additional remains are identified, they are returned to the family at a later time.

This can mean additional formal notification processes and additional possible burials that families may be unaware of when the news is first delivered. In addition to the family's personal funeral, military units typically have memorials for the service member that are followed by the burial. The family has the option of whether to have their special person buried in a Veteran's Cemetery or to be buried in a private cemetery. If the family chooses to bury their service member in a Veteran's Cemetery, there is often a waiting list and it may be days or possibly even weeks before their service member can be put to rest (Beard, Mathewson, Saari, & Campagna, 2008). This prolonged process can be difficult for adolescents as they attempt to return to "normal" and determine what their "new normal" may be. The typical challenges of adolescence, as well as adjusting to life within the family unit without that special person, can be exacerbated when everything is put on hold until the burial.

Media

An aspect unique to military children is the role that media can play in the grieving process. Circumstances surrounding military deaths may be very public and replayed on media outlets that can be viewed by young people. Difficulties can arise when the adolescent is repeatedly exposed to the accident or circumstances in which their service member died.

Military or graphic television shows, video games, and movies may also trigger an adverse reaction. For the military teen who wants to make a fresh start at a new school, classmates may find information about the death on the Internet, which creates difficulty for the teen who wanted to remain anonymous to "fit in" to his or her new environment.

Suicide

A growing number of child and adolescent military survivors are suffering a death of their special person by suicide. This type of death can lead to a tremendous amount of complications associated with their grief (Harrington-LaMorie, 2013). Common among struggles that face suicide survivors in their bereavement is the issue of guilt. Adolescents can contend heavily with profound guilt, thinking they somehow caused or contributed to the death of their family member or that they could have prevented the death. Guilt can come from the taboo feeling of "relief" when a family member dies by suicide. Children and teens may bear witness to violence, neglect, abuse, or the effects of invisible psychological injuries, such as post-traumatic stress disorder (PTSD), in their home. These survivors may feel relieved that their family is no longer living in an unhealthy environment as a result of the service member's suicide. It is not uncommon for military children to witness the suicide or find their special person who has died by suicide in their home. This adds an additional element of trauma.

In the past, the military has indicated that it was a sign of weakness to obtain mental health assistance. Although the military stance has shifted drastically on that standpoint, it is important to understand that some service members and their families do feel stigmatized when it comes to mental health and discussing mental health challenges in their families. The adolescent's parent or sibling who died by suicide may have been suffering from invisible psychological injuries, fighting a very different battle. For many who feel the stigmatization that may come with a suicide death of a family member, they often report experiencing that the circumstance of death eclipses their family member's military service (Harrington-LaMorie, 2013). This can lead to feelings of shame and disenfranchised grief.

Secondary losses

There are multiple secondary losses that can affect adolescents who have experienced the death of a parent or sibling in the military. Along with grieving the death of a service member, loss of the military lifestyle and what it encompassed for the family as a whole can be devastating after a death. This lifestyle includes a culture that is hard for many civilians to understand, one that requires a commitment from the whole family. For many children raised on or near a military installation, suddenly moving off the base or away from the community can be traumatic. It is a way of life and the only way of life that so many know, such as stopping to pay respect when *Reveille, Retreat,* and *Taps* are played over the loud speakers three times a day or seeing service members running in formation chanting cadences. A family living on a military installation has one year after the date of death to move, which usually includes changing schools. Children and adolescents often have problems coping with the adjustment of no longer being the "military brat" and living the military lifestyle, which can lead to a loss of identity and status. This may be additionally burdensome to teens, who are faced with identity challenges as part of normative adolescent development. Extended family members and friends may not fully understand the impact when the surviving family moves away from the culture to which they were accustomed; this lack of understanding can lead to a lack of support and isolation. Occasionally the bereaved military family may be faced with family and friends who have a differing political or social view of war and military service. Families can become estranged due to those differing opinions, which can lead to additional losses for these adolescents.

National Guard/Reserve components

National Guard and Reserve service members often have full-time jobs or are full-time students outside of the military and serve on drill weekends or when called to active duty. It is challenging for these families when these reserve and guard service members are called into active duty and die while deployed or away from home. There is often a lack of understanding of this military world in these communities, which can make the surviving adolescent feel "different" and lead to confusion or questioning about where they belong.

Changes in family dynamics and pride in service

Other issues that can arise are the change in family dynamics and what roles the young people take on after a death. The typical military family raises their family with discipline and respect. Boys at a young age can take on the role of a "little soldier," and when their father deploys these boys are told to take care of the family as they are now the "man of the house." Characteristically these boys take this role very seriously after the death and try to take care of their family. Many grieving young men in this situation will try to hide their grief, but it often may be seen in exhibiting psychosomatic complaints of stomach aches or headaches to get out of school to ensure mom is safe.

For military children, there is a pride associated in serving one's country that is not easily understood by their civilian peers. This can create a sense of turmoil as the young person suffers incredibly difficult grief reactions coupled with the immense pride that their loved one died in service to the country.

CONSIDERATIONS FOR WORKING WITH ADOLESCENTS FACING MILITARY LOSS

Supporting an adolescent who is suffering the death of a parent or sibling who was serving in the military can present challenges without understanding the military culture. While military adolescents have a vast amount of similarities, there are equally as many differences among them; whether the adolescent's parent was active duty and they were surrounded by the military daily or part of the reserve component, seeing their service member in uniform just once a month. A young person's exposure to that lifestyle would predict some of their background, but regardless the military is an important component of who these adolescents are and have become as they are establishing their identity. Below are considerations when working with this population to ensure the best possible care for these adolescents.

Considerations for clinicians

Above all else, when working with an adolescent who has suffered the death of a military service member, it is important to self-assess your own ideas on war and military service, making sure that this does not cause conflict with your clinical relationship. As working with anyone with a different culture than your own, it is important to be mindful of the cultural factors of the client; the military adolescent is no different. A practitioner must be able to learn as much as possible about the military culture prior to working with the adolescent and learn from them. Failure to do this could compromise the teen's well-being and further enforce that they are alone and not understood. Professionals who are not comfortable with incorporating a sense of military culture into practice should "do no harm" and refer them elsewhere. Because these cases can be very graphic, complicated, and often very public, it is important to understand traumatic grief as well (Harrington-LaMorie, 2011; Cohen & Mannarino, 2011). Organizations such as Tragedy Assistance Program for Survivors (TAPS), the Association for Death Education and Counseling (ADEC), National Alliance of Grieving Children (NAGC), and the National Child Traumatic Stress Network (NCTSN) can be sources for further education and training for professionals.

Considerations for educators

For educators, one of the considerations is to understand that multiple school days may be missed for various military ceremonies or events that honor that service member's service and sacrifice. Whether it is on Memorial Day, Veterans Day, or a special remembrance ceremony for a particular unit or base, it is important for families to have the opportunity to attend to honor their special person. As mentioned previously, there may be a longer than normal process for funerals or memorials due to the nature of the death and where the service member is being buried; there may even be multiple burials due to notifications of additional remains. Being understanding and lenient to the attendance policy for these teens and families can assist them in ways no one else can.

Another concern for educators to consider is understanding that some of the content of classes can be very difficult for a teen, especially in history or political classes. The opinions of others, even teachers, may be perceived as degrading to the military or to the wars in which their service member died fighting. It can be helpful to have clear communication and forewarning on lessons to be covered in these classes and consider what could be upsetting for an adolescent who has experienced a military death. If possible, alternative assignments can be offered and a designated place to go can be established if it does get too difficult in the classroom (for instance, to the guidance counselor's office or the library) (National Traumatic Stress Network, in progress).

Families often move away from a military installation after a death occurs, which can lead to teens feeling detached from their extended military family. Having a connection, whether it is a mentor program with prior military service (a teacher, volunteer in the community, or administrator) or just someone to talk to about "military" things when no one else understands, can be beneficial in their grieving process. In addition, it is important to understand that things associated with the military, whether it be the roar of a Humvee, the sound of a military helicopter overhead, or the rattle of firearm training at the range, can be sources of comfort and familiarity, reminding them that they are being kept safe. Be cognizant of jumping to conclusions when there are drawings or discussions of war-related items (National Traumatic Stress Network, in progress).

NORMATIVE GRIEF AND TRAUMATIC GRIEF

It is understood across the literature that military children and teens are at least as resilient, if not more resilient, than the general child population. However, exposure to unusual stressors with deployments, injury, and death can take its toll (Cohen & Mannarino, 2011). The service member is many times thought of as a superhero, and revered as strong and "larger than life." When the unthinkable happens and that person dies, the culture that binds them together is often fractured (Campagna, 2012).

While grief and bereavement after a death is normal, how the adolescent responds to the death is very individualized. Having a deep sadness for their special person, longing for and missing that person, and having positive memories of the deceased are all characteristics of normal grief. Adolescents coping with the death of a military service member may sleep or cry more, have an unrealistic guilt about having caused the death, engage in some risky behavior, take on adult responsibilities, worry more about their surviving parent, and hide their true feelings. While it is not a typical expected reaction to a traumatic loss, a small percentage of these children and teens experience Childhood Traumatic Grief (CTG). CTG is characterized by getting "stuck" on the traumatic aspects of the death, whether it is imagining the pain, picturing the real or imagined details of the death, or wishing for revenge. Children and teens experiencing CTG avoid reminders of the deceased person and react to the death in horror, fear or helplessness (Cohen & Mannarino, 2011; National Child Traumatic Stress Network, 2008).

The National Child Traumatic Stress Network (NCTSN) has additional resources about CTG (http://www.nctsn.org). It is important to understand the difference between normative and traumatic grief in children and adolescents and obtain additional support if needed.

MILITARY FAMILY CONSIDERATIONS

Sibling Loss

The adolescent sibling who has experienced the death of a brother or sister in the military has a different set of challenges in dealing with their loss. The sibling relationship is unique among relationships, as they share similar biological and familial characteristics as well as environmental exposure. This offers a special bond of closeness or shared experience that other members of a family do not share. Most adolescents view their older sibling as a role model. When this sibling dies, it can create turmoil and upheaval in their life and create distress in the sibling order. Often surviving siblings recreate the lives of their dead loved ones, modeling their military brother or sister, some even following in their military footsteps. Another factor in sibling military death is that the siblings do not receive benefits, unless they are named as next of kin; benefits generally go to the spouse or the parents. Siblings also are not privy to many benefits that a dependent child would have, including a military ID card and "privileges" on a base, which can compound feelings of being overshadowed by their brother's or sister's death. Sibling death is commonly experienced in both the civilian and military communities by surviving siblings as a type of disenfranchised grief. Society typically views parents and spouses as primary grievers when a son, daughter, or spouse dies, ascribing very little recognition to the grief and loss felt by a sibling.

For dependent children

The military is a way of life for teens who have a parent serving in the military. When that special person dies, the family often moves off post or away from a military installation. When you are a military family, you go where the military will send you and your family. After a death, the military will provide one move as a benefit and they will ask the dependent spouse where he or she would like to move. Ingrained culturally by the military, if "home is where the military sends you," then where is "home" when they aren't telling you where to go? This reality can create upheaval in the decision-making process for many surviving spouses during a time of stress and complex life decisions and often results in the family losing their ties to other peers who have a military connection.

INTERVENTIONS AND SOURCES OF SUPPORT

Interventions and support for adolescents who have suffered the death of their service member are important and often necessary. Remembering that the military culture is a very distinct culture that most civilians don't fully comprehend, it is important to ensure that these services are a good fit for a military adolescent based upon their own individual needs.

Bereavement counseling

Bereavement counseling is support to people experiencing emotional and psychological stress after a death. Bereavement counseling can include a broad range of transition services, including outreach, counseling, and referral services to families. While there are many providers available, the following are organizations that specifically serve families of service members.

The **Tragedy Assistance Program for Survivors (TAPS)** offers a full range of support for military families. Although TAPS does not directly provide bereavement counseling, TAPS arranges services and resources in the family's local area and provides a report on request for a military survivor based on their specified needs. A detailed list of providers at a no cost or sliding scale in their area can be provided, as well as available peer-based support groups in their local area.

The **Vet Center** through the **Department of Veterans Affairs (VA)** can be a source of support for those who have emotional and psychological stress after the death of a service member. These services are available to spouses, children, parents, or siblings of Armed Forces personnel and those who are reservists and National Guardsmen who die while on duty. Counseling is at no cost and is provided at Vet Centers that are community-based throughout the US. Be mindful to ensure that the Vet Center counselors are qualified to work with adolescents, as many are trained to work with adults only.

The **Give an Hour** organization is a nonprofit providing free mental health services to military personnel and families. This service includes anyone suffering the death of a service member and does not have to be a Department of Defense (DOD) listed dependent (for example, siblings and other family members are welcome, not just immediate family members). These providers are sensitive to military service and volunteer their time, however they may not have a direct understanding of the military culture.

Peer support

Peer support is the social support that the adolescent has from friends, classmates, and others within the same age group. Peer support has been found to be very helpful for adolescents who have experienced a death. Bereaved children report that friendships with other bereaved peers are more helpful and provide better support than nonbereaved friends who do not understand the loss (Worden, 1996). This need to be surrounded by like others can be found in bereavement support groups specific to adolescents. Support groups offer a model that helps the individuals cope with loss and grief by offering support to each other, which often helps the bereaved adolescent work through his or her own individual tasks of mourning.

TAPS has the only military specific peer-based support group for children and teens suffering the death of their special person while serving in the military or as a direct result of their service. The TAPS Good Grief Camps and Good Grief Camp Outs are offered throughout the country on a regional level (in one-day camps and overnight "camp outs"), as well as through two national Good Grief Camps. The National Good Grief Camp is held in Washington, DC, over

Memorial Day weekend where 500 children and teens join together; the other national program is specific to military suicide loss where approximately 150 children and teens gather together annually. While being with other peers who have experienced a similar loss, each young person learns that they are not alone, which allows them to normalize feelings, develop coping skills, and discuss support systems. The camps include military mentors, service members who go through background checks and training, and are paired with a child who has lost their special person while serving in the military. This aspect of the camp reinforces that neither they, nor their service member, have been forgotten by the military and that they will always be a part of the military family, an important reminder to these young people.

CONCLUSION

As a nation, we understand that war and military service have consequences. Oftentimes adolescents are the forgotten wounds of service. The military culture is a culture that is wrought with protocol, rituals, and a pride that cannot be fully understood unless one has lived it. Knowing the circumstances that surround the family after a death of a service member, coupled with the development of the adolescent and an understanding of the military culture, can create a place of healing for those families who need understanding. Having resources available for the adolescents to turn to and knowing when more help or resources are needed to assist them through their journey of grief are invaluable. There is no better way to honor the life and sacrifice of a service member than by caring for the family he or she left behind.

Heather R. Campagna, MA, EdS, FT, served as the National Youth Programs Director for the Tragedy Assistance Program for Survivors (TAPS) from 2005 to 2014, where she assisted families as well as children who have lost a loved one in the military, and served as a group facilitator for those children and teens at the regional Good Grief Camps. Heather is trained as a school psychologist and obtained her Education Specialist and Master's Degrees in school psychology from The Citadel. She is a Fellow in Thanatology through the Association for Death Education and Counseling and serves on the Board of Directors for the National Alliance for Grieving Children.

Tina Saari, BS, led the Fort Hood Survivor Programs for TAPS from 2004 through 2014. She also served on the Ft. Hood Special Victim Witness Multidisciplinary team (MDT), providing trial support and care to the families of the fallen after the November 5, 2009 shooting. Tina worked with TAPS' youth programs, including the National Annual Good Grief Camps and the USO/TAPS overnight and outdoor grief camps. Saari holds a BS from Texas A&M University and has also acquired an Early Childhood Education certificate.

Jill Harrington-LaMorie, DSW, LCSW, is currently the Senior Field Researcher on a Congressionally Directed Medical Research Project, The Impact of a Service Member's Death: A National Study of Bereavement in Military Families, being conducted at Uniformed Services University of the Health Services Center for the Study of Traumatic Stress, Bethesda, Maryland. Dr. LaMorie is the former Director of Professional Education at the Tragedy Assistance Program for Survivors (TAPS). Dr. LaMorie is one of the first published authors on the subject of Bereavement in U.S. Military Families. She is a member of the National Association of Social Workers and serves on the board of the Association for Death Education and Counseling.

REFERENCES

Balk, D. E & Corr, C.A. (2009). *Adolescent encounters with death, bereavement and coping.* New York: Spring Publishing Company.

Beard, B., Mathewson, J., Saari, T., & Campagna, H. (2008) Military children and grief. In K.J. Doka (Ed.), *Living with Grief: Children and Adolescents* (pp. 193-211). Washington, DC: Hospice Foundation of America.

Campagna, H. (2012, April). The military adolescent's journey of grief. *The Forum, (38)*2.

Cohen, J. & Mannarino, A. (2011). Trauma-focused CBT for traumatic grief in military children. *Journal of Contemporary Psychotherapy, 41,* 219-227.

Defense Manpower Data Center (2013). Military Casualty Information. Retrieved from http://siadapp.dmdc.osd.mil/personnel/CASUALTY/castop.htm

Harrington-LaMorie, J. (2013). Grief, loss and bereavement in military families. In J. Coll, R. Rubin, & E. Weiss (Eds.), *Handbook of Military Social Work*. Hoboken, NJ: John Wiley & Sons Publications.

Harrington-LaMorie, J. (2011). Operation Iraqi Freedom/Operation Enduring Freedom: Exploring Wartime Death & Bereavement. *Social Work in Health Care, (50)*, 543-563.

Holmes, A., Rauch, P., & Cozza, S. (2013). When a parent is injured, or killed in combat. *Future of Children, (23)*, 2, 143-162. A collaboration of The Woodrow Wilson School of Public and International Affairs at Princeton University and the Brookings Institution.

Lester, P. & Flake, E. (2013). How wartime military service affects children and families. *Future of Children, (23)*, 2, 121-142. A collaboration of the Woodrow Wilson School of Public and International Affairs at Princeton University and the Brookings Institution.

National Child Traumatic Stress Network. (In progress). *Childhood Traumatic Grief Tip Sheet for Educators*. Los Angeles, CA & Durham, NC: National Center for Child Traumatic Stress.

National Child Traumatic Stress Network. (2008). *Traumatic Grief in Military Children: Information for Medical Providers*. Los Angeles, CA & Durham, NC: National Center for Child Traumatic Stress. Retrieved from http://www.nctsn.org/sites/default/files/assets/pdfs/military_grief_medical.pdf.

Tragedy Assistance Program for Survivors (TAPS). (2013, September 3). *TAPS Fact Sheet & Statistics on Families of the Fallen (TAPS)* Retrieved from http://www.taps.org/uploadedFiles/TAPS/RESOURCES/Documents/FactSheet.pdf.

Worden, J. W. (1996). *Children and grief: When a parent dies*. New York, NY: Guilford Press.

Supporting Grieving Adolescents

Whatever losses adolescents experience, those adolescents merit and need support. Yet the nature of development may make adolescents reluctant to seek support. Adolescents may not like to show vulnerability to peers, parents, or teachers, and often will work hard to project normalcy.

Some sources of support are natural. Adolescents are digital natives, having grown up with the Internet and other aspects of social media. It is little wonder that they may turn to this media as they grieve. Carla Sofka's chapter reviews the ever-expanding ways that social media is used by adolescents to cope with grief. This includes not only seeking information and support as well as privately and publicly memorializing, but also using this media to bring about social change. Sofka also notes the limitations and dangers of this media. She advises counselors to question clients about their use of such resources. Sofka's chapter includes a number of recommendations that might stimulate debate. In the end, Sofka poses a provocative question: *In what ways do the new social media change the definition of what it is to be human?*

The next chapters explore the roles of educational institutions and resources in supporting grieving adolescents. Robert Stevenson's chapter begins with an excellent overview of the roles that death education can play in schools. He notes that death education can be preparatory, interventive, and used in postvention. Stevenson, a longtime pioneer in death education, offers an exceptional historical survey of death education from its earliest beginnings. Donna Burns reminds us that college students may grieve as well. Their grief may be unrecognized and unsupported in an environment of emerging adulthood. Burns recognizes both the many losses, aside from death, that can generate grief and underlines Sofka's point about the role of social media in the adolescent world. In addition, Burns provides an impressive overview of programs that support grieving college students as well as a very practical section on developing such support.

Charles Corr's chapter explores the value of bibliotherapy with grieving adolescents. Corr offers much here: a review of the role of bibliotherapy as a source of support, principles for the use of bibliotherapy with adolescents, and a host of recommendations of books that might be useful for and with adolescents. In his *Voices* piece, Justin Lewis reflects on the loss of his mother, a journey that takes him from early through middle adolescence. Justin's piece reflects the need of an adolescent to project normalcy and strength, one that limits the support that he is finally able to accept. Yet it also illustrates the support that can flow if unleashed by sensitive educators.

The value of bibliotherapy is that it provides a sense of validation, strategies for coping, and hope that one can overcome loss. This may ease the isolation of the grieving adolescent. Yet other strategies such as adolescent support groups and grief camps also can offer that validation, coping suggestions, and hope, as well as peer support. Donna Schuurman, the Executive Director of the Dougy Center, a ground-breaking organization that offers peer support to grieving children and adolescents, provides an extensive review of grief groups as well as guidelines for developing support programs for grieving adolescents. Jennifer Kaplan Schreiber and Cathy Spear continue this discussion with a valued examination of the role of grief camps. While firmly rooted in adolescent developmental research and literature, Schreiber and Spear also provide practical advice on a range of issues, from the structure of activities to deciding whether camps should be gender specific or mixed. Inherent in their chapter is that grief camps for adolescents are *camps*; they need both opportunities for play and respite and may suffer from the same issues as other adolescent camps including homesickness, behavioral issues, and, especially in coed camps, love triangles and unrequited romantic relationships.

The final chapters in this section address professional support. David Crenshaw begins his chapter on counseling adolescents with an affirmation that adolescents are resilient and a reminder that interventions ought to be targeted rather than generalized. While adolescents need grief support, not every adolescent needs grief counseling. His chapter integrates current thinking on grief and bereavement such as continuing bonds, attachment theory, disenfranchised grief, and neuroscience, with interventive strategies for counseling adolescents. Crenshaw notes how current neuroscience emphasizes the value of expressive approaches such as drawing, singing, or dancing.

Kora Delashmutt's *Voices* piece reaffirms many of Crenshaw's points, from the need to slowly build trust to the importance of creating a physical environment comfortable for the adolescent. Kora also addresses a range of losses, such as foster care placement, that adolescents may face. Finally, she reinforces the needs of adolescents, no matter what their circumstances, to project strength and normalcy.

Nancy Boyd Webb's chapter on expressive therapies follows. Webb again roots her work in developmental theory and is sensitive to the full range of losses that adolescents experience. Expressive therapies are wonderful ports of entry to the adolescent. They are natural, while conversing with an adult may seem forced and artificial. They are cathartic and projective, as adolescents cannot only express feeling and other reactions but may even project reactions of which they were unaware. Finally, expressive techniques are a bridge to the adolescent's culture and spirituality. Crenshaw's and Webb's rich theoretical models do not inhibit them from offering sound, grounded clinical technique.

Karla Helbert's chapter concludes this section. Helbert addresses the needs of an oft-neglected population, adolescents on the autism spectrum who may need professional support as they cope with loss. Helbert explores the ways grief may be manifested in this population, contrasting those reactions with their neurotypical peers. Like Crenshaw and Webb, she notes the value of expressive interventions and ritual and offers sound clinical strategies for working with this population.

CHAPTER 14

Adolescent Use of Technology and Social Media to Cope with Grief

Carla Sofka

D ue to the widespread use of digital and social media among adolescents in 2013, Montgomery's (2007) label, the "Digital Generation," remains accurate. The general appeal of technology among teenagers has been widely documented (Rideout, 2012; for a review of additional sources, see Sofka, 2012a). Data from the Pew Internet & American Life Project reported that 95% of adolescents spend time online and 74% have cell phones, 47% of which are smartphones (Madden, Lenhart, Duggan, Cortesi, & Gasser, 2013). In practical terms, almost 50% of teens have what Madden and colleagues refer to as "always-on connections" to at least one device.

In *Dancing with Digital Natives*, Manafy and Gautschi (2011) note that young people who have never known a world without these technologies "take the tools at their disposal and modify them to meet their personal, evolving needs" (p. xii). Digital immigrants (defined by Prensky in 2001 as those who were not born into the digital world but have, at some later point in life, begun to utilize some or most aspects of technology) are encouraged to "understand how the lifelong immersion in digital technologies (among adolescents) colors every aspect of their behavior" (p. xiii). Technology-mediated communication (TMC) has dramatically changed the speed at which teenagers learn about tragedies (Burrell, 2007) and how they deal with grief. Therefore, counselors and parents must become familiar with their use of "thanatechnology" (Sofka, 1997) for "digital grieving."

This chapter will summarize the types of technology and social media being used by adolescents to cope with grief and identify the potential benefits and risks of its use. Implications for counselors, parents, and researchers will be discussed. A tool designed to assess a bereaved adolescent's experiences with thanatechnology, social media, and digital social support (a teenager's social support "internetworks") is included (see Appendix A).

ONLINE COMMUNITIES OF BEREAVEMENT

Following one of the most public tragedies involving teens at Columbine High School in April of 1999, Linenthal (as quoted in Niebuhr & Wilgoren, 1999) noted that the creation of shrines following tragic deaths might indicate the desire to overcome feelings of powerlessness and to experience a sense of unity as a "community of bereavement." Since teenagers have grown up with technology, Atfield, Chalmers, and Lion (2006) recognized that adolescents would logically turn to cyberspace during times of grief, sometimes immediately after learning of a tragedy.

Teens can gain informational support on websites created by grief-related organizations such as the Dougy Center (http://www.dougy.org) and connect with other teens dealing with grief by joining an online Forum, such as one run by Comfort Zone Camp (http://www.hellogrief.org). While many virtual memorial sites commemorate individuals of all ages (deVries& Moldaw, 2012), some sites are designed specifically to commemorate teens. For example, the Teen Memory Wall is a living memorial to teens who have died in car crashes (http://www.teenmemorywall.com). This website, created by Allstate Insurance Company, also provides a "community" section where friends and family can pay tribute, reminisce, and share or participate in survivor advocacy efforts designed to prevent similar tragedies. Additional ways that teens can participate in online communities of bereavement involve posting on the personal Facebook (FB) page of a deceased friend, posting on Rest in Peace (R.I.P.) sites created after a person's death, or posting on a FB site that provides an opportunity for teens to memorialize a friend or family member whose death was related to a particular cause or circumstance.

In order to examine the coping strategies reflected in comments on social networking sites (SNSs) posted by bereaved adolescents, Williams and Merten (2009) analyzed the online social networking profiles of 20 adolescents for one year following each person's sudden death by a fatal accident or suicide. Utilizing Roberts' (2006) framework for identifying the functions of web memorials, the postings were categorized using the following themes: talking to the deceased (maintaining a continuing bond through acknowledgment of significant events such as holidays, major life events, and anniversaries of the death); comments with memorial sentiments or sentiments of loss; indicators of emotional or cognitive coping strategies; comments about current events; reminiscing; commentary regarding the act of posting on the deceased's website (metacommentary); comments about the cause of death; comments from peripheral friends or complete strangers; and comments about the funeral/seeing the body and the afterlife. These observations not only help us to understand how SNSs are being used by bereaved teens to discuss and process their experiences with sudden death and grief, but they also reinforce that there are predictable times when the social media activity of teens may increase as they experience STUG reactions (subsequent, temporary, upsurges of grief as defined by Rando, 2000).

Systematic searches on SNSs allow the gathering of anecdotal data to document death and grief-related postings. However, empirical research involving teens who utilize these online communities of bereavement is needed to document participation rates, factors that influence one's decision whether or not to visit or post on these sites, and the benefits and any negative consequences of their participation.

Super-Communication: Text Messaging and Social Media vs. E-mail

In 2007, Lenhart, Madden, Macgill, and Smith described a subset of teens, about 28% of the teen population, as "super-communicators:" those with multiple technology options ("multi-channel teens"). Their level of "mobile connectivity" has increased significantly, with Nielsen (2013a) documenting a 45% increase in smartphone use. Purcell (2010) reported that teens who are texting send an average of 112 text messages (TM) each day.

To what extent is texting being used by teens to seek support during times of grief? Is this type of communication effective? Although texting may be perceived as impersonal, Pascoe (2007) notes that teens who are texting are not rendered vulnerable the same way they are in other person-to-person interactions. Initially contacting someone via TM to begin a conversation may lead to increased intimacy in subsequent face-to-face communications. To date, no known empirical research has been conducted to explore these questions with bereaved teens.

New forms of social media are constantly being created, and examples of how they are being used in situations involving tragedy and grief are frequently described in the mainstream media. For example, prior to 2006, the word "twitter" was typically used to describe the vocalization of a bird, chattering among a group of people, or a fluttering movement (www.m-w.com). Now Twitter is best known as a free social networking and microblogging service that allows a user to "tweet" (share a brief message of 140 characters or less) with other users. In a period of 3 years, Twitter usage has risen from 8% of teenagers in 2010 (Lenhart, Purcell, Smith, & Zickuhr) to 24% (Madden et al., 2013). According to Carboneau (2013), Chris Syme, a trainer who educates companies and universities about social media, describes Twitter as a "newsroom" as opposed to Facebook, which is more like a "living room." While FB postings can be lengthy and viewed only by people of one's own choosing through the use of privacy settings, tweets are publicly-available and brief (140 characters or less). Some tweets contain a *hashtag*, a word or phrase preceded by the # symbol that allows someone to search for and identify all messages that contain a specific hashtag.

Twitter is being used by teens dealing with grief in a variety of ways. Following a car accident in December of 2012 that ended the lives of two high school seniors and severely injured two other students in a neighboring community, this author gained first-hand knowledge of the use of TM and Twitter by adolescents. Informal conversations with family friends whose teenagers attend this neighboring high school revealed that information about the accident was being shared within minutes via TM and other social media. Within 72 hours, teens (including my daughter) from our local high school (a sports "rival" of the neighboring school) were sending messages of support from the "518" (the area code for our geographic region, hashtag #518 or #518Family) such as "the best kind of rivalry is one where it goes away when something horrible becomes bigger than the rivalry ever could be." Friends of the survivors started Twitter campaigns designed to encourage the survivors' favorite athletes to call them in the hospital (#MissyCallBailey and #TebowCallMatt) that trended nationally (and both survivors received a call). The social media columnist from one local newspaper documented how reactions to this tragedy were being shared via social media (e.g., Barlette, 2012). One of the crash survivors is a prolific tweeter and has openly shared her grief journey on Twitter. Anecdotal data gathered by this author through the monitoring of publicly-available social media confirms that local teens are continuing to tweet their ongoing reactions to the deaths, with themes and timeframes similar to those described by Williams and Merten (2009). For teens who prefer quick and easy technology, Twitter is the answer.

With the rise in digital technology use, are teenagers still using "traditional" types of computer-mediated communication? According to a report from comScore (2012), web-based e-mail usage for teens 12 to 17 years old decreased 31% between December 2010 and December 2011. In 2007, Pascoe noted that e-mail had already fallen out of fashion among adolescents due to being "too formal" to use with friends and was reported by Lenhart, Madden, & Hitlin (2005) as something used to talk to "old people," institutions, or to send complex instructions to large groups. However, many adolescents may still use e-mail to communicate with teachers. While large-scale studies about the use of digital technology among adolescents have not specifically inquired about the use of various types of technology to cope with grief, anecdotal evidence has documented the use of e-mail to seek bereavement support from friends (Sofka, 2012a). A professionally-moderated support group sponsored by Griefnet.org that utilizes e-mail as the sole method of communication between group members (http://kidsaid.com) has been active and successfully supporting teens age 13 to 18 for many years (Lynn & Rath, 2012). Since e-mail may be used in the provision of online counseling with teens, its use as a potential resource for coping with grief merits consideration.

Instant messaging (IM) may also be used by teens without access to a cell phone with TM capabilities or by teens who use "chat" features on SNSs. This type of TMC occurs in real time and is interactive as opposed to TM, which may involve a delayed response if the recipient does not respond immediately. Blais, Craig, Pepler, and Connolly (2008) found that using instant messaging to communicate with best friends had a positive effect on the quality of these friendships. Pascoe (2007) also noted that some teens use IM to have important conversations that cannot be done via a traditional phone or cell phone without the risk of being overheard by a parent (Note: Teens will send a TM with the code "9" if a parent is within earshot).

Due to the rapid evolution of technology, it is tricky to know what new forms of TMC will evolve and capture the attention of teens during the next few years. Ask the teens in your life to keep you informed.

PLAYLISTING GRIEF

> *Life is not your own playlist where you*
> *can turn on the music you want!*
> *It's like a radio where you can't skip*
> *the song for listening [to] the next one.*
> ~Annie (posting #12156 at
> http://www.teen-quotes.com, 6/15/13)

Since 76% of teens own an iPod or other MP3 player (Rideout, Foehr, & Roberts, 2010) and report listening to music on this or some other type of device (radio, CD, smartphone, tablet, or computer) for up to 3 hours and 21 minutes a day (Nielsen, 2013a/b; Nielsen, 2012; McFerran, 2010), it is safe to assume that teenagers are listening to music that relates to events in their lives. Contrary to the quote introducing this section, teenagers truly can "playlist their grief" by organizing their digital music collections according to themes and using self-prescribed songs to lessen the power of stressful memories, regulate their moods, and alter their neurochemistry (Mindlin, Dourousseau, & Cardillo, 2012; Chanda & Levitin, 2013).

According to music therapist Katrina McFerran (2010), "The relationship between music and emotions is never clearer than when it comes to working with grief and loss. The capacity of music to express sorrow and mourning, as well as to capture stories and memories, makes music therapy a very relevant resource for young people" that is "utilized to access and express emotions, foster connectedness between grieving teenagers and their networks, and normalize young people's experiences of grief" (p. 217). When describing the ways that adolescents engage with music, McFerran (2012) reported that teens may be more attached to music that is significant at a particular moment in their life rather than music that is popular.

Counselors are encouraged to have conversations with grieving teens about their music preferences to foster an understanding of their feelings and provide opportunities for discussion (McFerran, 2010). Heeres (2013) noted that talking with someone about music is a nonthreatening, socially acceptable way of starting a conversation and opens the door to validating the griever's feelings and helping him or her to label emotions. Grocke and Wigram (2007) suggest asking specific questions about a teen's music preferences: Why do you like it? What does it mean to you? What do you think of when you hear it? Having these discussions over time allows for assessment of how the "playlist" (and his or her grieving process and coping strategies) may be changing.

Cushnie (2010) strongly endorsed the use of music with grieving adolescents: "Teens at Comfort Zone Camp never cease to amaze me with the ways music and song saturate their lives; how they use it to express their feelings, hopes and fears related to loss. They have taught me the power of music and song in navigating the grief journey. The music 'speaks to them'. Be courageous and listen to what they are listening to without judgment. If a conversation develops, that's great and if it doesn't that's OK too. They will know you paused to enter their world" (http://www.hellogrief.org/music-and-grief/; an extensive list of songs can be found in the comments below the blog entry).

Since quotes can be wonderful conversation starters, consider how you could use these quotes from teen-quotes.com: "When you're happy, you enjoy the music. And when you're sad, you understand the lyrics" (Posting #3557 by antoineaugusti dated 05/08/2012) or "I'm blasting my music so I won't hear my thoughts, but the lyrics just remind me of what I'm trying to forget" (Posting #4382 by clara dated 11/14/2012). It seems appropriate to conclude this section with a quote from www.motivationaltwist.com: "Life is like a piano; white keys represent happiness and black keys represent sadness. But as you go through life's journey, remember that the black keys make music too." Since you may be asked by a teenager if you "playlist your grief" during conversations about music, you are encouraged to consider how music relates to your own journey with grief and be prepared to share your observations (and your playlist). You can check for digital access to songs online via YouTube, Pandora, Spotify, and Vevo, with free digital downloads available through some local public libraries.

TECHNOLOGY AND CREATIVE EXPRESSION

Lenhart and colleagues (2010) reported that 38% of teens share self-created content online (e.g., photos, videos, artwork or stories), with 21% sharing material that they have found online and "remixed" into their own artistic creation ("mash-ups"), whether the original content consisted of songs, text, or images. Bell (2011) reminds us that digital natives are "devoted observers, collectors, sharers, and creators of video productions" (p. 355). Teens can become "digital curators" by compiling links from social media about a topic or theme on Storify. With the photo and video capabilities of smartphones and tablets, the availability of flip cams, and multiple online resources for posting their own creations (e.g., YouTube, Pinterest, Flickr, Vine, Tumblr, and Instagram), digital storytelling and the use of "do-it-yourself media" is common.

Although formal research has not documented the extent to which teens are posting grief-related content online, examples of their creativity abound, whether they are sharing their reactions to the death of a friend, family member, or someone they never met whose death has impacted them in a personal way.

Through a partnership between the Dougy Center and NW Documentary, several teens created short films about their grief and the people in their lives who died, giving the teens a chance to share their memories and tell their stories in a unique way (http://www.dougy.org/grief-resources/recording-resilience/). To locate tribute videos commemorating teens on video-based sites (e.g., YouTube), type keywords such as "In memory of" or "RIP"/"R.I.P." in the search box (e.g., RIP Brenda Gutierrez & Thalia Arredondo). Teens who wish to share stories, poetry, or artwork on a website can do so at GriefNet (http://kidsaid.com), designed to be "a safe place for kids to help each other deal with grief and loss."

The death of a celebrity who is popular among teens can precipitate an outpouring of grief for someone they never met. In the wake of *Glee* star Cory Monteith's death in July of 2013, young fans expressed their feelings through GIFs (Abad-Santos, 2013). A GIF (graphics interchange format) allows the sharing of images on numerous social media platforms, and fans shared GIFs of Monteith with his *Glee* co-star and real-life girlfriend Lea Michele (e.g., Lea Michele crying in Monteith's arms). Abad-Santos speculated that these "GIFed reactions" reflect how young people express their grief today: by personalizing the Internet experience.

Fans utilized multiple forms of social media to cope with this actor's death between July and mid-October. On October 10, 2013, 7.3 million people watched the tribute episode of *Glee* that acknowledged the death of Finn Hudson (Cory Monteith's character). Shortly before the start of the episode, FOX TV invited fans to "join us in lighting a candle in memory of Cory Monteith" at an online site and to spread the word via Twitter (hashtag #RememberingCory). Within 24 hours, over 428,000 tweets using this hashtag had been sent. Within one hour of FOX posting "To all the fans who lit a candle, shared a memory & watched last night's episode- thank you" on the *Glee* FB page, 103,538 people had "liked" and commented on the post.

Regardless of the relationship of the person for whom a teen is grieving online, parents and counselors are encouraged to ask tech-savvy teenagers about their use of technologically-based coping strategies. Researchers would be wise to partner with counselors to document the benefits that are gained through this type of creative expression, as well as the potential risks.

GOOGLING GRIEF

While posting to a blog on March 20, 2005, Laura at 11D noted that "maniacal googling" is a new aspect of grief (McKenna, 2005). Following the diagnosis of a life-threatening illness or during the grieving process, "informational support" or factual information about topics involving illness, death, or grief may be useful during the process of coping with these events (Sofka, 2012b).

How frequently do adolescents utilize the Internet to gain information about thanatology-related topics? Surveys estimate that between 31% and 49% of adolescents "cybersurf" for health-related information, including mental health issues, cancer, and other diseases (Borzekowski & Rickert, 2001; Lenhart, Madden, & Hitlin, 2005). While research has not documented the use of thanatology-specific sites among teenagers, it is important to be familiar with content related to illness, death, and grief that is targeted specifically for teens should they seek it out (e.g., http://www.dougy.org, http://www.teenhealthand wellness.com, http://www.teenadvice.about.com). To identify additional resources, type keywords such as "teen" or "adolescent" and the topic of interest into any search engine.

Be aware that keyword searches will also locate potentially inappropriate content unrelated to coping with loss. Due to the possibility that misinformation can easily be posted online, it is important to review a website's content before referring individuals to material posted online (see Sofka, 2012b). "Bouncing" (moving quickly from one resource to another without closely reading any material) is a common but potentially unproductive way for teens to utilize online resources (Bell, 2011), so adults should talk with teens about what they are reading to evaluate comprehension as well as the accuracy of the information.

In addition to sites for informational support, the World Wide Web also contains narrative sites that provide opportunities for grieving teens to read the personal stories of others or post their own story (http://www.hellogrief.org/ or http://www.teencentral.net). Adolescents may find it reassuring to discover that the thoughts and reactions of other teens are very similar to their own.

SOCIAL MEDIA AND SURVIVOR ADVOCACY: THE DRAGONFLY EFFECT

According to the Trauma Foundation (2001), some people who survive the traumatic loss of a loved one channel their grief into preventive action. They become "survivor advocates" who work to save others from experiencing a similar loss and trauma through raising awareness and policy change. For guidance regarding how to facilitate this type of change through the use of social media, readers are encouraged to consult the work of Aaker, Smith, and Adler (2010), who developed a model for enacting change called the "Dragonfly Effect." Since the small actions of a dragonfly can create big movements, their model is designed to guide "people who, through the passionate pursuit of their goals, hope to make a positive impact disproportionate to their resources" (p. xiii).

In addition to expressing their grief, teenagers are also participating in survivor advocacy through the use of social media. Following the suicide of a high school sophomore, fellow students utilized Twitter and Facebook to express their grief (Carboneau, 2013). They also posted stories and photos to a FB page (Makayla Guerriero Memorial Fund) that continues to raise awareness of teen suicide and solicit donations for the fund established in her name. Regarding the previously described December 2012 car accident, when the news media released information that the driver of the vehicle whose car struck the teenagers was allegedly intoxicated, the following request was tweeted: "Can we all make a pledge right now that WE WILL NOT DRINK AND DRIVE? RT [retweet] this if you're willing to MAKE and KEEP that promise." This message was retweeted by 247 people.

Many teens feel the need to "do something" following a loss, and digital technology makes it convenient and seemingly "effortless" to become involved. Research documenting the level of participation in survivor advocacy and social action by adolescents through the use of social media and the impact of using thanatechnology on the process of coping should be conducted.

POTENTIAL RISKS AND CHALLENGES IN CYBERSPACE

In addition to providing a comfortable, supportive environment where teenagers interact, digital media and online resources eliminate practical barriers such as the lack of transportation or scheduling conflicts. While these and the previously-noted benefits of adolescents' use of TMC are important to acknowledge, Steyer (2012) emphasized the need to balance the possibilities and the perils of this new digital landscape.

Some websites and social networking resources have generated concern about the appropriateness of the content (e.g., http://www. MyDeathSpace.com, the online discussion site/bulletin board with controversial postings of information related to accidents and murders; see Sofka, 2012a), or issues regarding safety. In 2007, Goodstein noted that while most postings by teens on SNSs and other types of social media simply record the events of the day or appropriately vent feelings of anger or frustration, some may raise a red flag (a cry for help) or have the potential to cause harm depending on the reaction of the intended recipient (e.g., Ask.fm, a site that has had postings linked to cyberbullying; see Jones, 2013).

Sadly, it is not difficult to find high-profile cases of *cyberbullicide,* defined by Hinduja and Patchin (2010) as suicide indirectly or directly influenced by experiences with online aggression. The most recent example prior to publication of this chapter involved Rebecca Ann Sedwick. After being cyberbullied for over a year (e.g., receiving messages saying "Why are you still alive?" "Can u die please?"), Rebecca changed her user name on Kik Messenger (a cellphone app) to "That Dead Girl" and delivered a message to two friends, saying goodbye forever before leaping to her death (Alvarez, 2013). It is interesting to note that over 700 comments have been posted online in reaction to a newspaper story about these events. When it comes to being the victim of a cyberbully, words do hurt; for some, words can kill (Edgington, 2011).

Counselors working with bereaved teens should routinely ask if they have had any negative social media experiences (see Appendix A). Sample "scripts" to facilitate conversations about cyberbullying are available at http://www.cyberbullying.us. Resources are available to assist with preventive efforts and appropriate responses when cyberbullying occurs (e.g., Kowalski, Limber, & Agatston, 2012; Patchin & Hinduja, 2012), and information about current laws regarding cyberbullying can be found at http://www.stopbullying.gov.

The literature about TMC documents additional "double-edged" swords. For adolescents who are typically shy or uncomfortable interacting with peers, online communication can provide a place for socialization (Hellenga, 2002). However, is it possible that adolescents who spend most of their time online will never develop the skills to be successful in face-to-face social interactions, such as reading nonverbal social cues or confidently using verbal skills? Is social support received online as effective as that provided in person?

Pascoe (2007) also noted that there are some subcultures online that may be a bit dangerous: "Kids who are marginalized can find community online…but for kids who are engaging in pathological behaviors… (the Internet) can be incredibly dangerous, because they can find other people who support that kind of behavior" (p. 8). While considering the impact of Internet use on mental health, Hellenga (2002) noted the need to investigate whether individuals who spend a great deal of time online may be doing so because they are lonely, maladjusted, or unhappy and may require professional help. Research on the co-occurrence of cyberbullying and suicide has also documented that many teens who died by suicide after being cyberbullied had other emotional and social issues going on in their lives (Hinduja & Patchin, 2010).

German and Drushel (2011) noted the need to consider the cultural and ethical implications of new technology that evolves at a dizzying rate: "Perhaps the most intriguing question is how the emergence of a medium affects the practice of what it is to be human" (p. 4). For the purposes of this chapter, consider the following question: Do today's teenagers approach the grieving process differently due to the types of digital media at their disposal? The previous examples illustrate that this may be the case. And since "most technologies evolve with applications that were never intended, bringing along with them the ethical quandaries that must eventually be addressed" (German & Drushel, 2011, p. 4), counselors and parents must be prepared to help teenagers navigate these dilemmas.

Safety online, what Bell (2011) refers to as "safe surfing" (p. 367), can be defined in a variety of ways. Parents need to remember that filtering applications can both underblock and overblock. Open communication about online activities between an adolescent and a parent or trusted adult is the best safeguard. It is important for adolescents to be educated about the differences between "public" and "private" in online environments and the potential risks of posting personal information in a public forum. An adolescent's physical safety can be compromised by sharing one's address or making arrangements to meet someone face-to-face who is a "virtual stranger" since it is not uncommon for children to pretend to be older and for some adults to pretend to be younger.

A teen's emotional safety can also be impacted by an unsettling phenomenon that occurs in the context of "memorial trolling/ RIP trolling": abusive remarks and insensitive images are posted anonymously on SNSs or shared through various types of social media. Interviews conducted with RIP trolls by Phillips (2011) revealed that fundamentally different beliefs about the appropriateness of publicly sharing one's grief, particularly by individuals who did not personally know the deceased, sometimes called "grief tourists," appear to be at the heart of this phenomenon.

While statistics regarding the incidence of cyberbullying and memorial trolling are not readily available, the reality of these inappropriate behaviors is a documented risk of participating in all types of resources in the digital world (Goodstein, 2007; Phillips, 2011). Those creating RIP/memorial sites must carefully weigh the pros and cons of allowing anyone to post vs. more restrictive privacy settings. Site administrators need to monitor these sites for egregious postings and handle any situations that arise appropriately. Raw emotions may also be shared in postings, and while they may not be intended to be offensive, it is possible that they may have a negative impact on some visitors to a SNS. Adolescents should be reminded to inform a trusted adult if they perceive or experience a threat to their safety as a result of online activities.

Those responsible for the oversight of discussion-oriented online resources must also consider the impact on a person seeking support or guidance if no one in the group responds to a member's posting. When members join a group, should they be prepared for the possibility that there are times when "traffic" on the site is slow, meaning that they may not get an immediate response to their posting (or perhaps no postings at all)? Should members also be reminded that others are depending upon them for support, even when they themselves do not actively need it? When someone has decided to stop participating in an online "community of bereavement," should they be asked to inform the group and say goodbye? These questions merit consideration by those responsible for communication about expectations for online group membership.

IMPLICATIONS FOR COUNSELORS AND PARENTS

In the past, the "digital divide" referred to differences in one's access to technology due to the lack of physical access to a computer or the inability to afford online services (see Gilbert & Massimi, 2012, for information about the evolving meaning of this concept). For death professionals and parents who are less connected to technology, "the digital divide is less about having access than it is about using the access that's available" (Dretzin, 2008, p. 9). The digital divide also remains if we do not learn about the technology being used by teenagers.

Bridging the differences in knowledge about and familiarity with thanatechnology involves a need for "digital literacy" for not only the digital immigrants but also for the digital natives. Parents, grief counselors, death educators, and researchers must spend time learning about digital technology in order to develop a common language for use with adolescents. In order to reassure parents and thanatologists that adolescents will not be harmed by use of these digital resources, teens have a need for "digital literacy," described by Pascoe (2007) as knowing how to keep themselves safe online (e.g., http://www.atg. wa.gov/InternetSafety/Teens.aspx), to think about the information they are putting out there, and the need to discuss these issues with their parents.

In addition to being digitally literate, parents and thanatologists must consider the best way to have open discussions with adolescents about these resources. (Resources to assist with these conversations include http://wiredsafety.org/ and books by Edgington and Goodstein, listed in the Reference section of this chapter). As Pascoe (2007) noted, forbidding the use of technology just shuts down communication, and teenagers will definitely find a way. Goodstein (2007) provides similar advice for parents: "Beginning a dialogue sounds a lot better than breaking and entering, online or off" (p. 50). Parents of minors should obtain passwords for all online resources that they will use only "in case of emergency" and discuss what should be done with a teen's SNSs in the event of a death (and how they would prefer for their friends in cyberspace to be informed). Counselors should also encourage similar conversations among family members who are dealing with the life-threatening or terminal illness of an adolescent.

Inviting adolescents to share tales of their adventures in the digital world, whether the genre of the tale turns out to be a drama, a comedy, or a horror story, is a useful way to help them process these experiences and to alleviate one's own worries or fears about the impact of digital technology on an adolescent's social and emotional well-being. Counselors are encouraged to utilize the tool for assessing the use of thanatechnology/social media and digital social support created by this author when working with bereaved teens (see Appendix A).

IMPLICATIONS FOR RESEARCH

Is "virtual grief" similar to or different from grief expressed without the use of thanatechnology? These and the many other questions posed throughout this chapter merit attention. Known studies documenting the online activities of young adults are limited to the analysis of publicly available information on social networking sites (Williams & Merten, 2009; Hiefjte, 2012) and a survey of college students following campus shootings to document participation in online activities and depressive/PTSD symptoms (Vicary & Fraley, 2010).

Thanatologists must identify ethically appropriate ways to collect data directly from bereaved adolescents, providing these "experts" with the opportunity to educate us about their experiences. While this process is challenging due to the ethical issues involved in conducting research on sensitive topics with minors, guidance for conducting research with bereaved minors as well as conducting research online is available (Cook, 2009; Cupit, 2012).

CONCLUSION

Rideout (2012) notes that for teens today, "social media are so intricately woven into the fabric of their lives that they don't really know what life would be like without them" (p. 27). In 2006, Greenfield and Yan encouraged us to see the Internet as a "new cultural tool kit" with an infinite series of applications (p. 392). Parents and counselors who want to effectively help bereaved adolescents should heed their advice and recognize that the list of devices and apps in teenagers' tool kits will continue to change. Keeping up with the constant evolution of digital and social media will require us to seek assistance from the adolescents we serve and to boldly explore resources that are available to help with this task (http://www.outboundengine.com/ blog/5-tips-on-how-to-keep-up-with-social-media/).

Adults who do not share adolescents' love of digital technology will be heartened to know that teens still prefer hanging out with each other in person; according to one survey respondent, face-to-face contact is "the only REAL way to be with each other. 'Moments' only happen in person" (Rideout, 2012, p. 15). Perhaps, with the assistance of bereaved adolescents who are creative and savvy about the technical aspects of digital media, thanatologists can help to develop new resources that merge the latest in technology with content specific to the experiences of bereaved teenagers (e.g., how to respond to friends when they are not being helpful during times of grief). In order to implement that tried-and-true counselor's directive to "meet the clients where they are at," working effectively with teenagers will require counselors to become knowledgeable about digital and social media. However, when talking with teens about their use of TMC, SNSs, and MP3s, it will always be important to remember to use some good old-fashioned TLC.

Carla Sofka, PhD, MSW, is a professor of social work at Siena College in Loudonville, NY. She co-edited the book Dying, Death, and Grief in an Online Universe *(Springer Publishing, 2012) about the use of technology and social media as a resource for death education and for coping with loss and has developed the term "thanatechnology" to describe this phenomenon. She has clinical experience with medical, psychiatric, and hospice social work and has conducted research on grief following public tragedy and how museums serve as "healing spaces." She served as president of the Association for Death Education and Counseling from 2011 to 2012.*

REFERENCES

Aaker, J., Smith, A., & Adler, C. (2010). *The dragonfly effect: Quick, effective, and powerful ways to use social media to drive social change.* San Francisco, CA: Jossey-Bass.

Abad-Santos, A. (2013, July 15). GIFs help teens express grief over Cory Monteith's death. Retrieved from http://www.theatlanticwire.com/entertainment/2013/07/how-gifs-help-teens-express-grief-cory-monteiths-death/67190/

Alvarez, L. (2013, September 13). Girl's suicide points to rise in apps used by cyberbullies. Retrieved from http://www.nytimes.com/2013/09/14/us/suicide-of-girl-after-bullying-raises-worries-on-web-sites.html

Atfield, C., Chalmers, E., & Lion, P. (2006, November 21). Safety net for grief – Anguished teens reach out across cyberspace. *The Courier Mail*, 9.

Barlette, K. G. (2012, December 7). Grief in the Shen/Shaker accident spread over social media. Retrieved from http://blog.timesunion.com/kristi/grief-in-the-shenshaker-accident-spread-over-social-media/52333/

Bell, M. A. (2011). Native knowledge: Knowing what they know – and learning how to teach them the rest. In M. Manafy & H. Gautschi (Eds.), *Dancing with digital natives* (pp. 351-372). Medford, NY: CyberAge Books.

Blais, J. J., Craig, W. M., Pepler, D., & Connolly, J. (2008). Adolescents online: The importance of internet activity choices to salient relationships. *Journal of Youth and Adolescence, 37*(5), 522-536.

Borzekowski, D. L. G., & Rickert, V.I. (2001). Adolescent cybersurfing for health information: A new resource that crosses barriers. *Archives of Pediatric Adolescent Medicine, 155*, 813-817.

Burrell, J. (2007, January 18). Electronic age changes face of grief: IMs, Facebook allow youths to connect without having to be face to face. *Contra Costa Times*.

Carboneau, A. (2013, July 15). In Brockton area and nationwide, grieving finds a place on social media. Retrieved from http://www.enterprisenews.com/answerbook/abington/x1293263745/In-Brockton-area-and-nationwide-grieving-finds-a-place-on-social-media comScore. (2013, February). U.S. digital future in focus 2012: Key insights from 2011 and what they mean for the coming year. Retrieved from www.comscore.com/ Insights/Presentations_and_Whitepapers/2012/2012_US_Digital_Future_in_Focus

Chanda, M. L., & Levitin, D. J. (2013). The neurochemistry of music. *Trends in Cognitive Sciences, 17*(4), 179-193.

Cook, A. S. (2009). Ethics and adolescent grief research. In D. Balk & C. Corr (Eds.), *Adolescent encounters with death, bereavement, and coping* (pp. 39-57). New York, NY: Springer.

Cupit, I. N. (2012). Research in thanatechnology. In C. J. Sofka, I. N. Cupit, & K. R. Gilbert (Eds.), *Dying, death, and grief in an online universe: For counselors and educators* (pp. 198-214). New York, NY: Springer.

Cushnie, B. (2010). Music and grief. Retrieved from http://www.hellogrief.org/music-and-grief/

deVries, B., & Moldaw, S. (2012). Virtual memorials and cyber funerals: Contemporary expressions of ageless experiences. In C. J. Sofka, I. N. Cupit, & K. R. Gilbert (Eds.), *Dying, death, and grief in an online universe: For counselors and educators* (pp.135-148). New York, NY: Springer.

Dretzin, R. (2008). What we learned. Retrieved online from www.pbs.org/sgbh/pages/frontline/kidsonline/etc/notebook.html

Edgington, S. M. (2011). *The parent's guide to texting, Facebook, and social media: Understanding the benefits and dangers of parenting in a digital world.* Dallas, TX: Brown Books Publishing Group.

German, K., & Drushel, B. (2011). Introduction: Emerging media: A view downstream. In B. Drushel & K. German (Eds.), *The ethics of emerging media: Information, social norms, and new media technology* (pp. 1-9). London, England: The Continuum International Publishing Group.

Gilbert, K. R., & Massimi, M. (2012). From digital divide to digital immortality: Thanatechnology at the turn of the 21st century. In C. J. Sofka, I. N. Cupit, & K. R. Gilbert (Eds.), *Dying, death, and grief in an online universe: For counselors and educators* (pp. 16-27). New York, NY: Springer.

Goodstein, A. (2007). *Totally wired: What teens and tweens are really doing online.* New York, NY: St. Martin's Press.

Greenfield, P., & Yan, Z. (2006). Children, adolescents, and the Internet: A new field of inquiry in developmental psychology. *Developmental Psychology, 42*(3), 391-394.

Grocke, D. E. & Wigram, T. (2007). *Receptive methods in music therapy: Techniques and clinical applications for music therapy clinicians, educators and students.* London, England: Jessica Kingsley.

Heeres, A. (2013). When talking is not enough. *Advances in Bereavement, 3*(3), 32-35. Retrieved from http://advancesinbereavement.org/2013may.php

Hellenga, K. (2002). Social space, the final frontier: Adolescents on the Internet. In J.T. Mortimer and R.W. Larson (Eds.), *The changing adolescent experience: Societal trends and the transition to adulthood* (pp. 208-249). Cambridge, England: Cambridge University Press.

Hieftje, K. (2012). The role of social networking sites in memorialization of college students. In C. J. Sofka, I. N. Cupit, & K. Gilbert (Eds.), *Dying, death, and grief in an online universe: For counselors and educators* (pp. 31-46). New York, NY: Springer.

Hinduja, S. (2009). Cyberbullicide. Retrieved from http://cyberbullying.us/cyberbullicide-the-relationship-between-cyberbullying-and-suicide-among-youth/

Hinduja, S., & Patchin, J. W. (2010). Bullying, cyberbullying, and suicide. *Archives of Suicide Research, 14*(3), pp. 206-221.

Jones, S. (2013, August 19). Ask.fm unveils new measures to combat cyberbullying after death of teenager. Retrieved from http://www.theguardian.com/society/2013/aug/19/ask-fm-cyberbully-hannah-smith-death

Kowalski, R. M., Limber, S. P., & Agatston, P. W. (2012). *Cyberbullying: Bullying in the digital age.* London, England: Wiley-Blackwell.

Lenhart, A., Purcell, K., Smith, A., & Zickuhr, K. (2010, February 3). Social media and mobile internet use among teens and young adults. Retrieved from http://www.pewinternet.org/Reports/2010/Social-Media-and-Young-Adults.aspx

Lenhart, A., Madden, M., Macgill, A. R., & Smith, A. (2007). Teens and social media. Retrieved from http://www.pewinternet.org/ Reports/2007/Teens-and-Social-Media/1-Summary-of-Findings.aspx

Lenhart, A., Madden, M., & Hitlin, P. (2005, July 27). *Teens and Technology: Youth are leading the transition to a fully wired and mobile nation.* Pew Internet & American Life Project. Retrieved from http://www.pewinternet.org/~/media/Files/Reports/2005/PIP_Teens_ Tech_July2005web.pdf.pdf

Lynn, C., & Rath, A. (2012). GriefNet: Creating and maintaining an internet bereavement community. In C.J. Sofka, I. N. Cupit, & K. R. Gilbert (Eds.), *Dying, death, and grief in an online universe: For counselors and educators* (pp. 87-102). New York, NY: Springer.

Madden, M., Lenhart, A., Cortesi, S., Gasser, U., Duggan, M., Smith, A., & Beaton, M. (2013, May 21). Teens, social media, and privacy. Retrieved from http://www.pewinternet.org/~/media//Files/ Reports/2013/PIP_TeensSocialMediaandPrivacy.pdf

Madden, M., Lenhart, A., Duggan, M., Cortesi, S., & Gasser, U. (2013, March 13). Teens and technology 2013. Report retrieved from http:// www.pewinternet.org/ reports/2013/Teens-and-Tech.aspx

Manafy, M., & Gautschi, H. (2011). *Dancing with digital natives.* Medford, NY: CyberAge Books.

McFerran, K. (2012). Music and adolescents. In N. S. Rickard & K. McFerran (Eds.), *Lifelong engagement with music: Benefits for mental health and well-being* (pp. 95-106). New York, NY: Nova Science Publishers, Inc.

McFerran, K. (2010). *Adolescents, music, and music therapy: Methods and techniques for clinicians, educators, and students.* Philadelphia, PA: Jessica Kingsley Publishers.

McKenna, L. (2005, March 17). The Google stage. Retrieved from http://11d.typepad.com/ blog/2005/03/the_google_stage.html

Mindlin, G., Dourousseau, D., & Cardillo, J. (2012). *Your playlist can change your life.* Naperville, IL: Sourcebooks.

Montgomery, K. C. (2007). *Generation digital: Politics, commerce, and childhood in the age of the Internet.* Cambridge, MA: MIT Press.

Niebuhr, G. & Wilgoren, J. (1999, April 28). Terror in Littleton: Shrines. Retrieved from http://www.nytimes.com/1999/04/28/us/terror-littleton-shrines-shock-violent-deaths-new-more-public-rites-mourning.html

Nielsen. (2013a, April 16). The teen transition: Adolescents of today, adults of tomorrow. Retrieved from http://www.nielsen.com/us/en/newswire/2013/the-teen_transitio--adolescents-of-today--adults-of-tomorrow.html

Nielsen. (2013b, September 4). Smells like teen spirit: How teens are using entertainment. Retrieved from http://www.nielsen.com/us/en/newswire/2013/smells-like-teen-spirit--how-teens-are-using-entertainment.html

Nielsen. (2012, August 14). More teens listen to music through YouTube than any other source. Retrieved from http://www.nielsen.com/us/en/press-room/2012/music-discovery-still-dominated-by-radio--says-nielsen-music-360.html

Pascoe, C. J. (2007). Interview conducted on July 17 and retrieved from www.pbs.org/wgbh/pages/frontline/kidsonline/interviews/pascoe.html

Patchin, J. W., & Hinduja, S. (2012). *Cyberbullying: Prevention and response – Expert perspectives*. New York, NY: Routledge.

Phillips, W. (2011). LOLing at tragedy: Facebook trolls, memorial pages, and resistance to grief online. *First Mind, 16*(12). Retrieved from http://firstmonday.org/ojs/index.php/fm/article/view/3168/3115

Prensky, M. (2001). Digital natives, digital immigrants. *On the Horizon, 9*(5), 1-6. Retrieved from http://www.marcprensky.com/writing/Prensky%20-%20%20Digital%20Natives,%20Digital%20Immigrants%20-%20Part1.pdf

Purcell, K. (2010). Teens, the Internet, and communication technology: A Pew Internet guide to online teens. Retrieved from http://www.pewinternet.org/~/media/Files/Presentations/2010/Jun/Purcell%20YALSA%20pdf.pdf

Rando, T. A. (2000). *Treatment of complicated mourning*. Champaign, IL: Research Press.

Rideout, V. (2012, June 26). Social media, social life: How teens view their digital lives. A Common Sense Media Research Study retrieved from http://www.commonsensemedia.org/sites/default/files/research/socialmediasociallife-final-061812.pdf

Rideout, V. J., Foehr, U. G., & Roberts, D. F. (2010, January). Generation M^2: Media in the lives of 8- to 18-year-olds. Retrieved from http://kaiserfamilyfoundation.files.wordpress.com/2013/04/8010.pdf

Roberts, P. (2006). From My Space to our space: The functions of web memorials in bereavement. *The Forum, 32*(4),1, 3-4.

Sofka, C. J. (2012a). The net generation: The special case of youth. In C. J. Sofka, I. N. Cupit, & K. R. Gilbert (Eds.), *Dying, death, and grief in an online universe: For counselors and educators* (pp. 47-60). New York, NY: Springer.

Sofka, C. J. (2012b). Informational support online: Evaluating resources. In C. J. Sofka, I. N. Cupit, & K. R. Gilbert (Eds.) *Dying, death, and grief in an online universe: For counselors and educators* (pp. 246-255). New York, NY: Springer.

Sofka, C. J. (1997). Social support "internetworks," caskets for sale, and more: Thanatology and the information superhighway. *Death Studies, 21*(6), 553-574.

Steyer, J. P. (2012). *Talking back to Facebook: The common sense guide to raising kids in the digital age.* New York, NY: Scribner.

Trauma Foundation. (2001). Moving through grief to survivor advocacy. Retrieved from http://www.traumaf.org/featured/7-01-survivor_advocacy.shtml

Vicary, A. M., & Fraley, R. C. (2010). Student reactions to the shootings at Virginia Tech and Northern Illinois University: Does sharing grief and support over the Internet affect recovery? *Psychology and Social Psychology Bulletin, 36*(11), 1155-1563.

Williams, A. L., & Merten, M. J. (2009). Adolescents' online social networking following the death of a peer. *Journal of Adolescent Research, 24*(1), 67-90.

Appendix A: Assessing Use of Thanatechnology / Social Media and Digital Social Support (Social Support "Internetworks")

Question #1: Have you ever used technology or social media in any way to cope with illness, dying, death, and/or grief?
____ No ____ Yes: If so, please place a check in front of each resource that you have used.

Facebook: ___ Individual page(s) ___ Other (describe): ___ RIP page(s)	
Twitter	Tumblr
Text messaging (TM)	Instant messaging (IM)
Skype	E-mail
YouTube (for non-music videos):	
MP3 player / iPod - Describe any songs(s) or playlist(s) related to grief/loss:	
Non-FB or MySpace memorial website(s) (describe):	
Online obituary: ___ I read it ___ I shared the link (where?)	
MySpace: ___ Individual page(s) ___ Other (describe): ___ RIP page(s)	
Pinterest	Instagram
Flickr	Spotify
Kik	Ask.fm
YouTube, Pandora, Vevo, etc. (access to music):	
Online discussion group or support group (describe):	
Online guestbook: __ Read the entries __ Added an entry	
Other (describe):	

Question #2: Have you ever learned about a death or a tragedy via technology or social media? _____ No _____ Yes   If yes, please answer questions 2a-2b:

2a) Please describe how and when you found out.

2b) Please share your reaction(s) to the way in which you first received the news.

Possible prompts: Was it helpful to receive the news in this way? (Any advantages to receiving the news this way?) Were there any disadvantages to receiving the news this way? (Any negative consequences as a result of receiving the news this way?)

Question #3: On a scale of 1-5, please describe how frequently you have used social media and/or technology to deal with illness, dying/death, or grief, with 1 = "Never" and 5 = "All the time".
Never =   1   2   3   4   5   = All the time

What do you think influences your level of use of these resources? (Possible prompts: Access? Comfort with? Level of familiarity with how these resources can be used to cope with loss?)

How has the use of these resources been helpful? A mixed bag? Any negative experiences (Cyberbullying/trolling)?

Question #4: Has the use of digital technology or social media had an impact on your ability to have face-to-face conversations about sensitive topics? (When you use these resources, is it easier or harder to have face-to-face conversations with someone later?)

Question #5: Is there anything else that you'd like to teach me about how technology/social media has influenced the way you deal with loss?

CHAPTER 15

Death Education and Adolescents

Robert G. Stevenson

S chools in the United States are charged with educating the "whole child" and, increasingly, to cover the full lifespan from birth to death. To carry out part of that charge, schools have developed units, full courses, and separate shorter programs and workshops to help young people, their families, and the entire school community cope with dying, death, grief and loss, since these realities touch every life. These programs and courses are referred to collectively as "death education." Death education is that formal instruction which deals with dying, death, grief, loss and their impact on the individual and humankind (Stevenson, 1984). Such instruction can occur at home with family, in religious instruction, and/or in schools. Age-appropriate school programs have been developed for high schools (grades 9 through 12) and middle schools (grades 6 through 8).

Death education begins in the home. Parents and family members are the first and most important teachers of children. They model coping behaviors as they try to cope with the losses they encounter in life. In an ideal situation, young people can go to family members for information and support in time of crisis, building on a foundation established early in life. However, emotional ties and concern about saying the "wrong thing" can hinder open family discussion of sensitive issues, such as the topic of death. If parental concern over possible "misstatements" is strong enough, such discussions may not take place at all. Parents may wish to protect the young person from an unpleasant reality, or they may want to preserve their own vision of the "innocence of childhood" for as long as possible.

Religious institutions also provide death education. Diversity of religious beliefs, or lack of such a belief, in our pluralistic society makes it difficult to generalize about the impact of religion in the education of young people about death. Christians may view death as punishment for sin and some attribute feelings of guilt to a traditional religious portrayal of death. On the other hand, their faith may also be a comfort in times of grief. When one feels hopeless, religion and faith can be a source of hope; hope that the deceased is now beyond this "vale of tears" and that those who mourn may one day be reunited with their loved one. Most religions offer a belief that life continues in some form after the event of physical death and such teachings may help the bereaved to move on with their lives.

The roles of family and religion must both be taken into account when working with grieving individuals. When death education is offered in schools it is not done in isolation. Teachers must be conscious of the many influences in the lives of their students. Instructors need to demonstrate a multi-cultural sensitivity so that cultural, regional and religious differences will be acknowledged if death education is to be truly responsive to the needs of students.

THE ROLE OF THE SCHOOL

Schools have developed death education programs that address three separate areas:

Preparation: This includes courses which present facts about the physical aspects of death, the psychosocial effects of death on the survivors, and methods of coping with dying, death, and grief. This information can prepare students to answer their own questions before a loss occurs.

Intervention: These programs offer guidelines for support in the midst of crisis. Response protocols would be included in this area.

Postvention: This includes programs which provide continued support for members of a school community after a loss occurs.

Death education does not include every course which mentions death. Hamlet's soliloquy or *Romeo and Juliet* may well be used in a death education context, but their inclusion in a curriculum does not, by itself, transform an English course into a death education curriculum. In a school setting, death education includes those courses, curricula, counseling programs, and support services which offer a structured approach to issues dealing with dying, death, grief, loss and their impact on the students, staff, their families, their friends and on society. As with every curriculum, it is important to provide information and exercises that are appropriate to the age and developmental level of the students involved.

Death education has been expanded and now includes losses other than death. In death education, bereavement is defined as the forcible loss of someone or something precious (Stevenson, 2002). It is a point in time and can include losses other than a death. This differs from general definitions of bereavement. Some say it involves "sadness after the death of a family member or friend" (Merriam-Webster, 2013); others define it as another term for grief (Gladding, 2011). In fact, any loss that is felt by the individual to be a major one can be called bereavement. Bereavement does not only occur due to a death. And, if the bereavement is because of a death, it need not be limited to the death of family and friends, as the Merriam-Webster Dictionary says.

After over forty years of death education in schools, the need for such courses and programs is clearer than ever. Although some cling to the illusion that death does not touch the lives of adolescents, the reality is quite different. Adolescents die each year. Each of those deaths affects not just the students at one school, but at schools throughout the area. One in 20 young people will lose a parent to death or divorce by their senior year in high school (Critelli, 1979). Sibling deaths, celebrity deaths (of adolescents' heroes or cult figures), and staff deaths (as the average age of school faculty grows older) also affect adolescents. Potentially, there are students trying to cope with their grief in every class in every middle school and high school in this country. Thus, the difference among adolescents in not whether or not they have been affected by grief, but in their degree of success in coping with that grief.

Grief can have a dramatic impact on the classroom atmosphere and on the learning process. Bereavement and the grief process can affect a student in a number of ways. Academically, it can cause a shorter attention span, difficulty in remembering facts, lower grades or a lowered level of self-confidence regarding school assignments. Behavior can be modified and some grieving students may exhibit disruptive classroom behavior, poor attendance, more frequent visits to the school nurse, increased absence due to "illness" or injury, a greater number of accidents, withdrawal from school sports or other school activities, or acting out. Those having the most trouble coping may even engage in punishment-seeking behavior or episodes of violence. The emotional impact can include greater need for teacher attention and support, apathy, a general loss of interest in school, altered relationships with staff and peers, greater feelings of anger or guilt, sadness, or an inability to enjoy life, including school (Stevenson, 1986).

A school or classroom can be turned upside down by the physical and emotional demands of the grief process and the disruption which even a few of the possible reactions listed above can cause; the larger the number of affected students, the greater the disruption of the educational process. A single death in a school community has the potential to impact every member of that community, including not only students, but faculty, staff, parents and others as well.

Further, there are some students who are more at-risk. Some bereaved students try to numb the emotional pain by self-medicating with alcohol or drugs. This attempt to cope with the pain of grief can be seen as the "cause" of problems instead of a symptom of unresolved grief. Some students are coping with the greater burden imposed by more than one loss. Multiple losses can involve personal losses of each individual, or they may be of the type which affect an entire community. Multiple losses are so common that they should be seen as the rule and not an exception.

COMMUNITY GRIEF

There are deaths which have an impact on an entire community. These present a special type of grief situation because an entire school, town, or region can be involved. This concept is not a new one. A set of guidelines for developing a protocol for a school's response to community grief was distributed in 1986 by the National Association of Secondary School Principals (Stevenson & Powers, 1986). The protocol was based on questions which must be answered when a school is faced with dealing with community grief. These questions include the following:

- Who should inform the student(s)?
- Who else should be informed?
- Where should the students be told?
- How should the students be told?
- How might the students react?
- What issues can complicate student reaction and/or student response?
- What support personnel are available to the school community? (Stevenson, 1994)

The process of developing a structured death education program and set of protocols within a school system can help prepare both students and staff to answer these questions and to respond more effectively to a loss.

In interviews with death education students, the two benefits most frequently identified were a lessening of fear and anxiety regarding death and improved communication by students with family, teachers and peers. Young people said that before taking a death education course, they believed they could not discuss the topic of death. This silence increased their fear of death and hindered communication with those, such as family members, who might have offered support. After taking a death education course, students spoke of bringing class materials home and of discussing death and grief with family members, often for the first time. As students spoke more openly on the topic, they felt that their fear and anxiety lessened. As one student said, "Before I took a death education course I thought about death all the time, but I couldn't talk about it. Since taking this course I talk about death with a lot of people...so I don't have to think about it" (Stevenson, 1984). The object here is *not* to eliminate a fear of death, but to bring it to a level which is less threatening to a student. Some say that "knowledge is power;" the intent is to provide knowledge about loss and grief and how people cope when these occur.

In addition to student grief, death education has come to play an important role in areas of prevention, including the areas of depression, suicide, violence, HIV/AIDS, and child abuse.

Death education curricula have been used as a means of informing students of warning signs of suicide and symptoms of depression. In Bergen County, New Jersey, suicide prevention programs were begun in the late 1980s. In the next decade, adolescent suicides steadily declined, while in three neighboring counties the number of adolescent suicides rose. The Adolescent Suicide Awareness Program (ASAP) succeeded so well that it was duplicated throughout the state.

Sexually transmitted diseases, including HIV infection and AIDS, continue to increase among adolescents. Today, almost all health education curricula address the means of HIV transmission and symptoms of AIDS. Death education curricula discuss related issues. Issues discussed in death education courses include dealing with feelings, confidentiality, and motives behind high-risk behavior such as drug use or unprotected sex. Death education students have even assumed a proactive stance in helping their school districts to develop policies related to HIV and AIDS.

The growing number of violent adolescent deaths has pushed this topic to the forefront of death education. High school age adolescents serving time for violent crimes in Bergen County, NJ, were five times more likely to have lost a parent through death or abandonment before age five. Unresolved childhood grief appeared to be a major source of their violence. As part of their rehabilitation, a death educator was called in to consult with correctional personnel in developing ways to facilitate the resolution of their grief. Death education curricula address the causes, risks, and consequences of violent behavior, social and psychological factors behind the increase in adolescent violence, and nonviolent alternatives to violence, such as peer mediation.

The degree of difficulty which a child experiences when coping with grief is directly related to how well the child's parents cope with their grief. Also, young children relate to death differently than adults. Death education curricula can help to prepare adolescents to better cope with loss, which could lead to their ability to help their own children someday understand and deal with this difficult topic.

QUALIFICATIONS OF DEATH EDUCATORS

Death educators are most often school counselors and classroom teachers. At this time, death education teachers are not required to have special certification, as they may need to teach health education or, in some states, psychology. Part of the difficulty in requiring special certification comes from the wide variety of sponsoring disciplines in the schools. Death education curricula have been developed in health, family living, English, social studies, and science departments. Death education teachers in public schools are certified as educators and have some background in child or developmental psychology but they often have no formal training in death education. They may have difficulty in finding such training, since teacher preparation programs have yet to recognize the need for preparing teachers to cope with the impact of death in the classroom. In private and parochial schools the preparation base is even more varied, since in most states less formal preparation is required of staff members than in public schools. In addition, there may be staff members who would be uncomfortable teaching death education curriculum because of unresolved grief in their own lives.

Staff development programs and workshops have provided an ongoing means of staff preparation for death education. Assisting students to cope with death is not a job for one or two staff members. The entire staff should be involved at some level since there are situations where they may be needed. Since bereaved students can likely be found in every class, all staff members should be aware of ways in which they can be of help. If not able to actively help, they should at least be aware of how to avoid inadvertently adding to the student's problems. The involvement of administrators is also important. It is these administrators who develop, and implement, school response protocols related to death and other crises, and may evaluate the performance of the staff members implementing death education curricula.

In response to a lack of standardized staff preparation or teacher certification requirements, the Association for Death Education and Counseling (ADEC) has developed a program for certification of thanatologists. To obtain certification as a thanatologist (one who studies death), a candidate is required to take a national certification examination. Having an accepted standard for preparation of death educators through this certification has been an aid to administrators and a comfort to the parents of students in death education courses.

The ADEC model has identified certain characteristics for thanatologists that are helpful in selecting teachers for death education courses. Teachers and counselors involved in such courses/programs need to be able to: actively listen to the thoughts and concerns of their students; have the appropriate knowledge and skills to teach the death education curriculum; be sensitive to social and cultural differences among students; and teach critical reading and effective problem solving (Wogrin, 2013). Additionally, such instructors need to demonstrate empathy for the emotional experience of their students.

High School Death Education Curricula

Setting standards for staff selection and preparation has been difficult but such standards now exist. Establishing standards for high school death education curricula has been an equally difficult task. Any curriculum is a statement of priorities. For that reason it is important that a curriculum be written by professional educators while its priorities reflect those of the community. The curriculum development process should allow input by parents and concerned community members. The final death education curriculum must be accepted by the district board of education. This open curriculum development process helps to establish lines of communication between home and school and allows educators to address possible community concerns regarding death education. Adolescents, although maturing almost daily, are not yet adults. They may be able to handle the intellectual requirements of college death education classes, but the emotional component of death education makes it important to remember that high school and middle school curricula must be age-appropriate in both content and methodology.

There are other decisions which must be made regarding death education in schools.

What will the subject area be that incorporates death education? The subject area in which death education takes place will shape what is taught and the manner in which it is presented. It must be determined whether death education will be placed in a single curriculum area or will be multi-disciplinary involving several academic departments. It will also determine who the evaluators will be and the standards by which the curriculum and teacher will be evaluated.

What will be the format for the death education curriculum? Some schools offer death education as a separate course while others have infused the death education curriculum into existing courses; some choose to have the program run by school counselors. Death education as a separate course, while still not the most common method, is more appropriate on a high school level. In middle school, shorter units focused on a single objective are more common and may be more easily delivered in a manner that is age appropriate to the students. It is also in middle school that school counselors are often the primary instructor for programs related to grief and loss.

Will this material be required? The content of death education curricula may well be important for all people at some time. This does not mean that every student will benefit from a course offered at a set point in their academic experience. This possible problem can be avoided by making death education courses, or units, elective in nature. If their personal situation makes it difficult for some students to participate in a standard death education class or unit, alternatives can then be made available to such students.

Are there risks in death education? Counselors are told in their training that any technique or theory that holds the potential to be of help also holds a similar potential to hurt if misused or delivered to people unable to accept its message. Supporters of death education would agree that there are "risks" in any course with content that holds such potentially strong emotional impact. What must be determined is the extent these risks can be addressed in advance and possible negative effects avoided. It is also important to differentiate between real areas of concern and the "myths" about death education propagated by demagogues who have used death education as a scapegoat to further a political agenda.

Some critics of death education have manipulated a few anecdotal stories to play on fears of concerned parents. However, the model used by death educators seeks to reinforce the family as a positive support for students. Open home/school communication encourages parent-teacher cooperation to benefit the young adults in schools. The counseling dimension of grief support involves certified school personnel. Knowing when to make appropriate referral of students who need additional support is part of the responsibility of every counselor and teacher.

Positive criticism of death education came from English researcher Sonja Hunt. She pointed out that there are events and processes in life which leave a distinct mark on an individual. Death is such an event and grief is such a process. She cautioned that educators need to be aware of the possible consequences of their work before attempting instruction which could affect the grief process. She also asked educators to clearly identify why schools would be an appropriate place for such interventions (Stevenson, 1984).She cautioned educators to examine death education lessons and their possible effects before implementing such lessons in the classroom. She also cautioned educators to maintain ongoing programs of evaluation of death education curricula and professional development programs. The last thirty years have shown the wisdom of her critique. Professional journals such as *Death Studies* and *Omega* regularly publish research results evaluating the effects of death education. Professional organizations regularly offer workshops, symposia, and extension courses to develop and enhance the skills needed by death educators.

Is there one preferred type of death education curriculum? This answer is a simple one: no, there is not. Death education curricula have developed a variety of models. The needs of a particular district or school must be taken into account when choosing to implement one or more of these models.

Models of High School Death Education Curricula

Death education was introduced into high schools beginning in the late 1960s. The first curriculum materials available to educators were divided into two categories: prepared units (with supplementary materials) which were fully developed, ready-to-use lesson plans, and unstructured "learning opportunities" with objectives to be used by educators in developing their own lessons. *Perspectives on Death* (1972) by Daugherty and Berg is an example of the former, while *Discussing Death* (1976) by Mills, Robinson, Vermilye, and Reisler, is an example of the latter. Both types saw death education as a series of discrete topics aimed at answering student questions about death and its effects. Both included outside experts, such as funeral directors, doctors, nurses, or clergy, coming into the classroom to supplement the work of the teacher.

As more information became available about dying, death, grief, and loss, curricula became model-centered. A lesson would typically start with a psychological model, such as the Five Stages of Death and Dying developed by Elisabeth Kübler-Ross. The model provided a way for students to look at an experience which was new to them. The structure of a model made the topic seem less confusing and gave a basis for comparing loss experiences. Additional stage models of grief soon appeared; Westberg offered one of the first in 1961, using ten stages. Other models came from Kries and Patti (1969), Kavanaugh (1972) and Davidson (1975) and these just scratch the surface (Metzgar, 1988). One drawback of these models was that as they were used more frequently they came to have a life of their own. In extreme cases, the integrity of the model actually became more important than the individual experience it was intended to describe.

Within each curriculum, there is a variety of themes. Some appear in almost every death education course. Others are used selectively, depending on subject area and instructor. Three widely used curricula (Zalaznik, 1992; O'Toole, 1989; Stevenson, 1990) are representative of those used in death education. These three curricula contain the following themes: Age; Change as Part of Life; Understanding Death; Life-Threatening Illness; Communication and Language; Cultural and Historical Perspectives; Definitions of Death; Economic and Legal Issues; Euthanasia and the "Right to Die;" Family as Support; Emotions; Grief and the Grief Process; Permanent versus Temporary Loss; Religious and Philosophical Views of Death; Rituals of Death and Mourning

(Funerals); Suicide and Suicide Prevention; and Views of Life After Death. The amount of time spent on an individual theme varies based on the needs of the students and on significant current events.

The first free-standing high school course on death education started in 1972 and was taught until 1999, after its creator retired. If we were to summarize the development of death education by the changes that took place in that course, *Contemporary Issues of Life and Death,* over the decades it might look like this:

1970s: Major themes in this death education course were consumerism and control. Jessica Mitford's book, *The American Way of Death*, became popular reading among young people. The book took a hypercritical view of American funeral practice and the denial of death in American culture. Students wanted to know more about the cost of death; from there, the students' questions moved to other areas. They asked the most questions when they studied the topics of dying, death-related rituals, and beliefs about spirituality and the afterlife. A theme that ran through these questions was control. Starting with the control exercised by an informed consumer, students looked at the whole of death education and each of its individual topics with a desire to have a feeling of greater control over their own lives and emotions. They learned that knowledge about the grief process could not prevent a future loss. That also learned that, by lessening the fear of the unknown, such knowledge could help the pain of the loss from being greater than it might otherwise have to be. In reading *On Death and Dying* by Elisabeth Kübler-Ross, students became acquainted with her five-stage model. They used it to look at issues of loss in their own lives and gained a greater feeling of control related to those losses. Garner and Acklen (1976) spoke about death education in middle schools, but educators were slower to start implementing formal instruction at that level and there were few materials and less training available at that time.

1980s: A new perspective was added to courses in "parenting" in high school. Students wanted to know more about a child's understanding of death, so they read Nagy's chapter from Feifel's *The Meaning of Death*. They also learned about the work of Myra Bluebond-Langner (*The Private Worlds of Dying Children*) and Sylvia Anthony (*The Discovery of Death in Childhood and After*). Once they had some understanding of the way in which children learn about death, they next looked at ways that they could help the child acquire a clearer understanding of death and the feelings that accompanied it.

They read children's literature with a reading list that often began with Joan Fassler's *Helping Children Cope*. Picking out some of the classic children's books, the students learned about *bibliotherapy*, therapy carried out with stories and related discussion. The components of bibliotherapy include: *identification*, seeing aspects of oneself in the characters or of the characters in oneself; *privacy*, the ability to explore feelings while reading the story without worrying what others will think; *catharsis*, a "cleaning out" of thoughts/feelings that have previously been held in; *normalcy*, the idea that others have felt as they do or have had similar experiences; and *insight*, the ability to apply lessons from the book in one's life.

Students read children's books to answer three questions:
- What were the author's purposes in writing this book?
- To what extent did the author succeed?
- If you were a parent, would you read this book to your child?

As they discussed their stories and conclusions, they had many of the same experiences they hoped that their children might one day have.

Death education was also tailored for specific groups of students. An example of such a curriculum can be seen in the work of Noland, Richardson and Bray (1980) who designed a death education curriculum for ninth-grade girls.

The 1980s also saw controversy arise. Much of it came from a political lobbying group, The Eagle Forum. The group distributed a video that pointed out what they saw as the dangers of death education. Perhaps the greatest danger was that the Eagle Forum sought to polarize parents and teachers by telling parents that a goal of teachers was to discover information about families and to turn children against their parents and family values. Fergus Bordewick wrote an article in *Atlantic Monthly* that looked at death education. The article was balanced in its presentation and led to a one-hour show produced by David Wilcock for the BBC. It was called *The Facts of Death*. Both the article and the television show came down strongly on the side of death education courses in secondary schools. There were additional shows in Japan, on NHK television, and on several of the American news networks. The overall tone of these stories was positive. Death education educators and their classes received requests for the curriculum from educators in Europe and Asia.

The final piece to be added in the 1980s was Suicide Prevention and Depression Awareness. The South Bergen Mental Health Center, led by Diane Ryerson, developed and piloted the Adolescent Suicide Awareness Program (ASAP). In a short time it was implemented in every high school in New Jersey and was replicated in schools throughout the United States and Canada. There was already a "suicide" unit in a death education course, but this program took that information to the entire community both within and outside of the school. It developed further into a middle school program for dealing with loss and grief (Stevenson & Downham, 1990).

1990s: There was a reexamination of the title "death" education. After all, what was being studied was less about death than it was about grief and the larger issue of coping with many types of loss. Educators wanted to resolve some of the negative connotations connected to the word "death." Increasingly, the courses now took on variations of "loss education" in their titles. Educators also realized that these courses had a broader scope than had first been envisioned. To issues of death, dying, loss, and grief were added communication and problem solving. Communication skills were being added to overall district goals, so death and loss education was already on the cutting edge. In follow-up questionnaires about the course, students reported that they were now better able to speak with their parents and others about sensitive issues as a result of their discussions in class.

Problem solving occurred in response to questions directed to the students concerning adolescent thoughts and feelings on dealing with issues of death and grief in school settings. The students carried out the research and attended graduate seminars. High school death education students had several of their studies published in *Illness, Crisis and Loss* and *Archives of the Foundation of Thanatology*. Students came to understand that if they were capable of helping others, they could also help themselves. They said that by helping others, they felt greater control when problems arose. This control extended even to feelings. When they had strong emotions, they felt less anxious and more tolerant of them.

There was an effort to find a place in the school curriculum for courses on death and loss. Once topics such as death, dying, grief and loss had been shown to have a place in the curriculum, people began to ask where, and in which department, these courses belonged.

There were death education units in English, social studies, home economics, and health education departments. The topic was dealt with in courses as diverse as literature, history, sociology, psychology, family life, and biology. There were even self-contained death education courses. Because of the differences in sponsoring disciplines there had been differences in content and a lack of clear standards regarding evaluation. It was clearly stated, however, that death education was not therapy. After all, as one teacher stated, when we teach a course, all we "cure" is ignorance.

ADEC has provided lists of "core knowledge" that express key ideas, identified by experts in the field. ADEC has also offered a revitalized certification program for death educators, and the number of qualified death educators increased. The basic text for educator certification is the *Handbook of Thanatology 2nd edition*. It contains a set of chapters by the leading people in the field and is intended to be an essential body of knowledge for the study of death, dying and bereavement (Meagher & Balk, 2013).

DEATH EDUCATION IN THE 21ST CENTURY

Those who try to look ahead and see what the future holds for death education can identify four themes. These are: the "passing of the guard," the influence of new death education programs outside of North America, the initiation of units on grief and loss in the middle school curriculum, and a broader focus for courses dealing with death and grief.

Passing of the guard

Many of those who have been involved in death education are retiring or moving on to new and different interests. Men and women who spent most of their careers in school classrooms, or who developed the materials that these educators use, are no longer as accessible to offer their support and advice to others in the field.

When the BBC did their investigative report in the 1980s on death education in the United States, the producer, David Wilcock, asked me if this sort of course was primarily academic or "pastoral." He also asked if it was a course that only a few people, with a combination of interest and special ability, could teach. While there is a strong affective component in most death education courses, they are more academic than religious, or "pastoral" (as used by Wilcock). If they are to be part of a public school curriculum, with the United States' emphasis on separation of church and state, this is essential. His second question seemed equally clear at that time. I answered that this was not a course that only a few people could carry on. At that time, it seemed clear, however, at many schools with long-standing death education courses, a change in faculty whether from transfer or retirement often saw the course disappear. The end was immediate in some cases and after a year or two in others. The first separate death education course in the United States, one that was taught for almost three decades, was gone within two years of the retirement of the educator who designed and taught it. All of the needed materials and the curriculum were in place. The students, parents and PTO were supportive of the course. The department chairman decided to teach the course himself and had an orientation. It made no difference. If other educators are to avoid the same fate for their courses, they will need to have alternate instructors available who have knowledge of the curriculum content and classroom techniques before such a need arises. In the short term, schools with similar curricula could become "partner schools." If one school's instructor becomes unavailable, there would be another educator close by with a detailed knowledge of the curriculum.

Influence of death education courses outside North America

Education related to death, loss, and grief now exists in many countries. One of these programs is *Merimna* in Athens, Greece. This program, with initial funding from the European Union, assists grieving children and their families. It has drawn on programs in other countries and adapted those to suit the Greek culture. Earlier, the Japanese demonstrated a great desire for such courses in their country. Their work was aided by the courses taught by Alfons Deeken, a German priest, at Sophia University in Tokyo. A group of Korean graduate students, with private funding, traveled to the United States and visited many of the leaders in death education to begin to develop similar programs in their country. It will be interesting to see what new information and interventions may be started in other areas of the world as they develop their programs.

Middle school curriculum

In the early 1970s, death education was offered in courses in American high schools. Some were uncertain if the subject, already taught in many colleges, could be successfully taught to adolescents at the high school level. The positive impact of such courses has been resolved and they are still being studied to identify and maintain their focus and effectiveness. The same questions once asked about high school courses are being asked as the topic of loss and grief is being introduced in middle schools (Garner & Acklen, 1976). At this level, there are not separate courses but units with specific objectives aimed at younger students. With younger adolescents, involvement of the students' families is essential. If families see this as something that undermines their relationship with their children, the program is almost certain to fail. If they see themselves as allies with the educators (both teachers and counselors) in helping their children, the success of such programs is almost assured.

Broader focus

Since their beginnings in public secondary schools, new units have continually been added to death education courses. In recent years, the broader concept of "loss" has come to replace "death" in many places in the curriculum. The belief is that if psychological models can also be used in dealing with losses other than a death, perhaps the focus should be on loss in general, rather than a focus chiefly of the grief that follows death. Models are, after all, not "real." It is the person/client/student who is real and models are only useful if they help that person and those who work with him or her to understand what he or she is going through. Researchers such as Neimeyer (1999), Stroebe and Schut (1999, 2008), and a host of others have developed such models that counselors, therapists and educators have found useful in explaining and helping others to understand grief in its broader sense.

Also, issues such as "communication" (whether parent-child, student-student or student-teacher) have developed a larger role in the curriculum. Students have repeatedly said that once they spoke about one difficult, or "taboo" topic such as death, they were more able and more likely to speak about others.

The latest approach to death education involves reintegration of life and death as part of a natural cycle. Stories, rather than psychological or behavioral models, are used to provide a new focal point for lessons in death education. Stories have long been used in primary school classrooms and are now being used in middle schools and high schools. These stories allow educators to bring a multicultural perspective to death education. Lessons can blend psychological models with traditional stories, symbols and rituals that have brought comfort to bereaved individuals literally for centuries. The rituals of storytelling allow an educator to move easily into an explanation of the rites of passage which have helped previous generations to cope with the same issues these students now face. Repeating the stories heard in class to parents and others continues the process of communication and brings other people and their unique points of view into the educational process. As students become more comfortable telling the stories they have learned, they are more likely to begin to piece together the stories of their own lives and to share those stories with others. This allows them to build a view of life and death upon a foundation which incorporates their personal stories. Shaping and telling their personal stories has become a new method for dealing with personal grief, as it has in narrative therapy (where clients rewrite their life stories to help themselves understand their own lives). Robert Neimeyer speaks of *meaning reconstruction* through narratives following a death. He sees theories using narratives and stories as having some points in common: skepticism about a predictable trajectory for the grief process; increased emphasis on continuing healthy bonds with the deceased; increased emphasis on the meaning-making process in mourning; greater awareness of the impact of major loss on the individual's self-identity; increased awareness of the possibility of "posttraumatic growth" as one recovers and uses lessons learned in the process; and a focus on groups beyond the grieving individual, such a family or community (Neimeyer, 1998, 1999).

CONCLUSION

Students cannot be shielded from the reality of death in their lives. School can play a positive role in preparing adolescents to cope with the reality of dying, death, and grief. Such preparation has come to be called death education. When a school wishes to implement such a program the following points need to be remembered:

- The process of implementing a death education curriculum should be open and input should be sought from students, parents and community members.
- Death education instructors must be qualified, both academically and emotionally.
- Death education curricula must be age-appropriate and sensitive to the culture and background of individual students.
- Ongoing programs of course evaluation and professional development should be established.
- Death education instructors can be valuable resources in times of crisis. A crisis response plan needs to be developed for this to happen.

- Death education courses can impart knowledge, assist students in coping more effectively with dying, death and grief, and develop communication and parenting skills.

Physical illness can strike an individual at any time. For that reason society recommends and may even require immunization to lessen the pain and suffering caused by such illness; treatment after the fact is often more difficult. Death and grief can also strike at any time. Death education can be viewed as a form of immunization. Experience and research have shown that it can help adolescents to face the pain and suffering such events can cause. It will not prevent pain, but it may help to moderate it, offsetting the pain that can be greater due to fear of the unknown.

Robert G. Stevenson, EdD, MA, MAT, is a professor at Mercy College in New York. He has published over 60 journal articles and book chapters and edited/authored several books. His most recent is Final Acts: End of life, hospice and palliative care *(2013). He developed the first independent high school course on death education, teaching it for 25 years. He is a member of the International Work Group on Death, Dying, and Bereavement and the Association for Death Education and Counseling. He received the 2013 Robert Fulton Founder's Award from the Center for Death Education and Bioethics for lifetime achievement in death education. He co-founded a community grief support center (Jamie Schuman Center) in Hillsdale, NJ. He worked as a counselor in Paterson, NJ, for five years with parolees reentering society from state prisons and adolescents in recovery and with the NY Guard in the aftermath of 9/11.*

References

Anthony, S. (1972). *The discovery of death in childhood and after.* New York, NY: Basic Books.

Berg, D. W. & Daugherty, G. G.(1972). *Perspectives on death.* Baltimore, MD: Waverly Press.

Bluebond-Langner, M. (1978). *The private worlds of dying children.* Princeton, NJ: Princeton University Press.

Critelli, C. (1979). *Parent Death in Childhood.* Paper presented at the Columbia-Presbyterian Medical Center Symposium *The Child and Death*, New York City, NY.

Fassler, J. (1978). *Helping children cope.* New York, NY: Free Press.

Feifel, H. (1959). *The meaning of death.* New York, NY: McGraw-Hill.

Davidson, G. W. (1975). *Living with dying.* Minneapolis, MN: Augsburg Fortress Publishing.

Garner, A. E. & Acklen, L. (1976). Does death education belong in the middle school curriculum? *NASSP Bulletin, (1)*60, 403, 98-102.

Gladding, S. T. (2011). *The counseling dictionary: Concise definitions of frequently used terms 3rd edition.* Upper Saddle River, NJ: Pearson Education.

Kavanaugh, R. (1972). *Facing death.* Los Angeles, CA: Nash Publishing.

Kries, B. & Patti, A. (1969). *Up from grief: Patterns of recovery.* New York, NY: Seabury.

Kübler-Ross, E. (1969). *On death and dying.* New York, NY: Macmillan.

Meagher, D. K. & Balk, D. E. (2013). *Handbook of thanatology 2nd edition.* New York, NY: Routledge.

Merriam-Webster.com. (2013). *Merriam-Webster Online Dictionary.* Retrieved from http://www.merriamwebster.com

Metzgar, M. M. (1988). *Crisis in schools: Is your school prepared?* Seattle, WA: Margaret M. Metzgar.

Mills, G. C., Robinson, A., Vermilye, G., & Reisler, R. (1976). *Discussing death.* Palm Springs, CA: ETC Publishing.

Mitford, J. (1963). *The American way of death.* New York, NY: Buccaneer Books.

Neimeyer, R. A. (1998). *Lessons of loss: A guide to coping.* New York, NY: McGraw Hill.

Neimeyer, R. A. (1999). Narrative strategies in grief therapy. *Journal of Constructivist Psychology, 12:65–85.*

Noland, M., Richardson, G. E. & Bray, R. M. (1980). The systematic development and efficacy of a death education unit for ninth-grade girls. *Death Education, (4)*1, 43-59.

O'Toole, D. (1989). *Growing Through Grief.* Burnsville, NC: Mountain Rainbow Publications.

Schlafly, P. (1988, April 13). Death education comes into the open. *The Brooklyn Spectator.*

Stevenson, R. G. (1984). A death education course for secondary schools: "Curing" death ignorance. Doctoral Dissertation. Teaneck, NJ: Fairleigh Dickinson University.

Stevenson, R. G. (1990). Contemporary issues of life and death. In John D. Morgan (Ed.), *Death education in Canada.* London, Ontario: King's College.

Stevenson, R. G. (1986). Measuring the effects of death education in the classroom. In G. H. Paterson (Ed.), *Children and death.* London, Ontario: King's College.

Stevenson, R. G. (2002). *What will we do? Preparing a school community to cope with crises 2nd edition.* Amityville, NY: Baywood Press.

Stevenson, R. G. and Downham, S. (1990). *Getting to know me.* Hackensack, NJ: Bergen County Task Force on Youth Suicide Prevention.

Stevenson, R. G. and Powers, H. L. (1986). How to handle death in the school. In *Tips for Principals.* Reston, VA: National Association of Secondary School Principals.

Stevenson, R. & Stevenson, E. (1996). *Teaching death education in schools.* Philadelphia, PA: Charles Press.

Stroebe, M. S. & Schut, H. (1999). The dual process model of coping with bereavement: Rationale and description. *Death Studies, 23,* 197-224.

Stroebe, M. S. & Schut, H. (2008). The dual process model of coping with bereavement: Overview and update. *Grief Matters: The Australian Journal of Grief and Bereavement, 11,* 1-4.

Westberg, G. E. (1961). *Minister and doctor meet.* New York, NY: Joanna Cotler Books.

White, M. & Epson, D. (1990). *Narrative means to therapeutic ends.* New York, NY: W.W. Norton.

Wilcock, D. (1989). *The facts of death*. London, England: British Broadcasting Corporation.

Wogrin, C. (2013). Professional Issues and Thanatology. In D. K. Meagher & D. E. Balk, *Handbook of thanatology, 2nd edition*. New York, NY: Routledge.

Zalaznik, P. H. (1992). *Dimensions of loss & death education, 3rd edition*. Minneapolis, MN: Edu-Pac Publishing Company.

CHAPTER 16

Supporting the Grieving College Student

Donna M. Burns

A s a professor I have a front-row seat in witnessing the ways in which college students navigate the tricky waters that ebb and flow between personal and academic life. Students dutifully attend classes, study, work on projects, and commiserate with fellow classmates while simultaneously tending to their lives outside of academe. Particularly challenging for college students is coping with loss:

> *...I never discussed this in class, as it's a pretty major and sensitive experience for me, but in October of last year, my significant other's older brother, 21 at the time, committed suicide, and we both found him...*(male graduate student)

This excerpt, a portion of a lengthy communication between me and one of my bereaved students, poignantly underscores the necessity for college administrators, counselors, and faculty to recognize, acknowledge, and support grieving students. Additional segments of this communication will be interspersed throughout this chapter.

In order to effectively address the needs of grieving students, college personnel must not only be skilled at identifying students affected by loss, but possess the competencies to provide timely and appropriate services. Toward that end, this chapter examines: types of losses and their effects; social media influences; support for student grievers; an overview of existing college programs; and recommendations for implementing grief support programs on campuses.

TYPES OF LOSSES

Culled from research studies, clinical observations, and anecdotal reports obtained from various academic environments, Balk (2008) asserts that a significant number of college students, ranging from 22 to 30 percent, are grieving the death of a loved one or friend within a year of the loss. Other researchers concur with these statistics, substantiated by their own studies (e.g., Battle, Greer, Ortiz-Hernandez, & Todd, 2013; Cooley, Toray, & Roscoe, 2010; Hedman, 2012; McCusker & Witherow, 2012; Neimeyer, Laurie, Mehta, Hardison, & Currier, 2008; Pennington, 2013). Results of a study conducted by Hardison, Neimeyer, and Lichstein (2005) revealed that on an initial survey, 508 bereaved college undergraduate participants indicated they experienced the death of a family member or close friend within two years. The prevalence of bereaved college students is concerning since the grieving process may be disruptive to both daily functioning and academic success (Servaty-Seib & Taub, 2008). During the college years, the death of a friend or loved one can be life-altering, as bereaved students attempt to understand both the loss and their responses to that loss. Further, in coming to terms with such losses bereaved students must also contend with the strong emotions that death elicits, deal with the grief responses others may have to the same loss, and try to restore a sense of purpose and direction as they assimilate the loss into their lives (Neimeyer et al., 2008). The words of Scottish poet and author Anne Grant succinctly capture the tumultuous emotions that many bereaved students feel:

> Grief is perhaps an unknown territory for you. You might feel both helpless and hopeless without a sense of a 'map' for the journey. Confusion is the hallmark of a transition. To rebuild both your inner and outer world is a major project (n.d.).

EFFECTS OF LOSS

Grief manifests itself in a variety of ways and the range of responses may vary considerably from person to person. The stressful demands of college life are further compounded when coping with loss. As a former bereaved college student, completing the final quarter of a semester while simultaneously tending to a multitude of personal and family issues was physically, cognitively, and emotionally draining:

When I was a graduate student my father died suddenly and unexpectedly. I was the one who discovered his body, and my world was turned upside down. Returning to school one week after saying goodbye to the most influential person in my life was challenging at best. There was a yawning emptiness and ache that could not be assuaged. I felt fragile - as though energy had been siphoned from my body. I was unaware of any services that may have been available that provided support to grieving students. (Author)

The effects of sadness, yearning, and sleep disturbances can consume a bereaved student. This may result in a more negative overall educational experience (Wandel, 2009). Several broad areas affected by loss and identified in bereavement literature (e.g., Balk, 2008; Servaty-Seib & Taub, 2008) include physical, behavioral, interpersonal, cognitive, emotional, and spiritual effects. Individual responses within each of these categories are influenced by, but not limited to, such factors as the griever's personality, his or her relationship to the person or event being grieved, and prior experiences with loss (Burns, 2010).

The nature of the death and the relationship of the griever to the deceased affect responses; unanticipated or traumatic deaths often evoke complex grief reactions (Burns, 2010). Responses associated with complicated grief (CG) are distinguished from the trajectory of typical or "normative" loss experiences in that the process is often debilitating and prolonged (Neimeyer et al., 2008; Schnider, Elhai, & Gray, 2007). Difficulty accepting the death, agitation, insomnia, and impaired academic and social functioning are some of the identifiable symptoms of CG (Neimeyer et al., 2008; Schnider, Elhai, & Gray, 2007). These sudden, traumatic, or violent deaths often leave the survivors reeling:

... He had hung himself from a tree in the front yard, and we were both very actively involved in getting him down, doing CPR, and following the ambulance to the hospital, where they were unable to revive him. (male graduate student)

One of the many challenges faced by those grieving tragic loss is making sense of the death. Neimeyer et al. (2008) contend that supporting grieving college students in an effort to help them make sense of a tragedy is an important step in the griever's ability to reconcile the loss and move ahead in their lives. It is imperative, however, that those providing support during a stressful time be non-judgmental and sensitive to the needs of the griever:

> *I was in therapy for a short time after the event, but ended it prematurely due to the therapist's extreme lack of sensitivity and his really uncomfortable approach to me being gay.* (male graduate student)

An unfortunate consequence of this therapist's inability to compassionately and objectively support the student in his grief resulted in a protracted period of bereavement. Although the student ended his sessions with the counselor, he grappled with not only the tragic death of his friend, but the subsequent separation from his partner:

> *In my mind, I have adjusted pretty well from everything, and do not find the experience majorly affecting my everyday life. But, given that it will be a year since the incident next week, I have been thinking about it a lot more lately, and since I am no longer dating my boyfriend and have no connections to his family, I feel a little lost as to who I can talk to about this. Like I said, I am dealing with things pretty well, and am reasonably happy right now, but feel that I would still benefit from some therapy, given that it has been on my mind a lot more lately with the year anniversary coming up.* (male graduate student)

Embedded in this excerpt are elements of non-finite, disenfranchised, and secondary losses. In one year this student experienced a traumatic loss, separated from his partner, became estranged from his partner's family, and was rebuffed by his therapist.

While death is recognized as the ultimate loss, non-finite and disenfranchising events represent losses that evoke emotional responses that parallel and sometimes exceed reactions to death (Burns, 2010). Losses come in myriad forms and multiple factors contribute to how each individual expresses his or her grief. Awareness of the multi-faceted nature of loss is essential in providing support to grieving college students. In a stratified-sampling study of 118 college students conducted by Balk, Walker, and Baker (2010), grieveable events cited included losses of: pets, physical function, jobs, material possessions, ideals, self-respect, ability, parental divorce, relationships, friendships, and separation. Cooley et al. (2010) cited similar events and included other non-death losses experienced by college students, such as: academic failure, being disowned by parents, abortion, arrest, and being raped. Participants completing the Loss Events Scale identified non-death losses "as the most significant loss they had experienced in the last 12 months" (p. 42). In reviewing studies investigating the ending of relationships, Field, Diego, Pelaez, Deeds, and Delgado (2009) found that "breakup distress" manifested in the forms of depression, sleep disturbances, anger, anxiety, and poor academic performance.

The death of a pet, a finite loss, along with several of the non-finite events referenced in the Balk et al. (2010) and Cooley et al. (2010) studies are often disenfranchising and those grieving such losses are disenfranchised grievers. Doka (1989) conceptualized disenfranchised grief as the "grief that persons experience when they incur a loss that is not or cannot be openly acknowledged, publically mourned, or socially supported" (p.4). Doka (2002) identified five ways in which grieveable losses are disenfranchising; when relationships, losses, grievers, circumstances, and expressions of grief are neither recognized nor socially accepted. Cooley et al. (2010) contend that non-death related disenfranchising losses may complicate the grieving process. Because these types of loss events are often disregarded, overlooked, or shunned, disenfranchised grievers may feel isolated as they struggle to find ways to cope with their grief (Burns, 2010):

> *I felt compelled a couple times to discuss my experience in class, but was worried it'd be an inappropriate place to do so.* (male graduate student)

The sentiments expressed in this student's desire to share his loss and grief experiences are no doubt echoed among a multitude of college students.

SOCIAL MEDIA

Among the ways many of today's students find support is through social media. One such popular forum is the website Facebook, often considered the predominant social network choice of college students

(Pennington, 2013; Wandel, 2009). Wandel (2009) investigated the perceived usefulness of Facebook as a means of communication for the bereaved. Some of the comments from focus group participants included: the ease of "checking in" and viewing profiles of deceased friends; appreciation of postings from those who, although not directly affected by the loss, reach out to find meaning and offer condolences; knowing that those grieving were in people's thoughts and prayers; and the ability to communicate with others in their hometown (Wandel, 2009). An important aspect of coping with loss, according to Pennington (2013), is finding support within social networks. Through Facebook, bereaved students can maintain a connection to the deceased as they cope with and process the loss. This is accomplished by maintaining "friend" status via a page that has been created by the grievers (Pennington, 2013). This practice is not without controversy, however. Discussions about who maintains the site, how long it should remain available, privacy settings, and perhaps most importantly, deferring to the wishes of members of the deceased's family, are all issues requiring thoughtful consideration.

One undeniable fact is that Facebook, Twitter, and other online social networking sites are deeply embedded in our technologically progressive culture. It is likely that bereaved college students and others will continue to express their grief and seek support through these online communities. Although convenient and beneficial, these cyber venues cannot provide the level of support that is offered through thoughtful, personal, and well-designed programs. The charge for colleges, then, is to develop, implement, and foster visible and ongoing programs and services that are sensitive and responsive to the needs of grieving students.

SUPPORTING STUDENT GRIEVERS

With the availability and ease of access to numerous online support networks, it is understandable that students will turn to these venues. One thing that these forums cannot provide, however, is in-person support that is sensitive to the individual needs of the griever. Particularly helpful to grieving college students would be responsive and understanding faculty and peers. Hedman (2012) asserts that faculty who are empathetic and willing to listen to the needs of grieving students are more likely to provide accommodations if they are struggling academically. Faculty, inclusive of adjuncts and teaching assistants (TAs), alongside student peers, including resident assistants (RAs), have direct and ongoing contact with students and, with training, could provide valuable assistance to grieving students (Hedman, 2012; Fajgenbaum, Chesson, & Lanzi, 2012; McCusker & Witherow, 2012; Tedrick Parikh & Servaty-Seib, 2013; Servaty-Seib & Taub, 2008).

Although faculty and peers are ideal candidates for partnering with bereaved college students, many are not adequately schooled in issues of loss and may not be comfortable providing support to grieving students (McCusker, 2012). Still, students will often seek support from those with whom they feel they have a connection, and could provide them with guidance:

> *I've been meaning to get in touch with one of my professors regarding some personal issues, and thought that given your background, you'd be the best.* (male graduate student)

Providing bereavement training for faculty, RAs, and other staff members would ensure that grieving students are effectively supported. Servaty-Seib and Taub (2008) suggest that workshops for faculty members and RAs include training in: observation and questioning techniques; development of listening skills; use of validating statements; offering tangible support; and referring out to additional service providers, if necessary.

EXISTING COLLEGE PROGRAMS

A variety of support services are currently available throughout campuses nationwide that are designed to ameliorate some of the effects that grief has on college students. One such program, born from students' requests for bereavement support on campus, was developed by Battle et al. (2013) and implemented at a large university in New England. Entitled *Reflect*, the program is comprised of structured bereavement support groups, informal coping with loss workshops, campus awareness-raising, and resource and referral services. The primary goal of the program, offered at no cost to students, is to facilitate their bereavement experiences in healthy and supportive ways as they move toward acceptance and meaningful integration of that loss into their lives (Battle et al., 2011).

An alternative to traditional bereavement counseling, proposed by Vickio (2008), is the implementation of grief workshops for students, which can be facilitated by counseling staff along with other trained personnel. Vickio (2008) contends that the function and benefits of such workshops include:

- Providing students with a conceptual framework for understanding their loss;
- Normalizing and legitimizing students' grief-related thoughts and feelings;
- Enabling students to interact with other bereaved individuals and thereby feel less isolated by their grief experience;
- Helping students identify options for coping with their grief;
- Directing students to other resources (p. 42).

Yet another program that is garnering attention and support is National Students of AMF. This program "...was created by grieving college students to support their fellow grieving students" (Fajgenbaum et al., 2012, p. 99). What distinguishes this program from others is that the National AMF has Campus Chapters that are student-led, with each chapter comprised of a Support group, Service group, and Mentoring program. Each group provides different functions. Support groups are student-led in a relaxed open forum; Service groups are open to all students and are encouraged to volunteer and raise awareness for a variety of causes important to members; Mentoring programs align students and faculty members for support on an as-needed basis (Fajgenbaum et al., 2012). Other events and activities that the National AMF participates in include National College Student Grief Awareness Week and the National Conference on College Student Grief. Their website (http://www.studentsofamf.org) also lists numerous other grief-related activities. As of this writing there are 43 university-recognized Campus Chapters; college campuses nationwide are encouraged to start their own chapters.

IMPLEMENTING COLLEGE STUDENT BEREAVEMENT PROGRAMS

Given the number of college students who are grieving at any given time, and based on information from studies, observations, and reports gleaned from both researchers and those who are bereaved, campuses should create and implement programs tailored to meet the needs of their grieving student population. A synopsis of several program recommendations (e.g., Balk, 2008; Battle et al., 2013; Taub & Servaty-Seib, 2008) includes, but is not limited to:

- Needs assessment to ascertain student preferences and examine bereavement services that may already be in place;
- Formation of a focus group comprised of bereaved students, administrators, faculty, counseling staff, and others to identify program goals;
- Maintaining a collaborative relationship among administrators, faculty, and students to ensure program goals are realistic and attainable;
- Appointment of a coordinator to oversee the program once it is established;
- Providing bereavement training to faculty, RAs, staff, and others who have direct contact with students;
- Establishment of guidelines requiring counseling staff to be trained in bereavement facilitation;
- Maintaining grief workshops where grievers are supported by other students who are bereaved;
- Sensitivity to cultural and developmental differences in grieving and mourning practices;
- Follow-up and program evaluation;
- Establishment of a center on campus that focuses on bereavement research, intervention, and education.

Envisioning, designing, organizing, and implementing a bereavement program must reflect the needs of the students and be championed by the college. It is also important that all members of the campus community be proactive and knowledgeable of the services available to bereaved students; a simple gesture such as pointing a grieving student in the right direction for assistance shows care and compassion. A struggling student burdened with grief can be lifted by a singular act of kindness:

> *I would really appreciate any suggestions you could make, and with some names and numbers, would obviously be more than willing to try and set something up myself. Thank you so much for your help!* (male graduate student)

Donna M. Burns, PhD, holds a doctorate in Educational Psychology and is an educator, author, and consultant. She is a professor in the Department of Educational and School Psychology at The College of Saint Rose, Albany, New York. She teaches courses in developmental psychology and specializes in issues of grief and loss. She has designed and taught undergraduate and graduate courses in death, dying, and bereavement and conducts seminars and workshops for school districts, institutions, and non-profit organizations. She has presented papers on various aspects of grief and loss at local, regional, national and international conferences and has created a conceptual framework that examines the multi-faceted nature of responses to loss. Dr. Burns coordinates and oversees the children's program for the annual New York State Police Survivor's Tribute Weekend and provides educational training and support to bereaved military families. She is the author of the book, When kids are grieving: Addressing grief and loss in school (Corwin Press, 2010).

REFERENCES

Balk, D. E. (2008). Grieving: 22 to 30 percent of all college students. *New Directions for Student Services, 21,* 5-14. doi: 10.1002/ss.262

Balk, D. E., Walker, A. C., & Baker, A. (2010). Prevalence and severity of college student bereavement examined in a randomly selected sample. *Death Studies, 34,* 459-468.

Battle, C. L., Greer, J. A., Ortiz-Hernandez, S., & Todd, D. M. (2013). Developing and implementing a bereavement support program for college students. *Death Studies, 37,* 362-382.

Burns, D. M. (2010). *When kids are grieving: Addressing grief and loss in school.* Thousand Oaks, CA: Corwin Press.

Cooley, E., Toray, T., & Roscoe, L. (2010). Reactions to loss scale: Assessing grief in college students. *Omega, 61,* 25-51.

Doka, K. J. (1989). *Disenfranchised grief: Recognizing hidden sorrow.* Lexington, MA: Lexington Books.

Doka, K. J. (Ed.). (2002). *Disenfranchised grief: New directions, challenges, and strategies for practice.* Champaign, IL: Research Press.

Fajgenbaum, D., Chesson, B., & Lanzi, R. G. (2012). Building a network of grief support on college campuses: A national grassroots initiative. *Journal of College Student Psychotherapy, 26,* 99-120.

Field, T., Diego, M., Pelaez, M., Deeds, O., & Delgado, J. (2009). Breakup distress in university students. *Adolescence, 44,* 705-727.

Grant, A. (n.d.) Anne Grant quotes. Retrieved from http://evi.com/q/what_did_anne_grant_say

Hardison, H. G., Neimeyer, R. A., & Lichstein, K. L. (2005). Insomnia and complicated grief symptoms in bereaved college students. *Behavioral Sleep Medicine, 3,* 99-111.

Hedman, A. S. (2012). Faculty's empathy and academic support for grieving students. *Death Studies, 36,* 914-931.

McCusker, K. M., & Witherow, L. B. (2012). Bereavement on the college campus: Establishing an effective ritual for the classroom and beyond. *About Campus/March-April.* doi: 10.1002/abc.21068

Neimeyer, R. A., Laurie, A., Mehta, T., Hardison, H., & Currier, J. M. (2008). Lessons of loss: Meaning-making in bereaved college students. *New Directions for Student Services, 121,* doi: 10.1002/ss.264

Pennington, N. (2013). You don't de-friend the dead: An analysis of grief communication by college students through Facebook profiles. *Death Studies, 37,* 617-635.

Servaty-Seib, H. L., & Taub, D. J. (2008). Training faculty members and resident assistants to respond to bereaved students. *New Directions for Student Services, 121.* doi: 10.1002/ss.266

Schnider, K. R., Elhari, J. D., & Gray, M. J. (2007). Coping style use predicts posttraumatic stress and complicated grief symptom severity among college students reporting a traumatic loss. *Journal of Counseling Psychology, 54,* 344-350.

Taub, D. J., & Servaty-Seib, H. L. (2008). Developmental and contextual perspectives on bereaved college students. *New Directions for Student Services, 121.* doi: 10.1002/ss.263

Tedrick Parikh, S. J., & Servaty-Seib, H. L. (2013). College students' beliefs about supporting a grieving peer. *Death Studies, 37,* 653-669.

Vickio, C. J. (2008). Designing and conducting grief workshops for college students. *New Directions for Student Services,* 121. doi: 10.1002/ss.265

Wandel, T. L. (2009). Online empathy: Communicating via Facebook to bereaved college students. *Journal of New Communications Research, 4,* 42-52.

CHAPTER 17

Bibliotherapy with Adolescents

Charles A. Corr

This chapter explores the use of bibliotherapy with adolescents and offers guidelines for such activities. In turn, this chapter covers: the meaning and nature of bibliotherapy; some comments on adolescents who are coping with death-related situations; principles for bibliotherapy with adolescents; a case in point for validation and guidance; and selected examples of useful books for bibliotherapy with adolescents grouped under topical headings.

BIBLIOTHERAPY

In the first edition of his book, *Grief Counseling and Grief Therapy*, Worden (1982) introduced an important and useful distinction between "grief counseling," understood as helping interventions for facilitating coping with uncomplicated grief, and "grief therapy," described as specialized techniques to help people with abnormal or complicated grief reactions. This distinction points to some differences in ways the word "therapy" and its analogues are used. Strictly speaking, *therapy* is a treatment designed to alter or cure a deviant state of affairs. It applies, for example, to psychiatric interventions, psychotherapy, and therapy groups for those with mental problems. By contrast, the adjective *therapeutic* has a much broader range of application, including remedial, restorative, or beneficial forms of support for those who are dealing with difficult, but not abnormal life situations. Worden's understanding of grief counseling is an example of a therapeutic intervention, but one that does not rise to the level of formal therapy.

Confusingly, many forms of what Worden might call "counseling" are today designated by some as forms of "therapy." Examples include art therapy, music therapy, play therapy, and bibliotherapy. But bibliotherapy is not normally intended for those coping with abnormal reactions to life-threatening illnesses, dying, or bereavement. On the contrary, bibliotherapy is an intervention that employs books to try to help individuals whose life situations may be unusual among their everyday experiences but are not abnormal. Coping with anticipated death or postdeath bereavement is a difficult experience for many adolescents, one that may not be familiar to most. However, it does not represent a psychiatric illness and may be helped by companioning, befriending, and support of many types.

This chapter explores one type of that support, an intervention that uses books to offer assistance to individual adolescents or groups of adolescents who are coping with death-related situations. More specifically, Berns (2004, p. 324) defined bibliotherapy as "the use of any kind of literature by a skilled adult or other interested person in an effort to normalize . . . grief reactions to loss, support constructive coping, reduce feelings of isolation, and reinforce creativity and problem solving."

Some people may think that contemporary adolescents no longer read books, but that is incorrect. Many of these young people are, indeed, familiar with books and can make use of them as tools in helping them cope with death-related challenges. They may find these books in hardcopy or paperback formats, or in electronic versions that can be read on computers, tablets, e-readers, or even smartphones. Furthermore, even adolescents who are digital natives may be willing to examine a traditional book if it is provided to them and they are shown the benefits it can offer.

ADOLESCENTS AND DEATH-RELATED SITUATIONS

For many—but certainly not all—contemporary adolescents, encountering a death-related situation is a rare occurrence, whether that involves their own life-threatening illness or the dying or death of someone close to them. Such lack of experience can add to or complicate challenges facing young people in a developmental period in which they are already struggling to establish a stable, personal identity. In our society, adolescence is an "in-between" or transitional period in human development between childhood and adulthood. It is a complex, evolving, and rather special developmental stage between the primary school years and the full recognition of adult status. Above all, adolescence is primarily a developmental period not directly congruent with the chronological markers of the teenage years. Not surprisingly, when death intervenes in the real world of an adolescent, in contrast with the fantasized realms of the entertainment media, that can present real challenges to what Erikson (1963) described as the principal virtue to be achieved in healthy adolescent development: fidelity or faithfulness to self, to ideals, and to others. Adolescence need not be characterized as a period of "storm and stress," turbulence and difficulties; established research has shown that "by and large good coping and a smooth transition into adulthood are much more typical than the opposite" (Offer & Sabshin, 1984, p. 101).

Nevertheless, adolescents do experience encounters with death, sometimes in their own lives, more commonly among their grandparents, parents, other cherished adults, siblings or peers, and occasionally among pets or companion animals. When any of these death-related events happen, their consequences depend largely on a foundation of sound values and good coping skills laid down earlier in the lives of the affected adolescents, as well as the availability and quality of the support they receive during the event and in its aftermath. The single most important factor when adolescents actually face what has been called a "double crisis" in their lives, one that brings together a confrontation with death and their own ongoing developmental challenges, is support from others. Adolescents can and will cope with death-related situations in healthy ways. They are often resilient even in the face of traumatic loss if provided with the information they need, effective communication with and support from others around them, and opportunities to be involved in constructive ways in what is happening in the circumstances. In particular, adolescents with high self-concept and positive developmental maturity have been shown to be able to address difficult death-related situations in constructive ways. They will, of course, experience psychological distress and other personal grief reactions, but that upheaval can be relatively transient and they can even achieve positive personal growth through "more introspection and more reorganization and/or restructuring of life values and priorities" (Mathews & Servaty-Seib, 2007, p. 1999).

So how can bibliotherapy contribute to an adolescent's coping processes that are likely to be both continuous and intermittent while also involving an extended period of time?

Principles for Bibliotherapy with Adolescents

As a general rule, prior preparation is always preferable, both for an adolescent and for an adult who wishes to help. Laying down a good foundation in both personal belief systems and sound coping skills is always desirable. Beyond that, some general guidelines for adults who seek to help are:

- Strive to be aware of an adolescent's concerns, to validate those concerns, and to accept the adolescent's feelings as real, important, and normal.
- Employ active listening, especially to the feelings underlying what is being said.
- Avoid efforts to solve the adolescent's problems; instead, help the adolescent to find his or her own solutions.
- Provide frequent opportunities to talk together and address issues in safe environments.

In using death-related books with adolescents, adults who seek to function as guides in the bibliotherapy process will benefit from adherence to the following specific principles:

- Evaluate the book yourself before attempting to use it with an individual adolescent or a group of adolescents; no resource suits every reader or every purpose.
- Select resources, topics, and approaches that correspond to the needs of the individual adolescent or group of adolescents, i.e., be purposeful.
- Be prepared to cope with limitations; every book like every other tool will have its own strengths and limitations.
- Match books to the capacities of the individual adolescent; this can relate to specific interests or situations, but it can also mean that some books may suit more advanced readers, while less challenging titles may work better for other individuals.
- Work along with individual adolescents, either by reading a book together or at least by discussing it together as often as seems appropriate; after all the book is only a vehicle or a catalyst for the interactive process that is the real aim of bibliotherapy

Validation and Guidance: A Case In Point

One book written by a 16-year-old author after the death of her father to cancer, *Weird Is Normal When Teenagers Grieve* (Wheeler, 2010), can serve both as a source of validation for bereaved adolescents and as a useful guide for adult helpers. As validation, this book confirms the wide range of grief reactions that adolescents often experience in anticipation of, or in the wake of, a significant loss in their lives. The author acknowledges the individuality of both grief and mourning during the adolescent years, as well as the varied and creative ways in which adolescents may express their grief. Wheeler correctly accepts the reality of "grief attacks" that occur in their own time and ways. She also affirms that, while life may never be the same after an important personal loss, there can be hope for better times ahead and it is possible to maintain continuing bonds with the person who died. While all of this may seem "weird" to some adults, all that means is that adolescents are likely to grieve in ways that are different from those of many adults. The standard of normality for adolescents is not to mimic adults, but to cope effectively with their losses and their grief reactions, while also finding constructive ways to go forward in healthy living.

As a guide for adult helpers, *Weird Is Normal When Teenagers Grieve* points out that adolescents have every right to walk their own paths in grief, that no loss is too small if it is significant to a particular adolescent, and that no adolescent has to grieve according to some adult's timetable or come to what someone else regards as a "suitable" outcome. Adults need to relax overly-strict expectations of when and how adolescents should react and respond to a major loss in their lives. Beyond that, adults can help adolescents see the value of reaching out to others in counseling relationships, support groups, and bibliotherapy.

These and other modalities facilitate building bonds with others who can help, but they have to be acceptable to the individual adolescent. In particular, perceptive adults can reach out to adolescents who may be overlooked when others around them are caught up in their own grief or when others don't know what to say or do to help. Sharing stories from books about bereavement can help adolescents open up when loss seems overwhelming or when some are afraid to show their grief. Venting in a safe context and with a trusted person can help relieve isolation and the pressures of trying to keep it all in, something that is never really possible or healthy in the long run.

SELECTED EXAMPLES OF BOOKS FOR BIBLIOTHERAPY WITH ADOLESCENTS

Numerous books can serve as useful tools for bibliotherapy with adolescents, from classics to more contemporary offerings. In this section, selected examples of such books are grouped around topical headings. Additional information about each of these books appears in the Appendix to this chapter. More information and other titles can be found in the appendices to *Death & Dying, Life & Living* (Corr & Corr, 2013, pp. 669-699). Note also that while only the original publication date is given in the text of this chapter, several of these books have had additional editions or been republished many times.

Although a number of these books were published many years ago, they remain compelling and useful resources because of their descriptions of grief and how they speak to young people. Interestingly, some recent books deal openly and directly with teenagers, illness, and grief, such as *The Fault in Our Stars* by John Green, (Dutton, 2012), which follows the friendship between two teens who meet in a cancer support group. But it can be argued that even some of the most popular young adult book series in the past few years, such as the *Harry Potter* series by J.K. Rowling and the *Hunger Games* series by Suzanne Collins, have underlying themes of parental loss and the impact that the bereavement process has as adolescents face life, even in a fantastical world. While these books might not seem obvious choices to use with bereaved adolescents, it can be useful to meet young people where they are by utilizing books that are popular with this developmental group. Such books can open up conversations that deal directly with the impact of death and grief.

Grief

This is a very broad topical heading, one that often overlaps with those that follow. While many books listed here were published many years ago, the classic stories and themes still resonate. *Beat the Turtle Drum* (Greene, 1976) describes multiple, different grief reactions in a loving family when one member suffers an accidental death. By contrast, *Annie and the Sand Dobbies* (Coburn, 1964) is a story in which elf-like characters called "sand dobbies" help a boy find solace in his grief arising from the deaths of both his young sister and his runaway dog. Comfort does not come easily in Judy Blume's *Tiger Eyes* (1981) when a young girl, her mother, and her younger brother try unsuccessfully to cope with their grief by physically relocating after their father/husband is killed. Eventually, they realize they need to face their losses directly by moving back home and working together to rebuild their lives. *Winter Holding Spring* (Dragonwagon, 1990) describes the great pain another girl and her father experience after the death of the mother/spouse. As they share their experiences and memories, however, they come to the realization that "nothing just *ends* without beginning the next thing at the same time" (p. 11).

Other books about grief for adolescents include: *Dicey's Song* (Voigt, 1982), in which a 13-year-old girl abandoned by her father and her institutionalized mother must hold things together for her three younger siblings and Gram; *A Grief Observed* (Lewis, 1976), based on the notebook jottings in which a world-renowned author wrote out his grief following the death of his wife; *Say Goodnight, Gracie* (Deaver, 1988), in which a girl is so disoriented when a drunken driver kills her close friend that she can hardly function until a wise aunt helps lead her to more constructive coping; and Pearl Buck's classic, *The Big Wave* (1948), in which a boy loses his entire family to a tidal wave only to realize after many years that loss is universal and inevitable: "To live in the presence of death makes us brave and strong" (p. 54), and "life is stronger than death" (p. 86). Finally, an unusual collection of short stories, *ZEBRA and Other Stories* (Potok, 1988), offers six different scenarios each describing a young person facing grief, trauma, and change.

All but the Lewis book in the previous two paragraphs are fictional portraits of grief, although their messages are no less real. Several books, however, reproduce or reflect the views of bereaved youngsters: *How It Feels When a Parent Dies* (Krementz, 1981); *Losing Someone You Love: When a Brother or Sister Dies* (Richter, 1986); *Teenagers Face to Face with Bereavement* (Gravelle & Haskins, 1989); *Death Is Hard to Live With: Teenagers and How They Cope with Death* (Bode, 1993); and *Flowers for the Ones You've Known: Unedited Letters from Bereaved Teens* (Traisman & Sieff, 1995).

There are also many books written by adults that offer advice to adolescents as to how they might cope with death-related situations. For those, see Corr and Corr, 2013, pp. 669-699. Finally, one unique book is aimed at children but will serve many adolescents and some adults equally well: *What Does That Mean? A Dictionary of Death, Dying and Grief Terms for Grieving Children and Those Who Love Them* (Smith & Johnson, 2006).

Grandparents

Deaths of grandparents are, perhaps, the most frequent type of death that most adolescents encounter. As such, they are the subject of books like: *So Long, Grandpa* (Donnelly, 1981); *Blackberries in the Dark* (Jukes, 1985); *The Last Dance* (Deedy, 1995); and *Sun and Spoon* (Henkes, 1997).

Parents

The power of the dying and/or death of a parent or substitute parent figure on the life of an adolescent is undeniable. It is portrayed in James Agee's Pulitzer Prize-winning novel, *A Death in the Family* (1969), when the aftermath of the accidental death of their father is not easy for two young children to accept without much help from the adults around them; in *There Are Two Kinds of Terrible* (Mann, 1977) when a boy and his "cold fish" father initially find it difficult to share their grief; in the sad portrait of two children who only learn that their father is dying by overhearing adult conversations in *Mama's Going to Buy You a Mockingbird* (Little, 1984); in *With You and Without You* (Martin, 1986) when four children struggle to cope when their father is told he will die soon as a result of an inoperable heart condition; in the grief that a child experiences after the death of her beloved foster mother in *Missing May* (Rylant, 1992); in the extreme disorientation experienced by one young girl in *Daddy's Climbing Tree* (Adler, 1993) who cannot believe her father is really dead; in the confusion initially experienced by a boy in *Black Jack Jetty: A Boy's Journey Through Grief* (Carestio, 2010) after his father is killed on active duty in Afghanistan and he is relocated to spend a summer with members of his dad's family whom he doesn't know; and when a girl learns that her mother has an incurable form of cancer in *Never Blame the Umpire* (Fehler, 2010).

Siblings and friends

Relationships with brothers or sisters and friends can take many forms. In some cases, the aftermath of the death of such a person can be puzzling or challenging as shown in *Ordinary People* (Guest, 1976); *Mick Harte Was Here* (Park, 1995); *Olive's Ocean* (Henkes, 2003); and *Sunflower Promise* (Hemery, 2005). In some cases, like *Ghost Brother* (Adler, 1990) and *Last Left Standing* (Russell, 1996), when older brothers are killed accidentally, their younger siblings try desperately to live up to their memory or find it problematical to go back to the way things were before. By contrast, *A Taste of Blackberries* (Smith,

1973) and *Bridge to Terabithia* (Paterson, 1977) both depict children who eventually find positive outcomes after the deaths of their friends. Unique historical reports in *Children of the Paper Crane* (Nasu, 1991) and *One Thousand Paper Cranes* (Takayuki, 2001), tell about a Japanese girl and her peers before and after her death from "A-bomb disease."

Life-threatening illness

Struggles with illness and dying in which adolescents are personally or closely involved (in addition to those noted earlier) are described in the words of young people themselves in: *Too Old to Cry, Too Young to Die* (Pendleton, 1980); *How It Feels to Fight for Your Life* (Krementz, 1989); and *Be a Friend: Children Who Live With HIV Speak* (Wiener, Best, & Pizzo, 1994). A father records his son's brave struggles with a fatal illness in *Death Be Not Proud* (Gunther, 1949). As well, sensitive novelists fill out the picture in: *A Season In-Between* (Greenberg, 1979); *Hunter in the Dark* (Hughes, 1984); and *Sky Memories* (Brisson, 1999). An exceptional piece of world literature worth mentioning here is *The Death of Ivan Ilych* (Tolstoy, 1960), in which a grave illness gradually leads a man to a growing appreciation of his own mortality and an awareness of how many one-time friends are gradually withdrawing from him, leaving only one servant and his young son who treat him with real compassion and candor.

Suicide

Suicide is a topic of great interest to many adolescents, puzzling in its apparent rejection of many common values, the sense of desperation often implied, and the wish that more help could have been offered to avert a fatal outcome. Many books for adolescents address this subject. They include: *Grover* (Cleaver & Cleaver, 1970); *Tunnel Vision* (Arrick, 1980); *The Sunday Doll* (Shura, 1988); and *Tears of a Tiger* (Draper, 1994), which communicates its story without any narrative. Three among many books that take a more analytic or didactic approach include: *Too Young to Die: Youth and Suicide* (Klagsbrun, 1976); *Dead End: A Book about Suicide* (Langone, 1986); and *Living when a Young Friend Commits Suicide—Or Even Starts Talking About It* (Grollman & Malikow, 1999).

Pets and companion animals

Adolescents often form close bonds with pets or companion animals. This can teach them important lessons about what is involved in caring for a living thing, but it can also mean that they are likely to encounter the death of animals that have shorter lifespans than a human. Situations like this are described in: *The Black Dog Who Went Into the Woods* (Hurd, 1980) when a boy tells other members of his family that his dog must have gone off alone to die; in *The Comeback Dog* (Thomas, 1980) when a boy believes his parents don't seem to care very much when his dog dies and when he takes in a stray dog who doesn't become his friend in the same way as the previous dog; and in *The Bravest Thing* (Napoli, 1995) when a girl experiences the deaths of almost every one of the babies born to her pet rabbit in the midst of other personal and family challenges.

For adolescents who can draw support from historical perspectives, four classic books tell about youngsters who experience the serious injury or death of a pet or companion animal in the midst of other family challenges: *The Yearling* (Rawlings, 1939); *Old Yeller* (Gipson, 1956); *Where the Red Fern Grows: The Story of Two Dogs and a Boy* (Rawls, 1961); and *Sounder* (Armstrong, 1969). Finally, perhaps the best known of all books about life, death, animals, and a young person is *Charlotte's Web* (White, 1952) in which a girl saves a pig named Wilbur from the butcher's knife with the help of amazing webs spun by a spider named Charlotte A. Caravatica whose legacies live on after her death in these accomplishments and in her offspring.

Activity books

These books take many forms and can be used in different ways with different adolescents. Most activity books encourage youngsters to draw or write on their pages in ways guided by specific themes. The goal is to help vent and process grief reactions to death-related events in safe and constructive ways. Some of these books describe therapeutic activities that go beyond the pages of the texts themselves. Others begin with a story that develops into a workbook with space devoted to creating a scrapbook or other form of memorial activity. Activity books with a specific focus on adolescents are: *The Last Goodbye II* (Boulden & Boulden, 1994); *Reactions: A Workbook to Help Young People Who are Experiencing Trauma and Grief* (Salloum, 1998); *A Teenager's Book About Suicide: Helping Break the Silence and Preventing Death* (Grollman & Johnson, 2001); and *Chill + Spill: A Place to Put It Down and Work It Out* (Lorig & Jacobs, 2005). Beyond these, *Remember Rafferty: A Book About the Death of a Pet . . . For*

Children of All Ages (Johnson, 1991) and *Anna's Scrapbook: Journal of a Sister's Love* (Aiken, 2001) both begin by describing a particular loss but then leave space for the reader to construct a memorial scrapbook to reinforce a continuing bond with the deceased individual. [Note that there is a larger group of activity books that focus more broadly on children but could be used purposefully with selected adolescents. For an annotated list of such books, see Corr & Corr, 2013, pp. 696-699.] Finally, *Fire in My Heart, Ice in My Veins: A Journal for Teenagers Experiencing a Loss* (Traisman, 1992) and *In My World: A Journal for Young People Facing Life-Threatening Illness* (Crawford & Lazar, 1999) provide prompts to encourage adolescents to make a record of their struggles with a death-related challenge.

Charles A. Corr, PhD, *is a member of the board of directors of Suncoast Hospice Institute, an affiliate of Suncoast Hospice in Clearwater, FL; the International Work Group on Death, Dying, and Bereavement; the Association for Death Education and Counseling; and the ChiPPS (Children's Project on Palliative/Hospice Services) E-Journal Work Group of the National Hospice and Palliative Care Organization. A frequent contributor to the Hospice Foundation of America's* Journeys: A Newsletter to Help in Bereavement, *Dr. Corr's publications include more than three dozen books and booklets, along with over 100 chapters and articles in professional journals. His most recent book is the seventh edition of* Death & Dying, Life & Living *(Wadsworth, 2013).*

REFERENCES

Berns, C. F. (2004). Bibliotherapy: Using books to help bereaved children. *Omega, Journal of Death and Dying, 48*, 321-336.

Corr, C. A. & Corr, D. M. (2013). *Death & dying, life & living* (7th ed.). Belmont, CA: Wadsworth.

Erikson, E. H. (1963). *Childhood and society* (2nd ed.). New York, NY: Norton.

Mathews, L. L., & Servaty-Seib, H. L. (2007). Hardiness and grief in a sample of bereaved college students. *Death Studies, 31*, 185-194.

Offer, D. & Sabshin, M. (1984). Adolescence: Empirical perspectives. In D. Offer & M. Sabshin (Eds.), *Normality and the life cycle: A critical integration* (pp. 76-107). New York, NY: Basic Books.

Worden, J. W. (1982). *Grief counseling and grief therapy: A handbook for the mental health practitioner* (1st ed.). New York, NY: Springer Publishing.

APPENDIX: BOOKS FOR USE WITH AND BY ADOLESCENT READERS

Adler, C. S. (1990). *Ghost Brother*. New York, NY: Houghton Mifflin. After his older brother and father both die in a car accident, 12-year-old Wally desperately wants to live up to his brother's memory. He seeks support and advice from the spirit of his ghost brother until he decides to enter a skateboarding contest in his brother's memory, which seems finally to meet his needs.

Adler, C. S. (1993). *Daddy's Climbing Tree*. New York, NY: Clarion. After her cat, Mimsy, is accidentally killed and the family moves from the only home 11-year-old Jessica had ever known, her father is killed in a road accident. Jessica refuses to believe he is really dead, but has no safe place to turn to avoid people and their expressions of sympathy. So she takes her 6-year-old brother and sets out to walk back to their old home where she thinks Daddy must be hiding in his favorite climbing tree. Only when she is high up in the tree does she finally accept that Daddy is dead and Mom truly does love her.

Agee, J. (1969). *A Death in the Family*. New York, NY: Bantam. This Pulitzer Prize-winning novel unerringly depicts the point of view of two children in Knoxville, Tennessee, in 1915 when they are told of the accidental death of their father. Agee skillfully portrays ways in which the children encounter unusual events, sense strange tensions within the family, struggle to understand what has happened, and strive to work out their implications with and often without the help of the adults around them.

Aiken, S. (2001). *Anna's Scrapbook: Journal of a Sister's Love*. Omaha, NE: Centering Corporation. The first six pages of this book tell a story about Anna and her little sister with whom she shared love and good times. One day, when Amelia had an accidental fall and died, Anna's grief was profound. After the funeral, Anna kept a diary, which fills the next 18 pages of this book. In the diary, Anna writes about her grief and describes a scrapbook she made of memories and photos of Amelia. Blank pages at the end of the book encourage a reader to make his or her own similar scrapbook.

Armstrong, W. (1969). *Sounder*. New York, NY: Harper & Row; often reprinted in paperback. Only the dog has a proper name in this tale of an African American sharecropper family in the late 19th century told from the point of view of the oldest son. After the father is arrested for stealing a ham to feed his family, their coon hound is shot and disappears. Angry and grieving, the son searches relentlessly for the dog and then for his father who is sent to hard labor in a prison camp. Eventually, the dog returns (but is too injured to hunt); later the father comes back (hurt by an explosion in the prison quarry), only to die shortly thereafter. The story captures a harsh life in hard times for people "born to lose."

Arrick, F. (1980). *Tunnel Vision*. Scarsdale, NY: Bradbury, Dell, 1981. After 15-year-old Anthony kills himself, his parents, sister, best friends, and teacher feel bewildered and guilty. They each ask what they might have done to prevent this awful event. Clues are evident in hindsight, but easy answers are not available. Anthony's suicide hurts everyone he loved. His mother asks, "Why did Anthony believe that death was the only kind of peace he could find?" (p. 173)

Blume, J. (1981). *Tiger Eyes*. Scarsdale, NY: Bradbury. After her father is killed during a holdup of his 7-Eleven store in Atlantic City, Davey (age 15), her mother, and her younger brother all react differently and are unable to help each other in their grief. Seeking solace, they decide to live temporarily with Davey's aunt. Only when Davey and her mother, first separately and then together, finally face the horrors of the night her father was killed are they able to make a decision to move back to New Jersey to go ahead with rebuilding their lives.

Bode, J. (1993). *Death Is Hard to Live With: Teenagers and How They Cope With Death*. New York, NY: Delacorte. Based on extensive interviews with teenagers and others, this book shows how teens experience death and how they can cope with their loss and their grief. The book mixes statements by teens, factual information from experts, cartoons, and pop art.

Boulden, J., & Boulden, J. (1994). *The Last Goodbye II*. Weaverville, CA: Boulden Publishing. This book offers exercises designed for adolescents at about grade levels 9-12 to process feelings and issues surrounding death. Topics like suicide and not acting in a destructive manner are also presented.

Brisson, P. (1999). *Sky Memories*. New York, NY: Delacorte. While her mother struggles with cancer and its treatments, 10-year-old Emily and Mom develop a ritual to celebrate and honor their relationship. Together they gather "sky memories," mental pictures of the ever-changing sky in all its variety and wonder, images that reflect both the phases of Mom's illness and the vitality of her soul.

Buck, P. S. (1948). *The Big Wave*. New York, NY: Scholastic. After a tidal wave kills his family and all the fishing people on the shore, Jiya chooses to live on the mountainside with his friend Kino's poor family instead of being adopted by a rich man. Later, Jiya marries Kino's sister and decides to move back to the seaside. Loss is universal and inevitable, but as Kino's father says, "To live in the presence of death makes us brave and strong" (p. 54) and "life is stronger than death" (p. 86).

Carestio, M. A. (2010). *Black Jack Jetty: A Boy's Journey Through Grief*. Washington, DC: Magination Press. Shortly after his father was killed on active duty in Afghanistan, Jack has many bad feelings. His mother takes him to spend the summer with his dad's family far away from their home. When people keep talking about his dad, Jack's aunt explains that they do this because they've been sad so long and need to think about happy memories. Playing with his cousins and searching for a famous treasure help Jack realize he is not a stranger; he belongs here in his father's old home connected to his dad and the family.

Cleaver, V., & Cleaver, G. (1970). *Grover*. Philadelphia, PA: Lippincott. When Grover was 11, his mother killed herself, thinking to "spare" herself and her family the ravages of her terminal illness. His father cannot face the facts of this death or the depth of his grief, so he tries to hold his feelings inside and convince his son it was an accident. Issues posed include whether one's chief duty is to endure life no matter what suffering it holds, whether religion is a comfort, and how one should deal with grief.

Coburn, J. B. (1964). *Annie and the Sand Dobbies: A Story About Death for Children and Their Parents*. New York, NY: Seabury Press. Key events in this novel occur when 11-year-old Danny encounters the deaths of both his toddler sister, Anne, from a respiratory infection and his dog, Bonnie, after he ran away from home and is found frozen to death. Earlier, a neighbor had introduced Danny to some imaginary characters called "sand dobbies" who are a little like elves or fairies. Later, he uses them to suggest that the deceased are safe with God.

Crawford, B. B., & Lazar, L. (1999). *In My World: A Journal for Young People Facing Life-Threatening Illness*. Omaha, NE: Centering Corporation. This 32-page journal is designed to help teenagers who are coping with a life-threatening illness make a record of their lives and give expression to thoughts, feelings, and worries they may find difficult to share with family members and friends.

Deaver, J. R. (1988). *Say Goodnight, Gracie*. New York, NY: Harper & Row. When her close friend is killed in an automobile accident, Morgan is so disoriented by the extent of her loss that she is unable to face her feelings, attend his funeral, or speak to his parents. Her parents are supportive and tolerate Morgan's withdrawal from the world, but only when a wise aunt intervenes is Morgan able to confront her feelings in a way that leads her to more constructive coping and to decide to go on with living.

Deedy, C. A. (1995). *The Last Dance*. Atlanta, GA: Peachtree. Ninny and Bessie enjoy a close friendship starting in childhood that extends throughout their lives together and even after Ninny's death. Before Ninny's grandfather died, they used to visit the graveyard with Oppa who taught them to tell stories, to sing, and to dance. After Oppa's death, the children pledge to each other that when one of them dies, the other will dance in the graveyard. They share a rich life together and their love endures even after death.

Donnelly, E. (1981). *So Long, Grandpa*. New York, NY: Crown. Ten-year-old Michael's close relationship with his grandfather is threatened because Grandpa has cancer and knows he only has a few weeks to live. In this story, Michael describes his grandfather's deterioration and eventual death, along with his own reactions to these events. He also tells about the way in which his grandfather had helped to prepare Michael by taking him to an elderly friend's funeral.

Dragonwagon, C. (1990). *Winter Holding Spring*. New York, NY: Atheneum/Simon & Schuster. At first, nothing is the same for 11-year-old Sarah and her father after her mother dies. Despite their pain, they gradually begin to share their experiences and their memories of Sarah's mother. Eventually, they come to realize that "nothing just *ends* without beginning the next thing at the same time" (p. 11). Each season somehow contains its successor; life and love and grief can continue together, for winter always holds spring.

Draper, S. M. (1994). *Tears of a Tiger*. New York, NY: Atheneum. Without any narrative, this book uses excerpts from official statements, newspaper articles, letters, diaries, homework, phone calls, and conversations to describe the aftermath of the death of Robert Washington, captain of the high school basketball team, in a fiery automobile accident. The car's driver, Andrew Jackson, cannot get over Rob's death and his feelings of guilt. Two other friends in the car do well, but Andy sinks gradually into a deeper and more desperate depression. Smiling on the surface, he offers lots of clues about his inner trauma, but his parents, friends, teachers, and even a psychologist do not realize what is happening until he eventually kills himself.

Fehler, G. (2010). *Never Blame the Umpire*. Grand Rapids, MI: Zonderkidz. Kate is 11 years old when she learns that her mother has an incurable form of cancer. Mama's illness and anticipated death overshadow all of Kate's varied activities. Kate struggles with her faith in God until Mama compares God to an umpire. Mama says we need umpires to control our games, so we shouldn't blame them even when they make mistakes. But Mama says God doesn't make mistakes, so we need to accept his decisions even when we don't understand or disagree with them. Kate is consoled by her faith and Mama's love.

Gipson, F. (1956). *Old Yeller*. New York, NY: Harper & Brothers; reissued by HarperTrophy, 1990. An ugly, yellow stray dog becomes a close companion of 14-year-old Travis in Texas in the late 1800s and saves some members of his family from various dangers. But when the dog is bitten by a rabid wolf, Travis must kill him.

Gravelle, K., & Haskins, C. (1989). *Teenagers Face to Face With Bereavement*. New York, NY: Julian Messner. This book explores the unique qualities of adolescent grief by drawing on the experiences of 17 teens who have experienced the deaths of parents, siblings, and friends. Topics include what happens at the time of death, feelings after the numbness wears off, putting the family back together, and moving on.

Greenberg, J. (1979). *A Season In-Between*. New York, NY: Farrar. Carrie Singer, a seventh grader, copes with the diagnosis of her father's cancer in spring and his death that summer. She draws on a rabbinical teaching that recommends turning scratches on a jewel into a beautiful design.

Greene, C. C. (1976). *Beat the Turtle Drum.* New York, NY: Viking; Puffin, 1994. This book describes a warm, loving family that is flooded with grief when 11-year-old Joss is unexpectedly killed in a fall from a tree. Conveying this sense of the many dimensions of bereavement is the book's strong point.

Grollman, E., & Johnson, J. (2001). *A Teenager's Book About Suicide: Helping Break the Silence and Preventing Death.* Omaha, NE: Centering Corporation. The topic of suicide is introduced here through brief text passages in boxes and spaces for readers to comment. The book includes writings by teens who have considered suicide or been affected by someone else's suicide, along with advice designed to dispel myths about this subject. Danger signals and warning signs are identified, and guidance is offered as to what a teen might do if he or she suspects someone is thinking about suicide.

Grollman, E., & Malikow, M. (1999). *Living When a Young Friend Commits Suicide—Or Even Starts Talking About It.* Boston, MA: Beacon Press. This book is intended to help adolescents by guiding them through typical reactions and questions after a friend dies by suicide. It offers suggestions for how to cope and how to help suicidal people. Also addressed are religious questions, popular misconceptions about suicide, and getting on with one's life. A final chapter lists helpful resources.

Guest, J. (1976). *Ordinary People.* New York, NY: Viking; Penguin, 1982. Readers gradually learn that a 17-year-old boy has many problems after his older brother drowns in a boating accident. Conrad's grief is compounded by the guilt he feels for not saving the life of his sibling. An overprotective father and a distant mother are little help, but a therapist eventually helps Conrad realize that he is not to blame for his brother's death just because he lived through the accident.

Gunther, J. (1949). *Death Be Not Proud: A Memoir.* New York, NY: Harper. Johnny Gunther was 15 when he was diagnosed with a brain tumor; he died 15 months later. Here his father describes Johnny's courageous struggle, alongside his parents and physicians, to maintain as much of a normal life as possible in the face of an incurable disease.

Hemery, K. M. (2005). *Sunflower Promise*. Omaha, NE: Centering Corporation. Willow and Davy are best friends in a small town in Ohio in 1948. One day as they are teasing, Davy accidentally tears the big, floppy, cloth sunflower off Willow's lovely new hat. She is furious and won't play with Davy any more even though he promises he will make it up to her some day. After Willow punches Davy on the arm, she is regretful when his bruises don't go away and he has to go to the hospital for testing. Will he never get better? Did she cause it? In the end, Davy dies, but not before arranging a surprise for Willow to fulfill his promise: a gorgeous crop of sunflowers in the field where they used to play.

Henkes, K. (1997). *Sun and Spoon*. New York, NY: Greenwillow Books; Puffin, 1998. Shortly after the death of his grandmother, 10-year-old "Spoon" Gilmore is searching for something special of hers to keep. At his grandfather's house, Spoon finds the deck of cards that Gram used in playing games with him and Pa; without asking, Spoon takes the deck. Spoon learns later that the same cards also are a source of solace to Pa; when Spoon returns the cards, Pa takes their reappearance as a sign from Gram. Spoon also discovers other items that seem to be special signs that he shares with Pa

Henkes, K. (2003). *Olive's Ocean*. New York, NY: Greenwillow; HarperTrophy, 2005. After a girl is killed by a car while riding her bicycle, her mother delivers a page from her journal to 12-year-old Martha in which Olive had written about her three hopes: to become a writer; to see a real ocean; and to become friends with Martha, "the nicest person in my whole entire class" (p. 5). Martha is puzzled because she hardly knew Olive. Coincidentally, Martha also secretly wants to be a writer and the next day her family is off to visit her grandmother at the ocean. When Martha decides to bring a small jar of seawater back to Olive's mother, she has a near-drowning experience (death can happen to anyone at any time).

Hughes, M. (1984). *Hunter in the Dark*. New York, NY: Atheneum. A boy with overprotective parents sets out to face life and death on his own by confronting threats at different levels: his leukemia and the challenge of going hunting in the Canadian woods for the first time.

Hurd, E. T. (1980). *The Black Dog Who Went Into the Woods*. New York, NY: Harper & Row. One day, Benjamin tells the disbelieving members of his family that their dog must have gone into the woods to die. Eventually Benjamin says: "I don't think we should look for Black Dog anymore . . . Black Dog doesn't want us to look for her" (p. 11). Father agrees: "Benjamin understands better than any of us. Animals sometimes do go into the woods, or someplace, by themselves when they know it is time for them to die" (p. 14). Later, each family member has a special dream about an event they shared with Black Dog

Johnson, J. (1991). *Remember Rafferty: A Book About the Death of a Pet . . . For Children of All Ages*. Omaha, NE: Centering Corporation; rev. ed., 1998. Rafferty is a sheepdog who becomes ill and has to be euthanized. A neighbor, Miss Bertie, who lives with Rafferty's friend, a cat named Four-Eyes, helps by sharing stories of the deaths of other pets and validating the importance of such losses. The book also contains two pages of suggestions for adults and eight pages for a memorial scrapbook.

Jukes, M. (1985). *Blackberries in the Dark*. New York, NY: Dell Yearling. Everything seems so different now when Austin visits the farm after Grandpa died. In previous summers, Austin and Grandpa would do things together, like go fishing or pick blackberries in the dark. This summer, Austin had looked forward to Grandpa teaching him to fly fish. Still, when Grandma joins Austin at the stream, they help each other learn to fly fish, pick blackberries, and begin their own new traditions.

Klagsbrun, F. (1976). *Too Young to Die: Youth and Suicide*. New York, NY: Houghton Mifflin; paperback edition by Pocket Books, 1977. A clear, informed, and readable introduction to the myths and realities surrounding youth suicide, with useful advice for helpers.

Krementz, J. (1981). *How It Feels When a Parent Dies*. Boston, MA: Little, Brown; republished by Knopf, 1981, 2004. Eighteen children and adolescents (7–16 years old) describe their reactions to the death of a parent and subsequent events. Photos of the authors accompany each essay.

Krementz, J. (1989). *How It Feels to Fight For Your Life*. Boston, MA: Little, Brown; paperback by Simon & Schuster, 1991. Fourteen children and adolescents (7–16 years old) describe their struggles with life-threatening or life-limiting conditions. Photos of the authors accompany each essay.

Langone, J. (1986). *Dead End: A Book About Suicide*. Boston, MA: Little, Brown. A medical reporter explores the subject of suicide in detail for mature young readers.

Lewis, C. S. (1976). *A Grief Observed*. New York, NY: Bantam. The author is well known for books like *Out of the Silent Planet* and *The Lion, the Witch, and the Wardrobe*. When his wife died, Lewis recorded his experiences of grief on notebooks lying around the house. The published result is an unusual and extraordinary document, a direct and honest expression of one man's grief that has helped innumerable readers by normalizing their own experiences in bereavement.

Little, J. (1984). *Mama's Going to Buy You a Mockingbird*. New York, NY: Viking Kestrel. Jeremy and his younger sister only learn their father is dying from cancer by overhearing people talk about it. They experience many losses, large and small, that accompany his dying and death, often compounded by lack of information and control over their situation. Their need for support from others is clear.

Lorig, S., & Jacobs, J. (2005). *Chill + Spill: A Place to Put It Down and Work It Out*. Seattle, WA: Art with Heart. This book is a therapeutic journal for teens and tweens. Colorful pages introduce 20 activities, each followed by blank pages to provide ways for self-expression in a creative (yet structured), comfortable (yet challenging) manner. Goals are to foster meaningful connections with caregivers, increase self-awareness and self-expression, enhance ability to manage emotions and stress, and make healthy, positive choices.

Mann, P. (1977). *There Are Two Kinds of Terrible*. New York, NY: Doubleday/Avon. Robbie's broken arm is one kind of terrible, but it ends. His mother's death leaves Robbie and his "cold fish" father without any ending. They are together, but each grieves alone until they find ways to share their suffering and their memories.

Martin, A. M. (1986). *With You and Without You*. New York, NY: Holiday House; paperback by Scholastic. Family members struggle when the father is told that he will die soon from an inoperable heart condition. Before his death, each member of the family tries to make the father's remaining time as good as possible; afterward, each strives to cope with his or her losses. Two lessons emerge: no one is ever completely prepared for a death, and each individual must cope in his or her own way.

Napoli, D. J. (1995). *The Bravest Thing*. New York, NY: Dutton Children's Books; Scholastic, 2003. Even after Laurel's pet rabbit dies, she fights to get a new rabbit and arrange for her to breed. When a second litter is born and Bun Bun won't nurse, Laurel feeds the babies by hand and manages to save one of them while the other five die. Laurel learns that Mom's lengthy telephone calls with her sister are because Aunt Lizzie is being treated for bronchial cancer. Laurel is constantly reminded of the mortality of all living things.

Nasu, M. (1991). *Children of the Paper Crane: The Story of Sadako Sasaki and Her Struggle With the A-Bomb Disease.* Armonk, NY: M. E. Sharpe. Sadako was two years old when the atomic bomb exploded over Hiroshima; she died of radiation-induced leukemia 10 years later. Her story was first popularized in English in a book for children, *Sadako and the Thousand Paper Cranes* (Putnam's, 1977). It inspired a monument in Hiroshima Peace Memorial Park to honor all the children who died from radiation poisoning. This book is the first detailed account of Sadako's life, her family and classmates, her disease, and the grassroots movement to erect a memorial and make paper cranes as a peace symbol. (See I. Takayuki in this Appendix for a parallel version of this story.)

Park, B. (1995). *Mick Harte Was Here.* New York, NY: Knopf; Random House & Scholastic, 1996. Thirteen-year-old Phoebe recalls her younger brother, Mick, who died when he was hit by a truck while riding his bicycle without a helmet. Phoebe argued with Mick that morning; she describes memories of her relationship with Mick and her profound grief after his death. She very much wants to know where Mick is now; eventually she decides that if Mick is with God (as people keep saying) and God is everywhere, then Mick is everywhere, too.

Paterson, K. (1977). *Bridge to Terabithia.* New York, NY: HarperCollins. Jess and Leslie have a special, secret meeting place in the woods, called Terabithia. But when Leslie is killed one day in an accidental fall, the magic of their play and friendship is disrupted. Jess mourns the loss of this special relationship, is supported by his family, and at last is able to initiate new relationships that will share friendship in a similar way with others.

Pendleton, E. (Comp.). (1980). *Too Old to Cry, Too Young to Die.* Nashville, TN: Thomas Nelson. Thirty-five teens and young adults describe their experiences in living with cancer, including treatments, side effects, and interactions with hospitals, parents, siblings, and friends.

Potok, C. (1998). *ZEBRA and Other Stories.* New York, NY: Knopf. This collection of six stories for young readers focuses on youngsters facing loss, grief, trauma, and change. "Zebra," a nickname for Adam

Martin Zebrin, is positively influenced by an art teacher who has experienced loss; "B.B." is a girl facing the death of her little brother, the birth of a new sibling, and her dad's threat to leave; "Moon" has anger management problems but is touched by a the death of a boy in her community; "Nava," whose dad's life was saved by a comrade after a firefight in Vietnam, must defend herself against difficult schoolmates; "Isabel" struggles with intrusive dreams after her father and little brother are tragically killed in a car accident and further challenged a year later when her mother announces that she will remarry; and "Max" whose experiences are overshadowed by stories about his Uncle Max who died in Vietnam.

Rawlings, M. K. (1939). *The Yearling*. New York, NY: Charles Scribner's Sons; 50th anniversary ed.: New York: Simon Pulse/Simon & Schuster, 1988. This Pulitzer Prize-winning novel is a tale of a boy and his parents eking out a bare subsistence living in rural Florida in the early 20th century where the struggle to survive overrides everything else. Above all, young Jody wants a pet, something of his very own, and finds this in an orphaned fawn. Death-related events in Jody's life are numerous.

Rawls, W. (1961). *Where the Red Fern Grows: The Story of Two Dogs and a Boy*. Garden City, NY: Doubleday; reissued by Random House, 1997. Billy Colman saves for two years to get $50 to buy two registered coonhound pups. He trains them and they hunt raccoons together in the Ozarks of northeastern Oklahoma. There are numerous instances of hunting and killing coons, including one in which a boy trips, falls on an axe, and dies. After Billy buries one of his dogs, the other refuses food and dies at her sibling's grave. The money the dogs have earned enables the family to leave the hills, but as they depart they are comforted by the sight of a sacred red fern that has grown up at the dogs' gravesite.

Richter, E. (1986). *Losing Someone You Love: When a Brother or Sister Dies*. New York, NY: Putnam's. In their own words, 16 adolescents and young adults describe their reactions to a wide variety of experiences of sibling death. Photos of the authors accompany most of the essays.

Russell, B. T. (1996). *Last Left Standing*. Boston, MA: Houghton Mifflin; Puffin Books, 1998. After his older brother Toby is killed by a train, it's almost as if Josh is "in another dimension" (as a friend tells him). When Josh finds a cabin in the woods and meets people there who had known Toby, he does not tell them about Toby's death. Then he cannot tell his parents about the cabin and the lies pile up so quickly that it is almost impossible to keep up with them.

Rylant, C. (1992). *Missing May*. New York, NY: Orchard Books; Scholastic, 2003. After 6-year-old Summer's mother dies, no one really wants her. Eventually, Uncle Ob and Aunt May take her into their rusty old trailer; but when Summer is 12 May dies suddenly, and Summer and Ob have a very hard time coping. In the end, a memory of May opens the floodgates and Summer cries her heart out. That catharsis and Ob's love reminds them that May will always be with them.

Salloum, A. (1998). *Reactions: A Workbook to Help Young People Who are Experiencing Trauma and Grief*. Omaha, NE: Centering Corporation. This workbook allows young people to describe their loss and grief experiences and their implications at their own pace. The text offers prompts for writing, drawing, and answering questions. The book seeks to legitimize different reactions people may have to loss and to lead eventually to a reflection on what has been learned from these exercises as one moves into the future.

Shura, M. F. (1988). *The Sunday Doll*. New York, NY: Dodd, Mead. Thirteen-year-old Emily's parents exclude her from something terrible involving her older sister (which turns out to be the suicide of a boyfriend) by sending her off to visit Aunt Harriet in Missouri. Through these challenges, Emily gradually learns she has strengths of her own and, like the doll, can choose which face to present to the world.

Smith, D.B. (1973). *A Taste of Blackberries*. New York, NY: HarperCollins; paperback, HarperTrophy, 1988. Jamie is a showoff who loves surprises and playing tricks like stealing an apple from a farmer's yard or running on a forbidden lawn. One day he pokes a stick into a bee hive, is stung, and dies from an allergic reaction. Afterwards, his best friend (the book's unnamed narrator) reflects on this upsetting event: Did it really happen or is it just another of Jamie's pranks? Could it have been prevented? Is it disloyal to go on living when Jamie is dead?

Smith, H. I., & Johnson, J. (2006). *What Does That Mean? A Dictionary of Death, Dying and Grief Terms for Grieving Children and Those Who Love Them*. Omaha, NE: Centering Corporation. It is important to find the right words to use when talking with children and adolescents, especially when the subjects involve loss and death. This book identifies 71 key terms, explains how to pronounce each of them and what they mean, and offers guidance about how to use them in talking about death.

Takayuki, I. (2001). *One Thousand Paper Cranes: The Story of Sadako and the Children's Peace Statue.* New York, NY: Dell Laurel Leaf. This book retells the famous story, supplemented by drawings, photos, and other background information about the atomic bombing that eventually led to Sadako's death and the memorial erected in her memory. (See also Nasu in this Appendix for a parallel account.)

Thomas, J. R. (1980). *The Comeback Dog.* New York, NY: Houghton Mifflin/Clarion. A nine-year-old boy is angry because his dog died recently and his parents don't seem to care as much as he does. When he finds a dirty, wet, raggedy dog that is barely breathing, Daniel takes the dog home and talks the adults into letting him take care of her, even though they don't believe she will survive. With care from Daniel, Lady gradually grows stronger, but she doesn't act like his first dog. Eventually, Lady runs away; Daniel is angry, but when Lady comes back she lets him help her and ultimately it seems they might become friends.

Tolstoy, L. (1960). *The Death of Ivan Ilych and Other Stories.* New York, NY: New American Library. The title story is an exceptional piece of world literature in which a Russian magistrate in the prime of his life is afflicted with a grave illness that becomes steadily more serious. As his health deteriorates, Ivan begins to realize that glib talk in college about mortality does not apply only to other people or to humanity in general; now it is about him.

Traisman, E. S. (1992). *Fire in My Heart, Ice in My Veins: A Journal for Teenagers Experiencing a Loss.* Omaha, NE: Centering Corporation. This book is intended as a journal for a teenager who has experienced the death of someone he or she loved. A line or two of text on each page and many small drawings offer age-appropriate prompts for this purpose.

Traisman, E. S., & Sieff, J. (Comps.). (1995). *Flowers For the Ones You've Known: Unedited Letters From Bereaved Teens.* Omaha, NE: Centering Corporation. This collection presents unedited letters and poems in various handwritten and print formats from teens who have encountered the death of an important person. Also included are artwork and writing guides from experienced group leaders.

Voigt, C. (1982). *Dicey's Song.* New York, NY: Atheneum; Simon Pulse, 2002; Aladdin Paperbacks, 2003. At 13, Dicey Tillerman has multiple responsibilities. Her father disappeared when she was seven and her mother is now institutionalized, so Dicey takes her three younger siblings to live with Gram. Gram and the children need love, trust, and courage to face their many challenges. Overriding all else are the losses they all have suffered, including Momma's eventual death.

Wheeler, J. L. (2010). *Weird Is Normal When Teenagers Grieve.* Naples, FL: Quality of Life Publishing Co. This book was written by a grieving teen for grieving teens mainly to validate their experiences and resist adult "shoulds" and unrealistic expectations.

Wiener, L. S., Best, A., & Pizzo, P. A. (Comps.). (1994). *Be a Friend: Children Who Live With HIV Speak.* Morton Grove, IL: Albert Whitman. The vivid colors, drawings, and layout in this book seek to permit children living with HIV infection to speak in their own voices. The result is sometimes poignant, often charming, and always compelling.

CHAPTER 18

Voices
Holding Back

Justin Lewis

I was twelve when my mom was diagnosed with stage IV colon cancer. For the next twelve months, I deluded myself into an optimistic belief that her prognosis was positive. I can't blame my younger self for thinking this; I was still a kid, I had never dealt with a close loss before, and the last thought that should be on a twelve-year-old's mind is, "*How many more months until Mom dies?*" If someone had explained to me back then that the 5-year survival rate for a stage IV colon cancer patient is 6%, I would have told them, with full confidence, that my mom would be a member of those fortunate few.

My naïve understanding of my mom's situation made it more difficult for me when her illness took a turn for the worse. After responding positively to chemotherapy treatments for about eight months, my mom was severely injured in a car accident as a passenger. The severity of her broken bones forced her oncologist to halt further chemo treatments. As my mom's physical strength returned, so too did her cancer, with what seemed to be a renewed vigor. I remember visiting her at a rehabilitation facility when she was able to move around using a walker. I can't recall exactly what we spoke about, but that night was the last time I'd have a real conversation with my mom. That was the last time that I knew she understood what I was saying; the last time that my unnecessary assurance of "I love you" was met with, "I love you, too." Looking back, I'm glad that I said "I love you" so much, because I had to fit an entire lifetime's worth of "I love you" into thirteen years.

In a matter of days, my mom was in an ICU, unable to breathe without the assistance of a tube down her throat. A large portion of her digestive tract had been removed in emergency surgery, and she was in intense pain, unable to move or talk. It was at this moment that my family realized that this was the end of my mom's struggle with cancer, and the cancer had won. I visited my mom in the ICU every day, unsure of whether each time would be the last I saw her. Eventually, by nothing less than a miracle, she was able to work up the strength to breathe on her own. While this was a huge victory for her, it was only delaying the inevitable. Fortunately, my mom was able to move into a hospice facility, where the focus was on pain management and making her passing as comfortable for her as possible. I'll always be thankful for those last days that my mom was with us. She looked more relaxed than she had in months, and her family, friends, and I were able to say our goodbyes in a respectful, peaceful manner. After twelve days in hospice care, and just shy of a year after she was diagnosed, my mom passed away at the age of 45, five years short of when adults are advised to get screenings for colon cancer.

My mom's funeral was a few days later, and I gave a speech to the 400 or so family and friends who attended. I don't remember what I said on that day, but I do remember my primary goal: *don't cry.* Sure, I cried when she was first diagnosed, when I saw her in the ICU for the first time, and when she finally passed away, but for some reason, I took it upon myself to express little emotion in such a public setting. And for the next few years, that is how I coped with my mom's death: I pretended that I was fine.

High school started a few months after my mom passed away, and as a shy fourteen-year-old, I did not want to discuss my family history with the new students and friends I met. When someone who didn't know about my mom asked me a question involving her, I either changed the subject, or gave a vague, nondescript answer that didn't require me to explain that she was dead.

"*What does your mom do?*"

"*She used to be a teacher.*"

And I would leave it at that.

This attitude of avoidance and denial stuck with me until I was in the 12th grade. My school had chosen a colon cancer charity as that year's cause for a coffeehouse organized by my choir and theater department. Before the event, some volunteers from the charity came to our chorus practice to talk about the importance of getting screened for colon cancer when you turn 50. As they gave personal accounts of people's lives that were saved by these screenings, I became overwhelmed. *My mom was healthy, she was young, and yet she still died. It's not fair!* For the first time since my mom's death, I cried. I cried in front of my teacher, my friends, and my prom date. I left the room, feeling miserable, but as my classmates departed to their next classes, something unexpected happened. One by one, almost all of them came up to me, gave me a hug, told me that they cared about me, and offered to be there for me if I ever needed someone to talk to.

This event became a cathartic experience for me. From then on, I became much more open about my mom's passing, and now I don't mind discussing it with others. I commemorate my mom's birthday and the day of her death on Facebook every year, because writing and sharing my feelings is much better than hiding and repressing them. I hope that by sharing my experience, I can help teenagers who are going through what I've gone through. If I could concisely sum up what I've learned in these past five years: don't be afraid to talk, don't be afraid to share, and definitely, *don't be afraid to cry.*

Justin Lewis is a sophomore at the George Washington University in Washington, DC. He is studying political science and music, and hopes to one day become a lawyer. He enjoys video games, the Philadelphia Phillies, singing, and playing trombone. He lives in Cherry Hill, NJ, with his father and sister.

CHAPTER 19

Support Groups for Adolescents

Donna L. Schuurman

S ince the 1980s, hundreds of programs serving grieving children and adolescents have developed through hospices, hospitals, community health centers, and independent non-profits. Whether geared toward providing therapy, peer support, or both, all serve a broad common goal: to assist young people in their grieving following a death.

This chapter provides an overview of practical and philosophical issues related to running grief groups and camps, including types of services, principles, goals and objectives, guidelines, evaluative methods, and a review of efficacy studies.

SUPPORT GROUPS

The first program of its kind to run support groups for children and adolescents in the United States was The Dougy Center in Portland, OR, incorporated in1982 by former nurse Beverly Chappell, in tribute to Dougy Turno, a teenager who died of an inoperable brain tumor six years after diagnosis. When visiting Dougy in his hospital ward, Beverly observed his eagerness and ability to engage other young patients in discussions about their shared plights. He voiced his concerns about facing death, struggling openly with his peers and encouraging them to do the same: "Don't you think it's unfair we'll never get to graduate from high school? Do you think you'll get to kiss a girl before you die? What happens to us when we die? Will anyone remember us?" The adults around them were reluctant to join the conversations and often left the area in tears. Beverly and her husband, pediatrician Allan Chappell, opened their home to the first families in December 1981.

Through the support of community members, The Dougy Center was incorporated as a non-profit organization in 1982, moving into its own home, and opening its doors to children as young as three, up through age 18, and their parents.

In response to national exposure on ABC's *20/20*, *World News Tonight with Peter Jennings*, and *Good Morning, America*, the center was flooded with calls from around the country for help starting programs in local communities. In 1986 The Dougy Center initiated a training program for communities wanting to develop grief support services in their area. Fernside Center in Cincinnati, OH, now an affiliate of Hospice of Cincinnati, opened its doors in 1986, followed by the Center for Grieving Children in Portland, ME, in 1987. Over thirty years later, hundreds of grief support programs serve children, teens, young adults and their parents or adult caregivers throughout the US and beyond. Some are independent non-profit organizations, while others are affiliated with hospices, hospitals, or mental health agencies.

As programs grew and the interest in networking and sharing best practices evolved, a group of social workers, counselors, chaplains, and volunteers gathered in 1997 in Oberlin, OH, at the first Children's Grief Symposium, where the idea of a more formal alliance percolated. The symposium has been held annually ever since that first meeting, and the National Alliance for Grieving Children (NAGC) formalized as a nonprofit organization in 2004. The NAGC "promotes awareness of the needs of children and teens grieving a death and provides education and resources for anyone who wants to support them." Over 300 children's bereavement support professionals and volunteers gather at the annual symposium. The NAGC also provides online education, promotes national awareness on issues impacting grieving children and teens, and maintains a national database of children's bereavement support programs. The National Alliance for Grieving Children has been instrumental in gaining the designation of the third Thursday in November as "Children's Grief Awareness Day."

From its first national training to the present, The Dougy Center elected to provide training and technical assistance rather than franchise its name and program, advocating for local and cultural adaptation of its model, based on four principles.

Grief is a natural reaction to loss

Amid the current move toward pathologizing grief, evidenced in part by the push to include a grief-related mental disorder in the most recent *Diagnostic and Statistical Manual of Mental Disorders* (DSM-5) (American Psychiatric Association, 2013), one could easily lose sight of the reality that grieving losses of all kinds is a normal, human response, and a healthy one. Complicating factors may contribute to difficulties, including prior-existing family problems and mental illness, the frequent lack of positive social support systems, and a general lack of understanding about the needs of grieving people. Sometimes people will benefit from professional intervention through therapy and medication, but many professionals, including physicians, psychiatrists, school personnel, and psychologists, have received no formal training in understanding and responding to grieving patients or students. Grief is not a mental disorder or a pathology.

Within each child is the capacity to heal

We all have the capacity to heal from physical and psychological wounds, but this outcome does not happen in a vacuum. Sometimes our wounds need professional care. Sometimes they need to be covered and treated; other times they need to be exposed to the air. We also have better outcomes with the compassionate understanding of family and friends. Resiliency, the ability to cope with stress and adversity, is a combination of internal and external factors, about which much has been studied and written. While it is beyond the scope of this chapter to fully explore the resiliency literature, protective factors contributing to resilience include having an internal locus of control, strong social connections and problem-solving skills, and identifying as a survivor, not a victim (Cherry, 2013).

The duration and intensity of grief are unique for each child

Children who have experienced a loss through death are thrust into a new and unpredictable reality, including the knowledge that those they love (or hate, for that matter) may be taken away in an instant, or through a long period of intense suffering. Peer support groups and camps allow teens to articulate and express their intensely personal reactions to loss, as well as to know they are not alone. Ideally, these programs and groups create a sense of safety that enables young people to ably chart their own course through grief, rather than simply accommodating the wishes of others.

Caring and acceptance assist in the healing process

Teens often report that their friends and the adults around them don't understand what they're going through and say and do things that are not helpful. It's not uncommon for teachers to pressure students to perform at the same level as before the death, without acknowledging the toll grief takes on the ability to concentrate and complete tasks. Families find that after a brief wave of care and concern, the outside support starts to diminish. Peer support groups and camps work to provide this missing care and support in an environment that welcomes sharing about the challenges of living, learning, and connecting after the death. Teens are able to tell their stories as often as they need to without fear that they'll be criticized for continuing to process the impact the death has on their lives. They're also able to take a break from active grieving to laugh, play, and enjoy life without fear of being judged by others.

The types of support groups offered to grieving adolescents range from time-limited (usually in the 6, 8 or 12- week range), to open-ended, where youth participate for as long as they wish to attend. Groups are held in school settings, hospitals, hospices, community centers, and mental health agencies. Depending on the geographic reach and target audience, groups may be based on age, mode of death (accident, illness, suicide, homicide), and/or the relationship of the deceased to the teen (parent, sibling, grandparent, other relative, friend). They are generally staffed by a combination of professionals and trained volunteers, and the majority are offered at no cost to participating families. Most, though not all, include a parent or adult caregiver component, to provide support for the grieving parent as well as assistance in understanding and responding to the needs of the grieving child or children. The importance of including parents in grief support outreach is underscored by the seminal research of William Worden and Phyllis Silverman through their findings in the Harvard Child Bereavement study (Worden, 1996; Silverman, 2000). The findings of the research team in the Family Bereavement Program at Arizona State University strongly emphasize the importance of parent education and support (Wolchik, Coxe, Tein, Sandler, & Ayers, 2008).

Teen grief support groups may be structured or semi-structured. Time-limited groups tend to follow a curriculum for each group which is pre-set by the program administrators. Open-ended groups frequently provide a structure (opening circle, discussion or suggested activity, closing circle or ritual) within which the participants themselves determine the content of the group's discussion and activity. As in all human activities, there is no one-size-fits-all grief support group or model, and the group setting is not going to work for all teens. Some programs prescreen out participants with existing mental health issues, while others, like The Dougy Center, allow the teens to decide for themselves whether or not to participate.

GRIEF SUPPORT CAMPS

Leaving home and attending camp as a child or teen has a long tradition in the US. The American Camp Association (formerly the American Camping Association) was established in 1910 and currently includes 9,000 members, through whom their camp participants "...have the opportunity to learn powerful lessons in community, character-building, skill development and healthy living – lessons that can be learned nowhere else" (retrieved from http://www.acacamps. org/about/who-we/are).

Camping experiences specifically geared to children and teens grieving a death began, like peer grief support programs, in 1982, with Camp Amanda in Windsor Heights, IA, the first and longest running camp in the US for grieving children and teens. Another early entry was El Tesoro de la Vida ("The Treasure of Life"), a week-long resident camp for children 6 to17 who are coping with a death, under the auspices of Camp Fire USA First Texas Council.

The two largest grief support camps with national reach are Comfort Zone, founded in 1998, and Camp Erin, founded in 2000. Comfort Zone, for ages 7 to 17, "provides grieving children with a voice, a place and a community in which to heal, grow and lead more fulfilling lives" (retrieved from http://www.comfortzonecamp.org). Founded by Lynne Hughes in Richmond, VA, camps are now held in four locations (Virginia, California, Massachusetts, and New Jersey), with a goal of reaching all 50 states. The weekend camps provide year-round access, and Comfort Zone provides an online community through the website www.HelloGrief.org.

Camp Erin is a free weekend bereavement camp created and supported by The Moyer Foundation, a nonprofit organization founded in 2000 by former professional baseball player Jamie Moyer and his wife, Karen. Named in memory and honor of Erin Metcalf, a family friend of the Moyers who died of cancer at age 17, Camp Erin combines traditional, fun, high-energy camp activities with grief education and emotional support, facilitated by grief professionals and trained volunteers. The Moyer Foundation identifies and partners with health care and bereavement organizations in local communities to provide the camps at no cost to families. One of Jamie Moyer's original goals was to ensure a Camp Erin location in every Major League Baseball city in the US, and over a decade since the first camp was held in 2002, over 9,700 youth have participated in camps in 40 locations. Additionally the Moyer Foundation has sponsored a National Bereavement Camp Conference for several years, open to all who run or wish to run bereavement camps for children and adolescents.

Another national grief support camp program is offered through Tragedy Assistance Program for Survivors (TAPS), described as "America's only nonprofit Veterans Service Organization chartered solely to assist the surviving families of military members who have died while serving our nation" (retrieved from http://www.taps.org). TAPS holds "Good Grief Camps" for children as young as 18 months through 21 years old annually over the Memorial Day weekend. Much like the variety of grief support programs, grief camps range from day camps to weekend or weeklong. Some, like Camp Erin and Comfort Zone camps, are offered at no cost to families, while others are fee-based, usually offering scholarships based on need. Overnight camps tend to incorporate traditional camping activities with activities structured specifically around grief and memorialization in order to provide children with a unique chance to process their experiences in ways that are both fun and meaningful.

Clute and Kobayashi (2013) highlight the shared objectives of grief camps: providing a safe place for participants to share their feelings about their losses with peers; facilitating the child's expression of grief; and education around healthy ways to cope. The common aim is "increasing the psychological and behavioral well-being of the camp attendees through various activities, peer support, and support from trained professionals and volunteers" (p. 47).

Camps also provide a normative social experience for children who may feel different or isolated from their non-bereaved peers. As opposed to adults, children and teens tend to grieve in short bursts, so camps and retreats facilitate them being able to "take breaks from their painful feelings and experience a balance of fun and grief work" (Schachter & Georgopolous, 2008, p. 247).

GUIDELINES FOR ADOLESCENT GRIEF
SUPPORT SERVICES

Adolescence is a time when youth move into a more complex realm of thoughts and ideas, higher level questioning about the meaning of life, and more advanced reasoning. They are challenging assumptions of the adults around them, gaining more responsibility for and in their lives, developing competencies (and becoming increasingly aware of their incompetencies), and experimenting with interpersonal intimacy. The death of a family member or friend threatens, and sometimes shatters, the assumptions they may have made about the world and their place in it. The research of Tedeschi and Calhoun (1996) indicates that deep tragedy, while shattering assumptions, also provides great possibility for growth, a phenomenon they termed "post- traumatic growth."

Parental or sibling death places children at risk for negative outcomes, including mental health problems like anxiety, depression, somatic complaints, lower academic success and self-esteem, and greater external locus of control. Outreach goals targeted to grieving teens should help teens know they're not alone, provide opportunities to share with others and know their feelings are normal, and allow for opportunities for remembrance.

To date, North American youth grief practitioners have yet to develop a universally-accepted set of guidelines for principles and best practices, though a Work Group in the National Alliance for Grieving Children has set the goal to do so. In the United Kingdom, The Childhood Bereavement Network secured funds in 1999 from the Diana, Princess of Wales Memorial Fund to set up a nationwide network of support services for bereaved children and to develop standards and codes of good practice. Their model may serve as a good starting point, stating that "any information, guidance and support offered to children should:

- acknowledge the child's grief and experience of loss as a result of death;
- be responsive to the child's needs, views, and opinions;
- respect the child's family and immediate social situation, and their culture, language, beliefs, and religious background;
- seek to promote self-esteem and self-confidence, and develop communication, decision making, and other life skills;

- be viewed as part of a continuous learning process for the child, contributing to the development of the child's knowledge and understanding as they grow into adulthood; and
- aim, wherever possible, appropriate, and feasible, to involve family members, other caregivers, and any professionals working with the individual child in a wider social context. (retrieved from http://www.childhoodbereavementnetwork.org.uk)

EVALUATIVE METHODS

Many programs and camps have developed program evaluation tools to help assess the effectiveness of their program offerings, and most funding sources require them to do so. Generally these are self-report from participants.

The American Camp Association provides a wealth of resources, including a CAMP Program Quality Assessment (PQA) tool in both long and short forms. While the long form is "robust enough for reliable external assessment," the short form is for self-assessment purposes only, and includes a helpful checklist. Both include opportunities to assess "best practices of positive youth development" designed to help camp staff evaluate and improve the quality of camp. The Eight Best Practices include:

1. Staff friendliness and circulation
2. Emotional safety
3. Support for belonging
4. High expectations and good challenge
5. Active and cooperative learning
6. Camper voice
7. Planning and reflection
8. Nature

(retrieved from www.acacamps.org/sites/default/files/images/research/PQA-Assessment-short-form.pdf). For more information on the full Camp PQA and the Youth Program Quality Intervention, see the Center for Youth Program Quality website at http://www.cypq.org.

EFFICACY STUDIES

The increase in services for bereaved children and adolescents leads to the important questions of their efficacy. Although some progress has been made, program effectiveness has not received the quantity or quality of research the subject warrants. This is not for lack of interest on the part of programs or practitioners, but due in large part to the cost and expertise required to conduct quality research. Curtis and Newman (2001) reviewed nine studies of programs for bereaved children, concluding that the programs produced moderate positive effects. They underscored that methodological weaknesses hampered most of the studies, including small sample sizes, lack of control groups, high attrition rates, and short-term evaluation, among other issues. Currier, Holland, and Neimeyer (2007) conducted a meta-analytic review of controlled outcome research on the effectiveness of bereavement interventions with children, analyzing the paucity of studies. "Unfortunately, the fact that the total controlled outcome literature on bereavement interventions with children appears to consist of a mere 13 studies restricted the number of questions that could be legitimately examined in this review and reduced the level of confidence that could be placed in the results" (p. 258).

Similarly, while there is minimal research on the efficacy of bereavement camps for children, there are a growing number of studies. Clute and Kobayashi (2013) reviewed existing literature on child bereavement camps with the following selection criteria utilized: Studies had to include children up through age 18, a description of the study evaluation criteria, details of the findings of the evaluations, and publication in peer-reviewed journals. Eight studies met the selection criteria. "Overall, the literature described camp experiences as positive and of value to the children and their families" (p. 52); however, "Given the small sample size of this study, "the results cannot be generalized... in the professional literature, effectiveness of grief camps was found to be just emerging. It could be that small nonprofit programs may struggle to both offer services and provide evidence of effectiveness" (p. 53).

Nabors et al. (2004) conducted a pilot study of a weekend-long camp for grieving children. Their research indicated that children reported the art activities to be helpful avenues for expression and that being with other grieving children assisted them to feel less alone in their experiences. Bereavement camps offer children an opportunity to come together with others who are grieving to talk and express their grief through a variety of activities in an intensive time period. As Nabors and colleagues state, "The opportunity to share feelings of grief in a supportive environment among peers who have endured the death of a loved one may be one of the most powerful aspects of the camp experience" (p. 404).

McClatchey, Vonk, and Palardy researched a short-term, camp-based, trauma-focused intervention and found that it reduced the symptoms of trauma and post-traumatic stress disorder (PTSD) in parentally bereaved children (2008). Farber and Sabatino (2007), in a two-year theory-driven evaluation of a summer camp for grieving children, found camp contributed to participant's improved self-esteem and self-confidence, and fostered teamwork. Another study, by Fluegeman, Schrauben and Cleghorn (2013), conducted focus groups with camp participants 11 to17 years old, finding a decreased sense of isolation, increased coping skills (including asking for help from peers), and increased ability to express emotions.

Clearly more research would be helpful, but as Clute and Kobayashi pointed out, it is unlikely to happen with the funding and research expertise limitations of nonprofit agencies. Currier et al. (2007) conclude that for future research, "the first priority is to develop well-validated and clinically relevant measures of child grief. Second, researchers need to flesh out the theoretical underpinnings and the operational implementation of their interventions" (p. 258). Although their meta-analysis does not "support the assumption that the bereavement interventions with children have a significant influence on adjustment" (p. 257), the small number of research studies makes it difficult to be conclusive.

This state of affairs does not have to discourage those of us engaged in bereavement services for children, adolescents, and families. Increasing interest in the efficacy of grief support services to children, teens, and their families will inevitably lead to more research dollars and interest on the part of researchers. And while competing demands for funding increase the pressure to provide evidence-based practice, we ought not to sell short the power of practice-based evidence.

Donna Schuurman, EdD, FT, is Chief Executive Officer of The Dougy Center for Grieving Children & Families in Portland, OR, where she has served in various roles since 1986. She writes and trains internationally on children's bereavement issues and is the author of Never the Same: Coming to Terms with the Death of a Parent. *Dr. Schuurman served as president of the board of directors for the Association for Death Education and Counseling and received its Annual Service Award in 2003 and Clinical Practice Award in 2013. She is a member of the International Work Group on Death, Dying, and Bereavement, and a founding board member of The National Alliance for Grieving Children. She has trained the National Transportation Safety Board (NTSB) and FBI's Rapid Deployment teams, as well as medical personnel, NGO staff and caregivers following major disasters including the Oklahoma City bombing, 9/11, and Japan's 1995 Kobe earthquake and 3/11 tsunami.*

References

Curtis, K., & Newman, T. (2001). Do community-based support services benefit bereaved children? A review of empirical evidence. *Child: Care, Health, and Development, 27*(6), 487-495.

Currier, J. M., Holland, J. M., & Neimeyer, R. A. (2007). The effectiveness of bereavement interventions with children: A meta-analytic review of controlled outcome research. *Journal of Clinical Child and Adolescent Psychology, 36*(2), 253-259.

Cherry, K. (2013). Characteristics of resilience. About.com, retrieved from http://psychology.about.com/od/crisiscounseling/p/resilience-2.htm?p=1

Clute, M. & Kobayashi, R. (2013). Are children's grief camps effective? *Journal of Social Work in End-of-Life Palliative Care, 9,* 43-57.

Farber, M., & Sabatino, C. (2007). A therapeutic summer weekend camp for grieving children: Supporting clinical practice through empirical evaluation. *Child and Adolescent Social Work Journal, 24*(4), 385-402.

Fluegeman, J., Schrauben, A., & Cleghorn, S. (2013). Bereavement support for children: Effectiveness of Camp Erin from an occupational therapy perspective. *Bereavement Care, 32:2,* 74-81.

Haine, R., Ayers, T., Sandler, I., & Wolchik, S. (2008). Evidence-based practices for parentally bereaved children and their families. *Professional Psychology Research and Practice, 39*(2), 113-121.

McClatchey, I., Vonk, M. E., & Palardy, G. (2009). Efficacy of a camp-based intervention for childhood traumatic grief. *Research on Social Work Practice, 19,* 19-30.

Nabors, L., Ohms, M., Buchanan, N., Kirsh, K. L., Nash, T., Passik, S. D.,...Brown, G. (2004). A pilot study of the impact of a grief camp for children. *Palliative and Supportive Care, 2,* 403-408.

Schachter, S. & Georgopolous, M. (2008). Camps for grieving children: Lessons from the field. In K.J. Doka & A.S. Tucci (Eds.), *Living with grief: Children and adolescents* (pp. 233-251). Washington, DC: Hospice Foundation of America.

Schoenfelder, E., Sandler, I., Wolchik, S., & MacKinnon, D. (2011). Quality of social relationships and the development of depression in parentally-bereaved youth. *Journal of Youth and Adolescence, 40*(1), 85-96.

Schuurman, D. & DeCristofaro, J. (2010). Principles and practices of peer support groups and camp-based interventions for grieving children. In D. Balk & C. Corr (Eds.), *Children's encounters with death, bereavement and coping* (pp. 359-370). New York, NY: Springer.

Schuurman, D. (2008). Grief groups for grieving children and adolescents. In K. J. Doka & A. S. Tucci (Eds.), *Living with grief: Children and adolescents* (pp. 255-268). Washington, DC: Hospice Foundation of America.

Silverman, P. (2000). *Never too young to know.* New York, NY: Oxford University Press.

Tedeschi, R. & Calhoun, L. (1996). The Posttraumatic Growth Inventory: Measuring the positive legacy of trauma. *Journal of Traumatic Stress, (9)*, 455-471.

Wolchik, S., Coxe, S., Tein, J., Sandler, I., & Ayers, T. (2008). Six-year longitudinal predictors of posttraumatic growth in parentally bereaved adolescents and young adults. *Omega, 58*(2), 107-128.

Worden, J. W. (1996). *Children and grief: When a parent dies.* New York, NY: Guilford Press.

CHAPTER 20

The Magic of Grief Camps: The Impact on Teens

Jennifer Kaplan Schreiber and Cathy Spear

If you asked a roomful of adults whether they would want to go back and be adolescents again, the chances are that most would politely decline. They forget about the thrill of the first time behind the wheel, driver's license in wallet, or the awe after the first kiss, and the excitement of talking about it the next day with your close friend. What is remembered is the self-consciousness, the doubts, the pressures, the indecision…it leaves a jumbled, largely conflicted memory in most people's minds.

Adolescence is a time when so many tasks need to be accomplished. It lasts for years and encompasses growth in every single system: hormonal, metabolic, and muscular, to address the visible; and the social, familial, academic, and cognitive, addressing the unseeable. Adolescence requires anticipating the future, while holding onto the past and living in the present.

Now, throw into this bewilderment the painful and complex experience of grieving over the death of someone close. What system does that fit into? What system does that impact?

What system doesn't it?

An increasingly common setting in which adolescents can address their bereavement is camp. When we think of camp, we think of the sound of screen doors slamming, of joyful shrieks as motorboats pull children around a lake, of the crackling of marshmallows as they are readied for s'mores, of noisy dining rooms where plates are stacked to the cacophony of singing and cheering. We think of childhood.

How do the two fit together—the stabbing pain of knowing someone will never be seen again, and the joy of belly laughing with your friends?

That is the magic of camp.

The following depictions of closing rituals at Circle Camps and Manitou Experience, weeklong overnight camps for grieving girls and boys, respectively, highlight the power of grief camp.

Two hundred people, mostly girls, encircle a newly planted tree, each holding a rock in her hand. As though choreographed, four girls approach the tree from each corner of the circle and simultaneously place their rocks under the sapling. Each rock is inscribed with a message to a parent who has died. As the girls place their rocks, the silence is matched in solemnity by the vista of the mountains off in the distance.

Imagine a massive boulder sitting in the middle of a sacred old Indian village, with a campfire crackling in front of it. Over one hundred boys line up in silence, each waiting to light his candle in memory of his person who has died and place it on the boulder. Once all of the candles are lit, the boulder is covered in flickering flames, making a beautiful backdrop for the stories that are about to be told.

ADOLESCENT BEREAVEMENT

Young people mourn differently than adults, so their grief often goes unrecognized. In a National Poll of Bereaved Children & Teenagers (n=531) released in April 2012, 75% of the respondents reported the pervading emotion they currently feel is sadness, with feelings of anger, isolation, worry, and being overwhelmed by other primary emotions. Other highlights include: 39% have trouble sleeping; 45% said they have trouble concentrating on school work; 41% said they have acted in ways that they know might not be good for them; 47% believe their life will be harder than it will be for others; and 73% said that they think about their loved one every day (McNiel, 2012). Without adequate interventions, these children are at risk for negative outcomes, including traumatic grief (Mannarino & Cohen, 2011; McClatchey, Searles, Vonk, & Palardy, 2009), decreased school performance (Balk & Corr, 2009) and lower self-esteem (Haine, Ayers, Sandler, & Wolchik, 2008; Worden, 2009).

In the United States, although the vast majority of young people will not experience the death of a parent or sibling, the result can be devastating for those who do. Janoff-Bulman (1992) conceptualized "shattered assumptions," to describe an individual's loss of core assumptions about the world when encountered by a tragic loss such as the death of a parent or sibling. Inherent world assumptions such as "benevolent," "meaningful" and "worthy" (p. 6) may become shattered.

In adolescence especially, trying to "fit in" with peers is paramount, and many bereaved adolescents anecdotally report feeling different or experiencing a profound sense of isolation from their non-bereaved peers. The normative life transitions encompassing adolescence both influence and are influenced by the non-normative experience of parental or sibling bereavement. Balk (1991) reviewed research conducted in the 1980s on death and bereavement and concluded that for adolescents, "bereavement presents an extremely serious life crisis at a time when development is marked by significant physical, cognitive, moral, interpersonal and psychosocial transitions" (p. 8).

Adolescence, composed of biological, physical, behavioral, cognitive, and social transformations, represents the shift from childhood to adulthood, and is considered one of the most complex transitions in the lifespan. In Erikson's model (1963, 1968, 1994), the period of adolescence includes two developmental tasks. The first, *Identity versus Identity Diffusion*, involves the determination of how adolescents see themselves compared with how others may view them, and how they begin to differentiate self from other. This is similar to Elkind's (1981) concept of *egocentrism*, the adolescent's belief that people around him or her are as preoccupied with his or her behavior/appearance as he or she is.

Bereaved adolescents are developmentally challenged by their desire to "fit in" with peers, because the death of a parent or sibling leaves them feeling markedly "different" than their non-bereaved peers. Some adolescents avoid telling peers about a family death to avoid the perceived stigmatization they fear.

The second task described by Erikson (1963, 1968, 1994), *Intimacy versus Isolation*, refers to the adolescent's increased sense of self while learning to create and maintain satisfying personal relationships. Oltjenbruns (1991) noted that adolescents often use parents and siblings as a mirror to help define either perceived positive or negative aspects of self, which is problematic for those whose parent or sibling has died. While learning to recognize another's shortcomings is a natural part of learning to be in intimate relationships, oftentimes adolescents idealize a parent or sibling who has died. This idealization can interfere with establishing intimacy with others, as living relationships cannot compare to sentimentalized figures. Some bereaved adolescents have difficulty separating from the deceased or reallocating their emotional investment from the deceased to their peers due to such idealization.

As adolescents develop greater autonomy, their primary attachments move away from parents and siblings, and peers take on a significant role in their identity formation. Boys and girls are socialized to respond to their emotional experiences differently. Adams (2001) found that adolescent boys have grown up learning to hide or deny their feelings of grief more so than girls, as well as to display more aggressive behavior. Doka and Martin (2010), pioneers of masculine models of grief, found that grieving men find comfort in physical activity and problem-solving. No such evidence exists for bereaved adolescent boys; yet, expansive experiences suggest this is so. Manitou Experience incorporates rigorous physical activities in their camp, such as mixing cement to create garden memory stones.

CAMP AND YOUTH DEVELOPMENT

Limited research has been conducted on youth development and the camp experience (Garst, Browne, & Bialeschki, 2011; Gillard, Watts, & Witt, 2009; Henderson, Powell, & Scanlin, 2005; Thurber, Scanlin, Scheuler, & Henderson, 2007). In 2000, the American Camp Association (ACA) began to study the outcomes of camp experiences for youth and developed the Camper Growth Index for children (CGI-C) aged 8-14; in total, 92 accredited camps participated, with a total sample of 5,281 campers. The CGI-C consisted of 52 questions with 10 constructs, representing the four domains of Positive Identity, Social Skills, Positive Values & Spiritual Growth, and Thinking & Physical Skills. Reliability of the underlying constructs ranged from .63-.81, considered acceptable given the exploratory nature of the development of the instrument (Henderson, Thurber, Whitaker, Bialeschki, & Scanlin, 2006).

In a descriptive, naturalistic, longitudinal study measuring growth as a result of camp experiences, parents, children and camp staff reported significant positive change from pretest, posttest and six months later, more than would be expected from maturation alone (Thurber, Scanlin, Scheuler, & Henderson, 2007). In addition to the self-report CGI-C, parents completed a version of the Camper Growth Index for parents (CGI-P), and camp counselors completed a staff observation checklist for each participating camper they supervised. Results indicated that session length was not significantly correlated with growth, nor was gender or ethnicity. Children with low pretest self-report scores showed the greatest gains on the posttest, and older campers showed slightly more changes on some constructs than did the younger campers.

While research indicates that camps facilitate positive youth development, the variables that promote growth have not been well understood. Garst, Browne, and Bialeschki (2011) identified the following factors that promote growth: supportive staff-camper relationships; small staff-camper ratios; sense of belonging; opportunity to learn new skills in an emotionally and physically safe environment; a natural, restorative environment; camp norms and rituals; group living environment; opportunities for self-reflection and re-creation of self; leadership development; and the scheduling of primarily structured activities with limited amounts of unstructured times. Circle Camps and Manitou Experience incorporate all of the above-noted factors in each of their camp models.

How and Why Grief Camps Spin Their Magic

By conservative estimates, over 200 bereavement camps exist in the United States. Although the models of camp programs vary, their missions are similar: to help kids feel less alone in their grief. Just like kids, grief camps come in many shapes and sizes, determined largely by an available physical site, the sponsoring agency or program, the budget, or an overriding philosophy. They can be day camp, or run for one day, a weekend, or a week. Overnight camp can last one night, a full weekend, or several days, up to a week. They can be gender-specific or co-ed; if overnight, this is often determined by the way bunks or cabins are situated. They can have a wide age range or target a specific age group. Some camps have fewer than 30 campers; others have more than 150.

Perhaps it is easier to say what nearly all of the models have in common. First, they integrate grief-related activities into a traditional camp program. Why does this provide such a powerful experience, a "magical" time for so many of the campers, and most markedly for the adolescent population?

As discussed earlier, grief is isolating. Adolescents especially value and need the connection to peers, as developmentally they are transitioning away from family. By bringing these campers together, giving them time and space and permission in which to share their feelings and stories with others who "get it," a very compelling bond is created. The normalizing that occurs—*I am normal here, not the pitied kid whose parent died*—helps to enhance self-esteem. Since adolescents are so acutely aware of how they measure up to their friends, any way in which they veer too far from the norm is risky to their self-image, especially in the younger teen years. The value of giving them a time to be "just like all the other kids" cannot be overstated. As one camper stated, "I have made my very best friends at grief camp. I can be myself and everyone here understands."

The other key component that these camps offer is the chance to play. So many adolescents in grieving families are forced to grow up quickly and childhood may be replaced with premature and pseudo-adulthood. At camp, childhood is returned to them. From racing down a zip line to jumping into a cold lake on a hot summer's day, the inherent pleasure that sets in as campers relax back into childhood is visible. Many camps provide creative opportunities for campers to have fun in ways that may be completely unavailable to them anywhere else.

Additionally, camp may be one of the few places where young people are the focus of adult attention 24/7. No laundry to do, no bills to pay, no meals to prepare; the adults are there simply to care for the campers. The campers' needs come first at all times. Since a death in the family can shift how parental attention is given, often lessening the healthy attention given to children in the family, it is an incredible gift to young people at grief camps to be so consistently attended to by caring adults. Some camps, in their belief in the importance of this factor, assign each child an adult "buddy" who accompanies the camper throughout the day from activity to activity.

And as any camp professional knows, there is a special culture at camps that is all-encompassing and refreshing. The outside world is unavailable, the worries of home and school and grieving families are left behind, and all that is left is camp, in its own safe bubble.

THE ACTUAL CAMP

The physical site of the camp determines many elements of the program. What time of year, what the weather allows, how much of a focus on the outdoors or on athletics or on water activities; all these are essential to how the program will evolve. After a site is located and secured, the first task is to determine the camper population, which includes defining the population for the camp (i.e., by relationship between the camper and the deceased, camper ages, length of time since death, camper gender(s), or campers who may be able to return year after year). Further decisions include determining the geographic region the camp will serve, and whether campers are sleeping at camp or at home. Overnight grief camps offer a host of opportunity for growth, as they foster healthy separation from family, create a true sense of community that the camper may have lost due to the family loss, and allow the building of skills, both in recreational activities and in grieving. They also are often in more remote areas, frequently held at summer camps, so that travel arrangements need to be considered. Day camp programs have more site flexibility than overnight camps, as they can be held at schools, day camps, or campuses, and can be less costly and simpler to staff. Children or parents who feel anxious about separation from home are more likely to participate when the child isn't being asked to pack up and go off into the "unknown" for a few days. While day camps do not provide the "living together" aspect of an overnight camp, they certainly provide opportunities for community building and individual growth.

Let the grief activities begin

If the camp program were to be visualized, it typically might be described as having bookend activities. The opening is often a sharing group, or Circle Time, in which the campers share their stories of loss. In programs where campers return year after year, it can be astonishing to watch the growth in campers who, over time, expand the stories they tell and the comprehension they show about the impact of their loss. Such sharing times are best scheduled early on, as they foster the initial closeness that develops between campers.

The ending activity is often a memorial ceremony of some kind in which the deceased person is remembered through a ritual. There are numerous ways to do this, and again, it may depend upon the site where camp is held. Some examples include sharing stories at a campfire, floating wish boats on a lake, hiking up a mountain with a balloon release, or planting a tree that is surrounded by memorial stones. Campers and counselors alike describe these as poignant, meaningful, and pivotal parts of the program.

Between these two fundamental activities, and depending upon how much time is available, other grief activities can be planned as a way to normalize the complex feelings found in adolescent bereavement. Numerous activities can be planned that invite visual and creative efforts, and they can be individualized or camp-wide. These can be as varied as writing in journals, writing letters to the deceased, or creating a camp-wide literary magazine; or crafts activities such as making memory boxes or feeling masks, designing picture frames, designing a collage, making mosaic memory stones, or creating an all-camp quilt. It is important to consider the age of the campers when designing these activities; younger campers are going to be more concrete in their understanding, whereas adolescents can bring more abstract thinking to a task.

Other activities may have a focus on social support as a way to strengthen the bond felt among grieving campers, such as ropes courses, ball games, and hikes. Ice-breaking activities enable campers to get to know and connect with one another. For example, in "The Human Knot", campers grab hands with anyone in the circle other than the person beside him/her, and then they attempt to unknot themselves without letting go of one another's hands. At Manitou Experience, the familiarity of being tangled in a "knot" is used as a metaphor for grief, and then the campers brainstorm ways to "get out or loosen some of the knots." In Circle Camps, teens who had settled in and were feeling safe in sharing feelings were invited to use visual metaphors of climbing mountains or crossing lakes in drawings as representations of their challenging journeys through grief.

Other grief activities focus on coping strategies and self-awareness. Learning where and how emotions are felt in one's body is critical if one wants to feel more in control of one's emotions. For example, body tracings have been successfully utilized to help adolescents at Manitou Experience recognize their body cues when they have stressful or overwhelming feelings related to the death. This exercise empowers campers by normalizing feelings, and fosters meaningful discussions about coping strategies for when one feels less in control of one's feelings than preferred. At Circle Camps, an activity called "The Colors of Grief" has campers add drops of food coloring into a fishbowl of water, with discussion of what feelings each color might represent. As more and more coloring is added to the bowl, the water gets murkier, and the metaphor of the murkiness of grief is explored.

Small amounts of bleach, which gradually clear up the water, are then added to represent the "supports" that help in life and these are also discussed. One camper noted, looking at the clearer water once the "supports" were added, "You can see the sky again."

Since grief can interfere with sleep, mindfulness activities may be incorporated into sleep rituals. For example, a Manitou Experience camper reported that he has continuously had difficulty sleeping because "I shared a room with my brother and now I lie in bed for hours thinking about him." Many of his bunkmates reported similar challenges with sleep, so at bedtime a clinician led them through a visual imagery exercise and provided a printed copy of the exercise that the campers could use at home. Doing this exercise as a group (as opposed to individually) normalized the negative feelings associated with sleep challenges, as well as stereotypes that boys should not cry and should be strong; this process creates a bond and empathic connections between the boys and counselors.

And, of course, there is the age-old camp tradition of having evening campfires, where either in a formal way or spontaneously, campers and counselors can share their stories of life, loss, or the impact of the camp.

And the part that is just plain fun

Non-grief activities are obviously also a huge part of the experience for campers of all ages. Fun is an essential element of a grief camp. The skills of the counselors determine which activities may be offered, but active engagement and enthusiasm can make virtually any activity fun. One model of scheduling allows campers to select their own activities, thus enabling them to focus in on special interests they have or skills they wish to develop, such as tennis or sailing. An alternative model is for campers' schedules to be set ahead of time, with age determining which activities are assigned. When this latter model is used, care needs to be taken to make activities inviting to campers of all skill levels. Activities that use music or dance are wonderful at providing a sense of relaxation without any competitive feel. Adolescents may appreciate "special" activities that require stamina and responsibility, such as a challenging hike, a swim across the lake, a canoe trip, or tent camping expedition.

Both girls and boys need times during the day when they are really active. Camps for boys may benefit from more physical and movement-based activities than those for girls. Girls of all ages are, typically, more able than boys to sit for longer periods of time and talk about their feelings. Or they might be more content at an arts and crafts table than boys. (For these developmental reasons, boys at grief camps may actually do well with additional structured grief activities, as they are less likely to spontaneously jump into heavy conversations about their losses).

How to proportion the grief and non-grief activities is a challenge. Is the goal largely to provide a fun setting, in which grief work is encouraged, or is it to focus in on the "grief work" and make sure some fun activities are provided to foster a child-friendly setting? Each camp will arrive at its own emphasis. Young people of all ages will need to enjoy themselves at camp, so it is essential to incorporate plenty of fun into each day. It is likely that the relaxation, comfort, and sense of belonging at camp that emanates from play strengthens the capacity to make use of the actual grief work that goes on at camps. We do know that adolescents have a greater capacity to engage in the grief component than younger campers. Their cognitive and emotional development enables adolescents to share and reflect upon emotionally charged feelings with greater intensity and for longer periods of time. Scheduling more time for adolescents to explore their grief, especially in a multi-day camp, is helpful.

Counselor-in-training program

Adolescents who have previously participated often seek mentoring roles with younger campers. This can be fostered through the creation of Counselor-In-Training (CIT) programs. While the roles and responsibilities may vary from camp to camp, a commonality is that the adolescent campers are viewed as having valuable life experiences and gifts to share with younger campers. CITs are typically between the ages of 15 to 17; they come to camp knowing that their role will enable them to learn how to become leaders, and potentially, counselors at camp. Through the training component of the program, CITs will be assigned to specific campers, cabins, or activities. They can enjoy the status that comes with being respected by both campers and staff. Care is needed to ensure that CITs are not being used as babysitters; the point is to offer them enriching and fulfilling learning opportunities.

At Circle Camps, the CIT program is offered through an application process to rising tenth and eleventh graders who are Circle alumnae. Their days at camp are split; they spend mornings assigned to a younger cabin and afternoons with their own CIT group. The role they play with younger girls is esteem-building; they are seen as competent and successful, not to mention a lot of fun, as they accompany the campers to activities and help out wherever needed. In their afternoon time, they have the chance to do more sophisticated teen activities that often result in some of the strongest friendship bonds they have felt since the death.

The CITs at one of the Circle Camps have explored their grief in a very comprehensive way, and they often say that the program is the most important thing they have ever done. First, they participate in both their own CIT grief training, designed to help them think conceptually about childhood grief at different ages, which they can draw upon when talking to their younger campers. They then are given a venue in which to think back on their own grief journey, obviously impacted upon when the death occurred in their lives. They are also invited to participate in a formal dramatic presentation where together they create, through use of performing/visual arts, a performance, depicting aspects of the losses they've experienced. Girls have written poems, essay, and songs that they work on during the first days at camp; these are then put together as an evening performance for counselors at camp. (Because some of their pieces are very emotionally-laden, it has been decided not to invite other campers). For many girls, this event is the culmination of years of attending camp. Over time, they have shared more and more of their stories with their friends, as they have felt supported and understood by those around them. They are then able to offer back this creative rendition of their grief. To say it can be a powerful experience is an understatement.

At Manitou Experience, the CIT program consists of multiple summers, with increases in training and responsibilities every year, in order to smoothly transition campers into counselor positions. There are two CIT years, the first of which is open to new campers, followed by a junior counselor (JC) year. First year CITs will have finished 10th grade. The second CIT year and JC year are by invitation, based on previous year's performance. During the first year of the CIT program's development, the CITs were asked to help define their responsibilities and the goals of the program as much as possible. In particular, they were tasked with creating a list of core leadership values for the incoming CITs to use as a framework for the program going forward. Limited direction was offered to the CITs; this enabled them to work cooperatively, intentionally, and creatively. The outcome was amazing.

They took the concept of "head, shoulder, knees and toes" and created a symbolic representation of core leadership values that they felt lived within each of them. For each body part, they chose a word that exemplified how a CIT should act. For the head, they chose the word *"wisdom;"* for the shoulders *"responsibility;"* the heart was *"love;"* knees were *"agility;"* and feet *"balance."* When presenting it to the camp, the CITs took turns sharing the story of each core value and relating it to what they experienced or learned at camp. For example, the CITs described "wisdom" by being able to use their grief experiences as ways to relate to and support the younger campers. A perfect example of this was when one of the CITs stood up at the first night's campfire and shared his story of his loss, and how scared he was coming to camp. He talked about how he stepped onto the bus feeling scared and alone, and then stepped off the bus feeling part of a brotherhood. It was amazing to watch a 16-year-old open up to the entire camp because he wanted the new campers to feel like this was a safe place for them.

The question of gender

How to make the decision whether to use a gender-specific model or a co-ed model? The site where a camp is situated may lend itself to one or the other; if it offers separate housing areas, then a co-ed model is a possibility. However, the site is only one consideration. Gender-specific camps may offer the possibility for greater intimacy among campers due to the tendency in nearly all young people to be more open around those of their own gender. Generally speaking, boys are not eager to show their vulnerability in front of girls, and talking about loss can easily create a sense of vulnerability for even the most stoic boy. Overnight grief camps also offer the unique intimacy of sharing morning and nighttime rituals such as brushing teeth, reading by flashlights, hearing the bugle play *Taps*; these moments of togetherness organically contribute to the comfort and security most campers feel while at camp.

There is the reality, however, that a co-ed camp can be more convenient for families with children of both genders. Transportation is simplified, administrative details are streamlined, and even packing is easier, if both girls and boys are headed to the same place in the same vehicle.

One new model developed by Circle Camps and Manitou Experience was successfully implemented as a five-day, overnight, co-ed camp where boys and girls had activities scheduled and planned separately, meals served together with seating merely split in half in the dining area, housing at separate sides of the campus, and a sharing of the facilities and some auxiliary staff (doctor, nurse, social workers). Since two camps were involved, there was the benefit of sharing the cost of the camp rental, as well as sharing the myriad of tasks required to plan and carry out the camp programs.

To the knowledge of the authors, there is no research comparing the benefits of gender-specific versus co-ed grief camps. Anecdotally, both models report tremendous success and life-affirming experiences for campers. However, the practice experiences of the authors contribute largely to their respective camp philosophies to offer gender-specific overnight grief camps. Childhood, and particularly early adolescence, is developmentally a time when comparing oneself to one's peers is basic to one's self-image and when self-consciousness is at its height. When adolescent boys were surveyed at two overnight grief camps for boys as to whether they would feel as comfortable sharing their feelings in a co-ed environment, more than 90% of the boys responded "no." Clearly, this is just anecdotal, but it calls attention to the need for evidence-based research on the relevant factors of successful grief camps.

CAMP, CHILDREN, AND SAFETY

When a family has experienced a death, either suddenly or through a prolonged illness, there is inevitably a heightened awareness of risk. Surviving parents can be terrified of "letting" a child go to camp. Young people can be terrified of being away from the surviving family members. If a camp experience is successfully navigated, and it most always is, the success can serve as a huge boost to the family's wish to trust in life again. However, grief camps have an important responsibility to reassure families of their commitment to safety in all areas: certified instructors in certain activities, criminal background checks for all staff, sophisticated waterfront safety systems, nursing staff on site and medical intervention availability if needed, and trained bereavement specialists.

Physical contact with campers

Camps need to make sure campers are safe in other ways, too. It is customary now for adults to respect the "bathing suit guidelines" whenever touching a camper: never touch a child in places that a bathing suit would cover. Shoulder, upper back, and arms are the most acceptable places to be in physical contact, unless a medical situation warrants otherwise. Since being playful and affectionate are wonderful components of any camp experience, common sense is encouraged for all counselors living with children at camps. If it makes you uncomfortable, don't do it. If it makes the camper uncomfortable, don't do it.

Social media

An ongoing question is how and whether everyone in the camp community can, or should, stay in touch after camp has ended. Some camps have a policy prohibiting contact between staff and campers once the program has ended, a policy offered to protect both campers and staff against misinterpreted or overly self-revealing communications. With the added complexities of the social media world, this is not as easily enforceable as it once was. Adolescents especially can be very committed to social media and now almost universally use this as a primary means of talking and planning and staying in touch with everyone in their lives, whether they live five houses away or five hours away. One of the Circle camps did find that a comprehensive explanation to counselors about the rationale for the policy helped them fully understand and endorse it. A legal advisor can be consulted on how to determine the best policies regarding camper/ staff communication for a grief camp, and once a policy is determined, parents and guardians, as well as staff, should be informed. It is also helpful for any limits on contact to be explained to campers before they leave camp, so there is no sense of rejection if a social media "friend request" is ignored.

But the reality is that contact between campers is hugely popular and happens across the various social media platforms. Ongoing contact can actually be useful in diminishing isolation, keeping campers in touch during the time when they are not at camp, and providing one of the newer ways of being a community. Manitou Experience strongly encourages its campers, and counselors, to stay connected through a specific Facebook page, which offers a shared site to communicate and the ability for the staff to monitor communications if a concern arises. The response has been overwhelmingly positive for all involved and provides an opportunity to maintain bonds throughout the year, as well as building excitement for the following summer.

ENDINGS ARE IMPORTANT, AND SO IS HOLDING ON

Grief camps have an important responsibility in addressing the importance of goodbyes. For a variety of reasons, many campers were not able to have a final goodbye with the person who died. Part of the grief work encouraged at camp is to learn the importance of goodbyes. Saying goodbye to the camp experience, an experience that is undoubtedly intense for most campers, can serve as an example of the benefits of acknowledging endings. There are many ways to do this: the final night's campfire service, where so much can be shared about the time spent together and what was learned; a slideshow of pictures taken during camp that is played for everyone the last day; a final Circle Time in the cabin on the last day, where there is a goodbye said to the communal living that went on; even autographing camp t-shirts before leaving.

Whether camp is for one day, a weekend, or a week, whether it is a day program or overnight, each camp can find its own way to end the experience on a positive note. Because of the important and fun time that was had, acknowledging that there may be sadness at saying goodbye is also essential. Campers are known to say things like: "This is the only place I can be myself," This is the most fun I've had since my mother/father/sibling died," or "How will I wait another 51 weeks before I can come back again?"

A program component that can buffer the sadness of the ending is the idea of a reunion. Optimally, this can be held sometime mid-year, where campers and their family members can gather in a social setting and reminisce about the previous year's summer, as well as reestablish ties and create new ones. Scheduling this well in advance is helpful to families who may want very much to attend and would be disappointed if they are unable to due to lack of notice. Again, if this is for a boys' program, incorporating physical activities can be a good strategy, whether the campers are participating themselves, such as going bowling, or going as spectators to a sporting event. Girls are usually happy to just get together; adolescent girls especially are generally happy just to sit together and chat. Camp mementos can be displayed, and counselors in attendance may show their camp spirit by wearing camp garb.

Grief camps can be very powerful experiences. They can masterfully teach and support the importance of connections to others, as well as teach and support the importance of farewells. What a unique opportunity for adolescents who are moving ahead in their grief journeys.

Jennifer Kaplan Schreiber, MSW, LICSW, FT, is a doctoral candidate at Simmons College School of Social Work, teaches as adjunct faculty, and is a research assistant on a study exploring childhood concussion and depression. She is Executive Director for Jeff's Place Children's Bereavement Center, Inc. serving MetroWest Boston, and Clinical Director of Manitou Experience, overnight grief camps for boys in Maine and California. Schreiber has presented at state and national conferences on issues related to childhood loss. In 2011, she was the recipient of the Graduate Paper Award in memory of Richard Kalish at the International Annual Conference for the Association for Death Education and Counseling (ADEC). She is the author of Young Adults Coping with Death: You Are Not Alone.

Cathy Spear, MSW, LICSW, is Director of Camper Services at Circle Camps for Grieving Children, a non-profit organization that offers week-long overnight camp programs to bereaved girls in Maine, New Hampshire, and California. In that capacity, she developed the grief programs for campers of all ages, as well as established grief training programs for volunteer counselor staffs and for adolescents. She has a full-time private psychotherapy practice in Wellesley, MA, where her specialty area is grief and bereavement with teens, adults, and couples, as well as a general psychotherapy practice. She worked for many years as a senior social worker at a mental health clinic, was an instructor in Social Work Methods, and has also worked as a training and behavioral consultant to an overnight camp.

References

Adams, D. (2001). The grief of male children and adolescents and ways to help them cope. In D. A. Lund (Ed.), *Men coping with grief* (pp. 275-308). Amityville, NY: Baywood.

Balk, D. (1991). Death and adolescent bereavement: Current research and future directions. *Journal of Adolescent Research, 6*(1), 7-27.

Balk, D. E., & Corr, C. A. (Eds.). (2009). *Adolescent encounters with death, bereavement, and coping.* New York, NY: Springer.

Doka, K. J. & Martin, T. M. (2010). *Grieving beyond gender: Understanding the ways men and women mourn.* New York, NY: Taylor & Francis Group.

Elkind, D. (1981). *Children and adolescents: Interpretive essays on Jean Piaget* (3rd ed.). New York, NY: Oxford University Press.

Erikson, E. (1963). *Childhood and society.* New York, NY: W.W. Norton & Company.

Erikson, E. H. (1994; 1968). *Identity: Youth and crisis.* New York, NY: W.W. Norton & Co.

Garst, B. A., Browne, L. P., & Bialeschki, M. D. (2011). Youth development and the camp experience. *New Directions for Youth Development 2011, (130),* 73-87. doi:10.1002/yd.398

Gillard, A., Watts, C. E., & Witt, P. A. (2009). Camp supports for motivation and interest: A mixed-methods study. *Journal of Park & Recreation Administration, 27*(2), 74-96.

Haine, R., Ayers, T., Sandler, I., & Wolchik, S. (2008). Evidence-based practices for parentally bereaved children and their families. *Professional Psychology: Research & Practice, 39*(2), 1-15. doi:10.1037/0735-7028.39.2.113

Henderson, K. A., Powell, G. M., & Scanlin, M. M. (2005). Observing outcomes in youth development: An analysis of mixed methods. *Journal of Park & Recreation Administration, 23*(4), 58-77.

Henderson, K. A., Thurber, C. A., Whitaker, L. S., Bialeschki, M. D., & Scanlin, M. M. (2006). Development and application of a camper growth index for youth. *Journal of Experiential Education, 29*(1), 1-17.

Janoff-Bulman, R. (1992). *Shattered assumptions: Towards a new psychology of trauma.* New York, NY: Free Press.

Mannarino, A. P., & Cohen, J. A. (2011). Traumatic loss in children and adolescents. *Journal of Child & Adolescent Trauma, 4*(1), 22-33. doi:10.1080/19361521.2011.545048

McClatchy, I. S., Vonk, M. E., & Palardy, G. (2009). The prevalence of childhood traumatic grief—A comparison of Violent/Sudden and expected loss. *Omega: Journal of Death & Dying, 59*(4), 305-323. doi:10.2190/OM.59.4.b

McNiel, A. (2012). National poll of bereaved children & teenagers. Retrieved from http://childrengrieve.org/national-poll-bereaved-children-teenagers

Oltjenbruns, K. (1991). Positive outcomes of adolescents' experience with grief. *Journal of Adolescent Research, 6*(1), 43-53.

Thurber, C. A., Scanlin, M. M., Scheuler, L., & Henderson, K. A. (2007). Youth development outcomes of the camp experience: Evidence for multidimensional growth. *Journal of Youth and Adolescence, 36*(3), 241-254. doi:10.1007/s10964-9142-6

Worden, J. W. (2009). *Grief counseling and grief therapy: A handbook for the mental health practitioner* (4th ed.). New York, NY: Springer.

CHAPTER 21

Counseling Adolescents

David A. Crenshaw

Adolescents are a unique species. You can't begin to help or even to work with teens unless you appreciate the unique culture that youth inhabit. Teens speak their own language and dress (often specific to each generation of youth) in their own signature way, embrace their own music, and make their own statement regarding the world that their parents and previous generations are handing off to them. Often they are critical and severely fault-finding with their parents while idealizing the families of their friends, particularly if they perceive the parents of their friends as less restrictive. Adolescence is the most colorful, exciting, sometimes maddening, and often baffling of the developmental stages that people encounter through the life span. The old cliché that the job of the adolescent is to drive their parents crazy is humorous unless you are the parent(s). Some adolescents join gangs, some engage in reckless, dangerous behavior such as unsafe sex, drive cars at unsafe speeds, drink excessively, or abuse drugs.

Neuroscience reveals that part of the explanation for the impulsive, reckless, and risky behavior of teens combined with poor judgment is due to the incomplete development of the higher brain regions and the neuropathways that link the prefrontal cortex to the lower brain regions (Siegel, 2012). The adolescent brain is a work in progress not to be completed until young adult life. The delay in completing the neural circuits of the brain combined with the social, physiological, and cultural challenges of adolescence can be hazardous to the health of adolescents and those who surround them. I live in a predominantly rural area of upstate New York with narrow and winding country roads. Families here have experienced unspeakable heartbreak year after year as a result of inexperienced teen drivers traveling at unsafe speeds on these treacherous roads, leading to serious accidents and fatalities of the driver and sometimes others. While the memories of these terrible tragedies are etched in the minds of our local youth, in some cases young people insist on making their own mistakes and don't learn from the devastating mistakes of their peers.

Adolescence can be, but is not always, a time of great turmoil and upheaval. Yet their spirit is indomitable among many youth I've counseled. I love working with teens for that exact reason. Most people, in spite of the hazards, survive adolescence and there is reason to be optimistic that even those who experience considerable unrest in this challenging developmental passage will go on to live productive lives. The picture is somewhat less optimistic for those young people who develop persistent behavior and emotional problems in earlier stages of development. The younger these problems appear the more likely there are biological or genetic factors contributing to their functioning as compared to a temporary period of "insanity" brought on by the pressures endemic to adolescence.

When adolescents are confronted with death they may be particularly jolted by such an experience since they are at a stage of development when they are just beginning to take steps to claim and make a life of their own. The response to a death of a loved one is unique for each individual. Even an anticipated death of a grandparent can be deeply disturbing to an adolescent who viewed the grandparent as a rock of stability or a primary source of nurture. Over and over in grief counseling we are confronted with the fact that the meaning of the death for the survivor is a powerful factor in the shape that the grief process takes. Particularly shocking is the death of a peer as result of an accident or illness. Even though adolescents understand death as natural, universal, and inevitable better than younger children, they tend to feel omnipotent and don't view this as happening to them or a friend. Typically a death of a peer triggers in adolescents intense grieving and a desire to immerse themselves intensely in clusters of other peers, sometimes moving from house to house as they hang together to grieve the loss in the comfort and belonging of their friends. Parents are sometimes confused by this behavior because adolescents may be reluctant to turn to their families for support at such a time. The teen may feel, however that he or she can't risk turning back to their parents for emotional support because it would threaten the emerging autonomy they are trying to develop. Thus, they seek emotional support and comfort from their peer group.

IMPORTANT DEVELOPMENTS IN GRIEF COUNSELING FOR ADOLESCENTS

The field of grief counseling has been influenced by important research findings that have resulted in changes of the mindsets of grief counselors working with adolescents and profound implications for counseling strategies. One critical development is a new appreciation of the innate capacity for self-repair.

The power of resilience-based mindsets

An important recent trend in bereavement research is the recognition of the natural capacity for resilience based on the findings of George Bonanno (2010) that revealed that the most common reaction to a wide range of potentially traumatic events is resilience. The implications for grief counseling are huge. If we treat the death of a loved one or a good friend as traumatic, it can become a self-fulfilling prophecy. Likewise, if we recognize the natural and common innate source of resilience in a person that too can become a self-fulfilling prophecy. Robert Brooks (2010) has eloquently described the power of resilient mindsets. Obviously, the death of an important person in the lives of our youth can result in enormous suffering and sorrow. But we need not pathologize it.

If children are exposed to harsh conditions such as poverty, maltreatment, or neglect, they will be at high risk and more vulnerable to adversities that come later in life. It is important to not minimize the impact of such social toxic influences in the lives of children, but not all at-risk young people have poor outcomes. In addition, research summarized by Bonanno (2010) reveals that resilience is the norm, not the exception, in bereavement. Research by Ann Masten (2001) emphasized the innate self-repair and healing capacities of children and termed it "ordinary magic." Resilience viewed as "ordinary magic" represents a dramatic shift in the mindsets and approaches of counselors. As Bonnano (2010) pointed out, in the 1960s and 1970s when some at-risk youth were reported to be thriving, they were viewed as "invincible" or "super kids." Such youth were viewed as extraordinary and rare. The research by Masten has opened up new ways of thinking for counselors working with adolescent grief. While counselors should never minimize or trivialize the suffering of adolescents in grief (Crenshaw, 2010), the resilience research emphasizes the need to pay careful attention to strengths and signs of resilience, and to highlight and honor these assets in teens. Resilience-based questions such as the following should be asked:

- What people in your life have been helpful in getting you through the suffering?
- What strengths and resources in you have helped you keep going in this difficult time?
- Is there a miniature or figurine in the office that could symbolize your strength?
- What family members have you been able to gather strength and support from?
- Is there anything about the life of your loved one, words or deeds, or some cause that she or he stood for that inspires you and gives you strength?

These are simply sample questions that can be used as a springboard to focus the adolescent on both internal and external interpersonal resources that are sources of strength. Some adolescents will draw on spiritual beliefs or religious faith to negotiate a difficult time in their life. One study found that being able to draw on religious faith doubled the resiliency in a sample of former Ugandan child soldiers (Klasen et al., 2010). Perhaps no single study is more validating of the ordinary magic (innate resilience) of our youth than the study by Klasen and colleagues who evaluated 330 former child soldiers in Uganda who had been exposed to unspeakable atrocities. Nearly 88% of them had witnessed murder, over 43% lost both parents, and more than 52% had been forced to kill at least one person. Yet in spite of these unimaginable multiple trauma events of such severe nature, more than a quarter of the sample (27.6%) showed a resilient mental health outcome.

It is crucial that we respect and highlight innate self-reparative resources in our youth but that we not hold everyone to the same standard. Resiliency is an outcome of many contributing and interwoven factors. In the simplest terms there are assets on one side of the ledger and risk factors on the other side. Some adolescents will have encountered death with considerable prior vulnerability consisting of previous losses, preexisting psychiatric disorders, unstable or chaotic families, school failure and frustration, or peer rejection, to name just a few of the possible risk factors. Young people may show resilience in response to a major loss, such as the death of a close family member or a friend, but if the losses continue the resilience may be overwhelmed by the risk factors, particularly if they are also dealing with issues of poverty, school, or community violence. The risk factors as well as the assets can have a cumulative effect, either eroding strength and resilience or building and fortifying inner and outer resilience. Every youth we encounter in grief counseling is different and needs to be appreciated for the unique person that we seek to help. Above all we should never be judgmental in assessing their resilience or lack thereof. This point was made emphatically when Patrick Tolan (1996) studied the most violent neighborhoods of Chicago and summarized his findings in a paper called, "How Resilient is the Concept of Resilience?" In the worst examples of high crime neighborhoods, extreme poverty, and multiply stressed families, Tolan found no examples of resilient youth. Resilience in this study was defined as being no more than one year behind grade level in school and not requiring mental health intervention. Sometimes the social toxicity of social and community environments can overtake even the most resilient among our youth.

Targeted rather than generalized intervention

Since resilience is common rather than rare in the human population it is not surprising that not every bereaved teen needs grief counseling. In fact the percentage requiring mental health intervention may be considerably smaller than believed. A review of the research suggested that a subset of grievers, usually about 10 to 15%, who experience what is referred to as either prolonged or complicated grief, are the ones most likely to benefit from clinical intervention (Mancini, Griffin, & Bonanno, 2012). These are the teens who experience a high level of distress, consisting of intense longing and yearning for the deceased loved one, avoidance of reminders, intrusive thoughts or images, anger and guilt related to the loss, physiological hyperresponsiveness, or a sense of emptiness. These symptoms overlap with what is frequently considered traumatic grief (Cohen & Mannarino, 2004). Teens who undergo a more typical course of bereavement may experience considerable distress, but this tends to abate over time. These teens may need extra support from family, friends, and community, including any spiritual leaders or religious communities with whom they may be affiliated, but typically they do not need professional counseling. There are always exceptions, however, and each individual's needs have to be carefully considered.

In a study of parentally bereaved children and adolescents, more than half were showing few manifestations of grief after one year, but some experienced a more protracted course (Melhem, Porta, Shamseddeen, Payne, & Brent, 2011). Nearly 31% experienced a slower reduction of grief-related symptoms and 10.5% showed intense distress three years after the parental death. It is these latter two groups and particularly the last group that require clinical intervention.

The importance of meaning making to adolescents

The grieving process for all children, adolescents, and adults focuses to some degree on the meaning of it all (Neimeyer, 2001). Adolescents may need help to reconstruct their assumptive world following bereavement because loss has shaken the foundations of their world (Neimeyer, 2005). Neimeyer's research revealed that when people are bereaved by violent death, for example survivors of suicide, homicide or accident, the inability to make sense of the loss was the primary factor that sets them apart from those whose losses are more anticipated such as a serious illness in the loved one leading to death (Neimeyer, 2005). Bereavement, particularly when sudden, shatters assumptions about safety and security in the world. Adolescents particularly grapple with questions of *Why? Why me? Why my family? Why now?* Adolescents in contrast to younger children possess the abstract cognitive capacities to grapple with deeper meanings and mysteries of life and death. A 14-year-old girl told me about her fears of death and separation from loved ones. She noted that even if there is an afterlife, how could spirits possess the memory capacity to recognize their family and friends? These are questions that usually don't trouble younger children because they lack the cognitive capacities to ponder such questions. Once again there are exceptions. A father once told me about a conversation with his five-year-old daughter who asked him, "Is there another world?" The father said, "We don't really know." The little girl then said, "If there is another world, a little girl like me could be asking her father the same question in that other world." Most preschool children don't ponder such abstract issues but some precocious children do. One of the reasons that a sudden, unexpected death can be so devastating to adolescents is that developmentally they have the cognitive ability to appreciate death in a more adult way: that it is final, irreversible, and inevitable. But at the same time, they are also just beginning to emotionally move away from their families to claim more of a life of their own. When adolescents experience the sudden death of a peer, they are often reluctant to turn back to their families for emotional support because it threatens their budding autonomy. Teens are far more likely to turn to their peers and grieve in clusters, sometimes moving like nomadic tribes from house to house of their friends to grieve together in an intense way. Because their foundation of beliefs and security in the world is so profoundly shaken by an untimely death, adolescents especially seek to make sense of their world suddenly turned upside down.

Creating a trauma narrative in traumatic grief

A small subset of the overall bereaved population will suffer traumatic grief, usually in response to a sudden death of a family member or a close friend under circumstances that are horrific. Deblinger, McLeer, & Henry (1990) proposed the trauma narrative as an exposure intervention whereby repeated verbal expression, reading, and writing what happened during the trauma desensitized the child to trauma reminders. The use of graded exposure thus decreased the hyperarousal associated with trauma memories or intrusive images, thereby lessening PTSD symptoms. In addition the descriptions of the trauma events allowed for opportunities for the therapist to correct dysfunctional thoughts often taking the form of self-blame or excessive guilt. The Trauma-Focused Cognitive Behavioral Treatment (TF-CBT) model developed by Cohen, Mannarino, and Deblinger (2006) currently views the trauma narrative as not just to desensitize to trauma reminders and decrease the avoidance and hyperarousal that are core components of PTSD but also to enable the child or adolescent to integrate the traumatic experience into the totality of her or his life. In other words, another key function of creating the trauma narrative is to expand the adolescent's self-definition and world view to include far more than the trauma experience rather than crystalizing their identity around the trauma experienced. Clearly clinical judgment and an attuned sense of timing and pacing that can only come from clinical experience is needed in order to make the confrontation with the trauma events beneficial rather than deleterious.

Continuing bonds and remembering practices

The death does not sever the attachment ties that are timeless. The attachment described as "continuing bonds" by Klass and his colleagues continue (Klass, Silverman, & Nickman, 1996). They continue in memories of the person, dreams, and in their sense of non-physical presence in the lives of survivors. It is not unusual for adolescents to report that they "consult" their deceased parent at times when faced with critical problems or decisions. The goal of grief counseling is not to extinguish these bonds but to find ways to accept that the deceased is no longer in their lives in physical form but can be present in terms of the timeless attachment and continuing influence in their lives. Bowlby (1980), a pioneer in attachment theory, recognized that a continuing attachment with the deceased loved one was the norm rather than an anomaly.

Grief counseling today, whether in individual, group or family sessions, often contains components of remembering examples of the positive relationship with the deceased loved one. Even when the survivor had a negative or conflicted relationship with the loved one, there may be at least some happy memories that will provide comfort. Obviously this is not done with the goal of invalidating the actual experience of the griever. The adolescent griever may need someone they trust to hear their disappointments, anger, or other negative feelings such as betrayal in relation to the deceased. A way of achieving a realistic perspective would then be pursued in collaboration with the adolescent in grief.

Family and community are important

Adolescents bereaved by the death of a peer are drawn to the peer group community, including school friends, more than family because of the threat to their emerging autonomy. When the death occurs within the family, adolescents may turn more to their families for support and comfort. The research of Kissane, McKenzie, Bloch, and Moskowitz (2006) using a Family Focused Grief Therapy approach confirmed what clinical practice has repeatedly shown: that relationships with family are crucial in the grieving process. Interventions that strengthen family connections and open up the communication about the grief are of significant benefit. Often grief in adolescents can be inhibited out of a misguided belief that they must protect other members of the family. Other family members may be operating under the same misconception and thus the family is unable to talk openly about the loss or to support one another in their mutual grief. The larger community of which the family is a part that includes cultural, religious, professional or work groups plays an essential role in reducing the sense of isolation that a family might feel at a time of what is often experienced as unbearable pain. The show of support and validation of the worthiness of the life of the deceased family member is often comforting to adolescents who are sometimes surprised by the large turnout for the memorial services and the expressions of love and affection from the larger community. Of course, in stigmatizing deaths, such as suicide or traumatic deaths that overwhelm supporters, crucial support from the larger community may be lacking. Doka (1989) defined "disenfranchised grief" as "the grief that persons experience when they incur a loss that is not or cannot be openly acknowledged, publically mourned, or socially supported" (p. 4). Disenfranchised grief leads to loneliness, isolation, and often shame in the griever. This concept has been applied to the losses of children as well as to adults not only in the case of stigmatizing deaths but in cases of foster care children who frequently suffer multiple losses that are not honored or even recognized (Crenshaw, 2002).

Attachment security and vulnerability

Modern attachment theory as articulated by Schore (2012) and Siegel (2012) anchors the original theory of attachment articulated by Bowlby (1969/1980) and Ainsworth (1967) in the revolutionary findings of neuroscience and neurobiology. Schore's work has delineated the role of the right hemisphere in emotional regulation and in turn the crucial neural networks in the right hemisphere that reach deeply into the limbic system that are dependent on favorable early attachments. Schore pointed out that the right hemisphere in most people is dominant during the first three years of life, while the left hemisphere, the seat of language, linear, and logical thinking, doesn't come online until about 15 months of age. During this preverbal period, the most rapid period of brain development, the role of secure attachment is critical in the proper development of the right hemisphere. Those individuals who miss out on the secure base provided by adequate, sensitive attunement from the primary caregivers develop insecure attachment and will be more vulnerable to the stresses, adversities, and the inevitable losses that an ordinary human life brings (Schore, 2012; Siegel, 2012). Siegel (2012) stated, "Insecure attachments confer vulnerability because they fail to foster children's integrative self-organizational process" (p. 354). In contrast, Siegel (2012) explained, "Secure attachment involves both the differentiation of child from parent and the empathic and attuned communication between the two" (p. 354). It is important to realize that the therapeutic relationship is an attachment relationship that can serve an emotionally/developmentally corrective experience leading to advances in attachment security (Schore, 2012). An approach to traumatic grief based on the interpersonal neurobiological theory identified specific tasks for the griever to actively master (Crenshaw, 2007).

Neurosequential model of therapeutics

The work of Bruce Perry in the neurobiology of traumatized children has led to his development of a Neurosequential Model of Therapeutics (NMT) (Perry, 2009). Because the brain is still in the process of development during childhood and adolescence, there is a significant differential in the impact of a trauma event in childhood versus adult life. Children suffering a traumatic event achieve asymptomatic status only 33% over time versus adults who attained asymptomatic status 75% over time (van der Kolk et al., 2007). During highly emotional states, neuroimaging studies demonstrated increased activation of sub-cortical regions and significant reduction of blood flow to the frontal lobe (van der Kolk, 2006). Chronic conditions of trauma, often referred to as "complex trauma," results in alterations of the stress response system leading the brain to being set in a persistent state of fear or alarm. Youth with this clinical history will be likely not to benefit from traditional therapeutic interventions that are cognitively and verbally dependent because the lower brain networks are disorganized, underdeveloped or impaired (Perry, 2009). The NMT model stresses that it may not be as important what you do as when and in what sequence you do things in therapy. While complex traumatized individuals are a small subset of the overall bereaved youth, it is this group that is most likely to require clinical intervention from mental health professionals and counselors. To reorganize and modulate the regulatory neural networks of the lower brain requires what Gaskill and Perry (2012, 2014) call "bottom-up" interventions which include music, dance, walking, and drawing. William Steele at the Center for Trauma and Loss has developed a set of sensory-based drawing interventions with children and youth in grief and traumatic grief based on these brain-related concepts (Steele & Malchiodi, 2012; Steele & Kuban, 2013). Additional practical ideas are available in creative arts (Malchiodi, 2014); in play therapy (Crenshaw, 2014); in art therapy (Malchiodi, 2014); in music therapy (Robarts, 2014); in dance therapy (Devereaux, 2014); and in drama therapy (Gil & Dias, 2014).

CLINICAL CONSIDERATIONS FOR THE ADOLESCENT GRIEF COUNSELOR

Adolescents are known for their ambivalence and giving the adults who wish to help them mixed messages. When teens talk in a group about what they find helpful when grieving, some will say they want adults to notice and pick up on signs that they are hurting. The same teen later in the discussion will say, "I don't want to be singled out and made to feel different." The task for the grief counselor is complicated by these mixed signals. Grief counselors have to make sensitive judgments about when to reach out and pursue a reluctant griever and when to back off and leave them alone because they are not receptive at that time and pursuing may alienate them further.

The art of engaging adolescents

Engaging adolescents in therapy can be challenging but potentially rewarding. In grief counseling, as in all counseling, one of the key factors in engagement is the degree of choice the adolescents were given regarding participating. If they felt coerced or pressured to attend counseling by parents or schools or courts that is a formidable obstacle to overcome. More adolescents attend counseling by choice than younger children who typically have little say in such matters. But a sizeable proportion of the adolescent population attending therapy is there because someone else thought it was a good idea. I have known many adolescents in my clinical practice who would protest in a face-saving way about being coerced to one degree or another but then once in the office with the door closed would make maximum use of the experience. Some would even bring their best friends or boyfriends/ girlfriends to sit in the waiting room while they were engaged in their therapy session. While some teens were embarrassed and felt stigmatized about attending therapy, others would be completely open with their friends and in some cases also encourage their friends to seek therapy.

Finding portals of entry

Adolescents who feel pressured to take part in grief counseling, whether it takes the form of individual, group or family therapy, often can be engaged by finding the "portal of entry" that works for that particular youth to express his or her grief in natural and safe ways. Some teens will not talk but will draw, or make a picture with symbols in a sand tray or make figures out of clay or respond to storytelling strategies (Crenshaw, 2006, Crenshaw, 2008; Malchiodi, 2014; Steele & Malchiodi, 2012).

Therapeutic presence and sensitive attunement

While flexibility and patience on the part of the grief counselor, is valuable in finding natural portals of entry and creating a safe and trusting space where the work can take place, decades of psychotherapy research confirms that nothing the therapist does is as impactful as the quality of the therapeutic relationship. Sensitive attunement and therapeutic presence may encompass the qualities of warmth, genuineness, and empathy emphasized long ago by Carl Rogers (1957) which he identified as being so crucial in his early research on psychotherapy outcome.

Modality of therapy

Whether adolescents benefit more from individual, group, or family counseling has to be decided on a case-by-case basis. The group format is arguably the best fit developmentally given the central importance of one's friends and peer group in the lives of teens. Family counseling is perhaps the hardest modality for adolescents given their developmental trajectory away from the family and their healthy attempts to emotionally move away in small steps from their dependence on their parents. In the case of death in the immediate family, some teens will prefer the support of their family and gather strength by going through the grief process together with their surviving loved ones. Still other teens who are quite private or take pride in their independence may strongly prefer individual sessions. There is no right way to do it; it is a matter of best fit for a particular teen.

Practical and specific intervention strategies

The adolescents who are verbal and invested in grief counseling may need little or no prompting or structuring of their counseling sessions. These are the highly productive clients that every counselor wishes to see. Other adolescents who are not happy about even being in the company of the counselor, or adolescents who simply are unable to verbally express the emotions of grief, may need considerable structuring of the therapeutic context in order to communicate their thoughts and feelings. The Trauma-Focused CBT approach to grief and traumatic grief (Cohen, Mannarino, & Deblinger, 2006; Cohen,

Mannarino, & Deblinger, 2012) is highly systematized and available in manualized form, although these authors who are astute clinicians strongly urge clinical judgment and modifications of the protocol when indicated. Creative and expressive arts approaches are quite useful with adolescents who don't easily verbalize and can take many forms that include play, sand play, symbol work, drawing, painting, drama, dance and movement, and working with clay as well as other mediums and materials (Crenshaw, 2005, 2006, 2008; Malchiodi, 2012; Malchiodi & Crenshaw, 2014; Steele & Malchiodi, 2012).

Ethical Considerations

The Association for Death Education and Counseling (ADEC) Code of Ethics can be found in the *Handbook of Thanatology (2nd ed.)* (Meagher & Balk, 2013). Of particular relevance to working with children and adolescents is II. Competence (B) that states, "When called upon to deliver professional services, members accept only those positions and assignments for which they are professionally qualified" (p. 443). Many counselors who were trained to work with adults are not necessarily qualified or properly trained to work with children and adolescents. I once received a call from a young woman who had worked only with adults and she told me that the private agency she worked for was asking her to see adolescents. She said she had no experience or training in working with adolescents and asked if I would recommend a book she could read. I reminded her of the ethical code that all counselors and therapists are sworn to and strongly advised her not to proceed until she received the proper training and supervision. Unfortunately, I believe this situation is not that uncommon. Sometimes professionals feel that a workshop or two instead of an accredited program of training and supervision qualifies them to treat a different population. I don't think many Professional Boards of Ethics or State Licensing authorities would agree.

Another ethical issue that arises frequently in working with adolescents is confidentiality. In jurisdictions where there is a duty to warn or there is clear and imminent danger of suicide, the counselor may need to break confidentiality in order to avoid a tragedy. All of the exceptions to confidentially and privileged communication with the counselor need to be spelled out clearly and explained in writing in the form of an informed consent. The adolescent client and his or her parent or guardian are given the opportunity to ask questions and to sign the agreement; they should receive a copy to avoid misunderstandings and potentially a feeling of betrayal if an urgent life threatening situation occurs in the course of counseling.

How communications with parents or guardians are managed is also an important ethical and therapeutic issue. No adolescent will trust a counselor who has private communications without his or her knowledge and consent. Every counselor will need to work out with the adolescent and family how the issue is to be handled in a manner agreed to and understood by all parties. I typically have a family session on a regular basis even when seeing a teen individually, where the concerns of the family can be addressed openly and there are no secret or behind closed door meetings that will injure the trust of the adolescent. Some counselors allow one-way e-mail communications from the parents that are shared with the teen in session. Every counselor will need to grapple with this issue to keep the family informed of progress without destroying the trust of their adolescent client or violating their right to confidentiality. Readers are urged to be intimately familiar with the entire ADEC Code of Ethics.

CONCLUSION

Working with spirited adolescents in the midst of grief can be both challenging and rewarding. This chapter describes the shift in thinking that research in bereavement has brought about that has led to greater appreciation of strengths and resilience in the adolescents and their families. The correlated trend towards targeted rather than generalized intervention was discussed as well. The influence of modern attachment theory and trauma-informed therapy was also described and its influence on practice in the form of the Neurosequential Model of Therapeutics was also explained. Finally practical clinical considerations, strategies, and ethical issues were discussed that should inform the practice of any contemporary grief counselor.

David A. Crenshaw, PhD, ABPP, RPT-S, is clinical director of the Children's Home of Poughkeepsie, NY. He is a Board Certified Clinical Psychologist by the American Board of Professional Psychology, Fellow of the American Psychological Association (APA) and Fellow of APA's Division of Child and Adolescent Psychology. He is also a Registered-Play Therapist-Supervisor (RPT-S) by the Association for Play Therapy. Dr. Crenshaw is past president of the New York Association for Play Therapy as well as the Hudson Valley Psychological Association, which honored him with its Lifetime Achievement Award in 2012. He has published widely in the grief counseling field.

REFERENCES

Bell, M., Thornton, G., & Zanich, M. L. (2013). Resources and research in thanatology. In D. K. Meagher & D.E. Balk (Eds.), *Handbook of Thanatology (2nd ed.)* (pp. 411-428). New York, NY: Routledge.

Bonanno, G. (2010). *The other side of sadness: What the new science of bereavement tells us about life after loss.* New York, NY: Basic Books.

Bowlby, J. (1980). *Attachment and loss: Vol. 3. Loss: Sadness and depression.* New York, NY: Basic Books.

Brooks, R. (2010). Power of mind-sets: A personal journey to nurture dignity, hope, and resilience in children. In D. A. Crenshaw (Ed.), *Reverence in healing: Honoring strengths without trivializing suffering* (19-40). Lanham, MD: Jason Aronson.

Cohen, J. A., & Mannarino, A. P. (2004). Treatment of childhood traumatic grief. *Journal of Clinical Child and Adolescent Psychology 33*, 820-832.

Cohen, J. A., Mannarino, A. P. & Deblinger, E. (2006). *Treating trauma and traumatic grief in children and adolescents.* New York, NY: Guilford.

Cohen, J. A., Mannarino, A. P., & Deblinger, E. (Eds.). (2012). *Trauma-Focused CBT for children and adolescents: Treatment applications.* New York, NY: Guilford.

Crenshaw, D. A. (2002). Disenfranchised grief of children. In K. J. Doka (Ed.), *Disenfranchised grief: New directions, challenges, and strategies for practice* (pp. 293-306). Champaign, IL: Research Press.

Crenshaw, D. A. (2005). New clinical tools to treat childhood traumatic grief. *Omega: Journal of Studies of Death and Dying, 51*, 235-251.

Crenshaw, D. A. (2006). *Evocative strategies in child and adolescent psychotherapy.* Lanham, MD: Jason Aronson.

Crenshaw, D. A. (2007). An interpersonal neurobiological-informed treatment model for childhood traumatic grief. *Omega, 54,* 315-332.

Crenshaw, D. A. (2008). *Therapeutic engagement in child and adolescent psychotherapy: Play, symbol, drawing, and storytelling strategies.* Lanham, MD: Jason Aronson.

Crenshaw, D. A. (2010). Reverence in the healing process. In D. A. Crenshaw (Ed.), *Reverence in healing: Honoring strengths without trivializing suffering* (3-18). Lanham, MD: Jason Aronson.

Crenshaw, D. A. (2014). Play therapy approaches to attachment issues. In C. Malchiodi & D. A. Crenshaw (Eds.), *Creative arts and play therapy for attachment problems* (pp. 19-32). New York, NY: Guilford Press.

Deblinger, E., McLeer, S. V., & Henry, D. (1990). Cognitive-behavioral treatment for sexually abused children suffering post-traumatic stress: Preliminary findings. *Journal of the American Academy of Child and Adolescent Psychiatry, 29,* 747-752.

Devereaux, C. (2014). Moving with the space between us: The dance of attachment security. In C. Malchiodi & D. A. Crenshaw (Eds.), *Creative arts and play therapy for attachment problems* (pp. 84-99). New York, NY: Guilford Press.

Doka, K. J. (1989). *Disenfranchised grief: Recognizing hidden sorrow.* Lexington, MA: Lexington Books.

Gaskill, R. L. & Perry, B. D. (2012). Child sexual abuse, traumatic experiences, and their impact on the developing brain. In P. Goodyear-Brown (Ed.), *Handbook of child sexual abuse: Identification, assessment, and treatment* (pp. 30-47). Hoboken, NJ: Wiley.

Gaskill, R. L. & Perry, B. D. (2014). The neurobiological power of play: Using the Neurosequential Model of Therapeutics to guide play in the healing process. In C. Malchiodi & D. A. Crenshaw (Eds.), *Creative arts and play therapy for attachment problems* (pp.178-194). New York, NY: Guilford Press.

Gil, E., & Dias, T. (2014). The integration of drama therapy and play therapy in attachment work with traumatized children. In C. Malchiodi & D. A. Crenshaw (Eds.), *Creative arts and play therapy for attachment problems* (pp. 100-120). New York, NY: Guilford Press.

Kissane, D. W., McKenzie, M., Bloch, S., & Moskowitz, C. (2006). Family Focused Grief Therapy: A randomized, controlled trial in palliative care and bereavement. *American Journal of Psychiatry, 163,* 1208-1218.

Klasen, F., Oettinger, G., Daniels, J., Post, M., Hoyer, C., & Adam, H. (2010). Posttraumatic resilience in former Ugandan Child Soldiers. *Child Development, 81* (4), 1096–1113.

Klass, D., Silverman, P. R., & Nickman, S. L. (Eds.) (1996). *Continuing bonds: New understandings of grief.* London, England: Taylor & Francis.

Malchiodi, C. A. (Ed.) (2012). *Handbook of art therapy* (2nd ed.). New York, NY: Guilford.

Malchiodi, C. A. (2014). *Creative arts therapy approaches to attachment issues.* In C. Malchiodi & D. A. Crenshaw (Eds.), *Creative arts and play therapy for attachment problems* (pp.3-18). New York, NY: Guilford Press.

Malchiodi, C. A. (2014). Art therapy, attachment, and parent-child dyads. In C. Malchiodi & D. A. Crenshaw (Eds.) *Creative arts and play therapy for attachment problems* (pp. 52-66). New York, NY: Guilford Press.

Mancini, A. D., Griffin, P., & Bonanno, G. A. (2012). Recent trends in the treatment of prolonged grief. *Current Opinion in Psychiatry, 25*(1), 46-51.

Masten, A. (2001). Ordinary magic: Resilience processes in development. *American Psychologist, 56,* 227-238.

Meagher, D. K. & Balk, D. E. (Eds.). (2013). ADEC Code of Ethics. *Handbook of Thanatology (2nd ed.)* (pp. 441-450). New York, NY: Routledge.

Melhem, N. M., Porta, G., Shamseddeen, W., Payne, M. W., & Brent, D. A. (2011). Grief in children and adolescents bereaved by sudden parental death. *Archives of General Psychiatry, 68*(9), 912-919.

Neimeyer, R. A. (Ed.). (2001). Meaning reconstruction and the experience of loss. Washington, DC: American Psychological Association.

Neimeyer, R. A. (2005). Grief, loss and the quest for meaning. *Bereavement Care, 24*(2), 27-30.

Perry, B. D. (2009). Examining child maltreatment through a neurodevelopmental lens: Clinical application of the Neurosequential Model of Therapeutics. *Journal of Loss and Trauma, 14,* 240-255.

Robarts, J. Z. (2014). Music therapy with children with developmental trauma disorder. In C. Malchiodi & D. A. Crenshaw (Eds.), *Creative arts and play therapy for attachment problems* (pp. 67-83). New York, NY: Guilford Press.

Rogers, C. R. (1957). The necessary and sufficient conditions of therapeutic personality change. *Journal of Consulting Psychology, 21,* 97-103.

Schore, A. N. (2012). *The science of the art of psychotherapy.* New York, NY: Norton.

Siegel, D. (2012). *The developing mind (2nd ed): How relationships and the brain interact to shape who we are.* New York, NY: Guilford Press.

Steele, W. & Kuban, C. (2013). *Working with grieving and traumatized children and adolescents: Discovering what matters most through evidence-based, sensory interventions.* San Francisco, CA: John Wiley & Sons.

Steele, W., & Malchiodi, M. (2012). *Trauma informed practices for children and adolescents.* New York, NY: Routledge Taylor and Francis Group.

Tolan, P. (1996). How resilient is the concept of resilience? *Community Psychologist, 4,* 12-15.

van der Kolk, B. A. (2006). Clinical implications of neuroscience research in PTSD. *Annals of the New York Academy of Science, 107* (IV), 277-293.

van der Kolk, B. A., Spinazzola, J., Blaustein, M. E., Hopper, J. W., Hopper, E. K., Korn, D. L., et al. (2007). A randomized clinical trial of eye movement desensitization and reprocessing (EMDR), fluoxetine, and pill placebo in the treatment of posttraumatic stress disorder: Treatment effects and long-term maintenance. *Journal of Clinical Psychiatry, 68*(1), 37-46.

CHAPTER 22

Voices
What Helped and Didn't Help My Grieving

Kora Delashmutt

Editor's Note: Kora is a resilient and courageous young lady. As the oldest sibling, she stood up for her younger siblings to protect them from her father's abuse and in return suffered beatings herself. Kora tells her story of acute grief, shock, relief, and confusing feelings in her own powerful words in the immediate aftermath of being placed, along with her younger siblings, in foster care.

I walked towards the building with my siblings and the foster care staff. It seemed like a normal trip to the main house but something was telling me that it wasn't normal at all. Something was off but I just couldn't put my finger on what was amiss; as we approached the front entrance of the building, my stomach did a flip and butterflies fluttered in. With shaky legs I walked towards the hallway and my eyes immediately settled on my brother and mother standing in the living room. Immediately, I got the energy to run down the hall to them; they both looked so sad. It was like they were trying to hold their own sadness in and be strong for us. We sat down on the couch. There were strange people in the room that were all looking at us with sympathy. Our mother was trying to not shake and cry as she began to speak. She looked at all of us and began to say, "My babies, my babies, I'm so sorry to tell you that your father committed suicide this afternoon." Everything seemed like a blur after that; my mind shut down and I just sat there and cried.

I didn't know what to do. I didn't even know what I wanted; whether I wanted to scream, cry or just stare, so many emotions went through me all at once. Anger that he would kill himself and leave us here to clean up all the messes he made of our lives; sadness because, even though he put us through a lot of abuse he was a human being and didn't deserve to die like that; and questions, so many questions ran through my head. It was like a swirl of emotion and I was in the middle of it going faster and faster down the spiral. The only thing that made the swirl slow down was hugging my mother but eventually she would have to go home with my brother and leave us. I wanted to be with my mom and brother, to be home around familiar surroundings just to have something normal around me while I was trying to get the idea that it was all over through my head.

At first, when the news was setting in I didn't want to do anything or talk to anybody. Just sitting there with everyone while they did what they wanted was fine for me. But it didn't always work out that way; sometimes people would try to get me to talk. At that time it was still too fresh to me and I wasn't used to the idea of not having a father and worrying about abuse any more. My life went from the usual to unusual in one night and that's a lot to take on. The last thing that I needed was someone to get me to talk about it and explain what happened; that wouldn't have helped my situation. While I was grieving, I didn't want them to look at the papers they receive explaining the reason that we were removed from our home and think that they know everything there is to know. The papers don't explain the story in full perspective and sometimes the information can be wrong. I didn't like being judged because of what they read on a piece of paper.

If a person talked to me, I found out that it helped when they had a normal conversation with me and started off with small talk; that made it easier for me to find out whom I was and wasn't comfortable talking to. It helped me when the person trying to help me waited for me to start talking about why I am grieving, my past, and why I was there. There were times when I had to talk about my past, that I didn't have a choice whether I wanted to tell every little detail about my life. When I had to speak about my past and had no option on the matter whatsoever I felt angry and copped an attitude. I'm not making an excuse for my attitude but this stranger was invading every private detail of my life, and it ticked me off. It's a slow process building trust in someone when you are grieving and you just had your world ripped from under you.

Foster care was terrifying to me at first because there were so many new people and questions; everything seemed to be a fast blur of action. I was scared. All I wanted to do was go to my room, shut the door, and cry in my bed, not be put in a strange house filled with strange kids and adults. Even so, I did feel safe there even though it was a foreign place. I felt safe because the Group Emergency Foster Care (GEFC) house we were placed in looked like a normal house with sofas, TV, and kitchen, and the bedrooms looked homey as well. The setting was homey and made things seem safer and more comfortable, and that helped during my grieving process as well. The setting I was in helped with my nerves and the anxiety over everything that happened. The comfortable settings made me feel more at home. In contrast some settings I was in were too cold. The room was empty with a table and three chairs, no personality in the room at all. It made me uncomfortable like I wanted to fold myself back into my shell.

It's difficult when you are grieving; you don't know what you want and all your emotions are on high alert all day, every day. Sleeping is sometimes impossible and crying is unstoppable on some days, but eventually you start to heal and get stronger. It doesn't go away; the sadness will always be there over your loss. Yet, it does get easier to deal with as you get stronger and thrive as a survivor; you begin to be less and less sad. It's not gone but it's under control and locked away and your strength is the key that keeps it closed.

*When **Kora Delashmutt** was 17, she went into foster care. She is now 21 and loves her family more than anything in the world. In her free time she enjoys listening to music and drawing.*

CHAPTER 23

Expressive Therapies to Help Adolescents Cope with Loss

Nancy Boyd Webb

Adolescence has been depicted as the bridge between childhood and adulthood. It comprises approximately the period between the ages 13 and 19, during which time the young person undergoes extensive physical, cognitive, psychological, spiritual, and emotional changes along the path toward maturity. In the search to discover his or her identity the youth during this period begins to move away from parental and familial supervision and authority in favor of the wider world of peers and other influences outside the family circle. This shift produces both losses and gains, since the teen relinquishes the protective security of the family and trades this for the perceived advantages of joining and becoming part of a group of age mates. Of course many young people continue to value their familial roots, while at the same time experimenting with new ideas, relationships, and behaviors. However, family conflict during adolescence is quite common among American teens whose new friendships and changed behavior may provoke parental disapproval.

Adolescence has been described as a see-saw, push-pull, back-and-forth period in which the young person wavers between the wish for independence on the one hand, and the continuing comfort of the old and familiar on the other (Laser & Nicotera, 2011). The thrust to develop one's own identity, referred to as the "identity crisis" by Erikson (1968), can continue for many years beyond adolescence, but the task is at its peak during the teen years. This is when the young person struggles to come to terms with his or her strengths and weaknesses, likes and dislikes, relationships, plans for the future, and the critical issue of gender identity.

Because so many significant changes occur during the adolescent period, age must be taken into account in evaluating the teen's behavior. We know that a young person at age 19 is very different from his 13-year-old self. However, individual variations can result in the onset of puberty for some even before 13 years of age, while other teens mature later and may struggle with identity issues well into their 20s. The youth's cultural and religious background also influences his or her behavior, and sometimes these values conflict with those of the larger society, thereby leaving the teen with the difficult decision about which set of expectations to follow. The discussion here intends to portray the development of the average American teenager, with the caveat that individual variations always prevail over generalizations. In addition, fast-changing and differing customs and beliefs in our rapidly evolving world can make it difficult to determine with certainty the current norms of acceptable behavior.

This chapter presents an overview of adolescent development as the foundation for understanding how teenagers react to different kinds of losses. Expressive therapies can help teens discover and experiment with creative ways of coping with their feelings following various loss experiences. Several forms of expressive therapies will be discussed as they apply to adolescents. Many expressive methods can be employed in a group format, thereby appealing to young people who highly value and crave peer group involvement and acceptance.

THE MULTIPLE CHALLENGES OF ADOLESCENT DEVELOPMENT

Adolescents must tolerate and learn to adjust to the physical changes in their bodies at the same time they are struggling to come to terms with the turmoil of their evolving emotional, sexual, moral, occupational, spiritual, and social identities. The fact that the adolescent brain does not achieve full maturity until the mid-20s (Steinberg, 2009) seriously compromises the successful achievement of these major developmental tasks. When we consider the multiple stresses typical of the adolescent period, it is not surprising that it is fraught with so many hurdles.

High-risk behaviors and violence

Often teens want and need to experiment with different and extreme ideas and behaviors. Their egocentrism may lead them to believe that they are impervious to harm, and they may lack the caution that they will have later in their twenties in initiating new behavior. Adolescents may experiment with drugs and alcohol and engage in risky activities such as unprotected sexual activity, or driving at high speed or performing other dangerous feats. Sometimes the quest for popularity motivates such activities because the need for social approval is so strong among youth. The adolescent's poor judgment and belief that he or she is invulnerable (Balk, 2008) also contributes to their "wild" behavior.

Regardless of the reason, the facts indicate that accidents are the leading cause of deaths for adolescents ages 15 to 19, with the second being homicide, and the third suicide (FASTSTATS, 2013). Adolescent suicide is also a stark reality, accounting for approximately 4,600 deaths each year among 10 to 24-year-olds. This type of death carries a stigma of shame insofar as no one wants to talk about it, thereby contributing to the experience of disenfranchised grief (Doka, 2002) for the survivors.

The violent death of a peer by suicide or other means may generate a confusing blend of feelings among the circle of adolescent friends, ranging from the desire for revenge, to rumination about whether the death might have been prevented, and guilt because they did not intervene in some way. This complicated mixture of emotions seriously complicates the grief process and may contribute to depression or even compromise the youths' future developmental course. When professional intervention is available, the use of expressive therapies can help bereaved adolescents support and bond to each other in a helpful way.

Sexual orientation/gender development

Sexual orientation refers to a person's sexual attraction to individuals of a particular gender. This attraction does not always conform to society's expectations, even though we know that people may be attracted to individuals of the same sex (homosexual/ gay/lesbian), or even to both genders (bisexual) (Laser & Nicotera, 2011). Adolescents who identify as LGBT (lesbian, gay, bisexual, or transgender) may be subject to harassment by straight teens and they may be at greater risk for "emotional distress, isolation, depression, substance abuse, suicide, pregnancy, sexually transmitted diseases and internalized homophobia" (Morrow, 2006, as cited in Laser & Nicotera, p.185). These teens suffer ongoing and painful losses including the disapproval of society, their families and their peers; they clearly need support, which can be provided by some form of expressive therapies such as music, journaling, or art.

Bullying

The deliberate aggressive behavior of one or more persons toward another includes face-to-face intimidation or covert electronic confrontations (cyberbullying). All forms of bullying involve an imbalance of power between the perpetrator(s) and the target. Often other individuals witness the aggressive episodes of bullying without expressing any open disapproval of the behavior, either because they are afraid of the perpetrator(s) or uncertain about how to respond (Webb, 2011). Whatever the reason for the bullying, the youth who is bullied feels humiliated, unsafe, alienated, and isolated from his or her peers. He or she has lost a sense of safety as well as the company of other teens. Often families and the community at large do not understand or support an adolescent who is bullied and they may tell the teen to "just ignore it" or "fight back". When bullying occurs electronically on the Internet, the victim is especially helpless since the perpetrator(s) can be anonymous and the acts can be widespread, such as in sending uncomplimentary photos to hundreds or thousands of on-line viewers. The youth typically feels powerless and disgraced. The losses in a situation like this can be enormous, and some teens feel that they can never again regain any degree of self-respect or acceptance among their peers. Some teens may give up and take their own lives.

THE IMPACT OF LOSSES ON ADOLESCENTS

Numerous losses impact every adolescent's life and may include one or more of the following few examples:

- deaths;
- moving/change of schools/neighborhood/friends;
- the end of a significant relationship;
- parental divorce; or
- health issues for self or family members.

An implicit element in many of these occurrences, in addition to the loss itself, involves the end of a sense of safety, or predictability about the future. This can happen following an unexpected death or after the destruction caused by a natural disaster, as well as after a situation of human violence such as a mass shooting or exposure to family or other relational violence. Major crisis events such as these can lead to a loss of faith and/or the questioning of one's religious beliefs, with concern about how a loving God could permit such tragic occurrences. The expression "loss of innocence" sometimes applies to jolting experiences as well as to the loss of positive beliefs about the goodness of other people. This can occur after sexual experiences (either consensual, or due to force), or after the young person observes or hears about physical or sexual abuse situations among friends or others portrayed in the media. The adolescent sadly confronts the reality of the complex adult world in which people are not always kind to one another and in which deaths can occur to innocent people. After such losses, the young person may feel overwhelmed and have difficulty coping, either due to immaturity, lack of experience with how to respond, and/or a reduced capacity to marshal the necessary energy, thought, and consideration to deal with the upsetting event.

The response of any individual to a crisis is the result of the interplay of different factors including his or her personal history, the nature of the specific event, and the degree of support or lack thereof in the family and community. An assessment tool, *The Tripartite Assessment*, can be used to illustrate how a particular loss interacts with the background and current status of the responding individual, in conjunction with the quality of available support from the surrounding environment. (For more discussion about the use of the Tripartite Assessment in situations of bereavement and trauma see Webb, 2010 and 2007). The person's background, plus the nature of the stressful crisis or loss experience, blends with the type of support in the surrounding environment to determine an individual's unique response to a particular loss. This conceptualization helps professionals understand why different people who undergo the same or very similar crisis experience may have decidedly different reactions, varying from depression, to agitation, to quiet withdrawal or even acceptance. It is not the event, or the nature of the loss itself that determines specific reactions among those involved, but rather their personal histories and the environmental context in which the event occurs.

For example, teenagers (and people of any age) who were in a theater when a crazed adult began randomly shooting at the audience would be terrified and fearful for their lives. After the tragedy, many individuals would continue to have ongoing anxiety about whether this horrible behavior might be repeated in other locations by other deranged people; could it happen again? Some teens might continue to have bad dreams and agitation for several months related to their frightening experience, while others could return to their pre-crisis activities, feeling glad to be alive and determined not to permit this one horrible memory to continue to haunt their everyday psyches. What causes the difference between these two extreme reactions?

At the risk of oversimplifying, professionals should consider the backgrounds of the different victims, especially their temperamental characteristics, and their past histories of abuse, experiences with violence, and typical ways of dealing with stress. The differing nature of their family environments and the amount of support available either in the nuclear family or in the community must also be considered. For example, an adolescent living in a family characterized by alcohol or drug abuse, where disagreements often ended in physical conflict, was told to "man up" following the movie shooting. Compare this teen with another of the same age who comes from a supportive family that expressed appropriate concern and empathy about his frightening experience. Although it is never possible to predict with certainly the precise nature of anyone's reaction to stress, it is more than likely that the youth from the supportive family would respond with fear and anxiety, and that the youth from the harsher family background would try to repress his feelings of fear, but might feel jumpy, irritable, and angry with other people who would be oblivious as to the reasons for his hostile reactions. Both adolescents in this situation experienced a severe loss of security and control, but each one responded according to his unique life history.

Even people in the same family who experience the same loss (such as the death of a father) will react differently, and professionals must be prepared to assure the family that there is no *one* right way to grieve. Temperamental differences and distinctive personal characteristics may cause one adolescent to withdraw to his room and lose interest in participating in previously valued activities such as soccer or playing the guitar, whereas a sister two years younger in the same family can carry on her regular activities and calmly accept an invitation to join a hospice support group of other bereaved teens.

EXPRESSIVE THERAPIES TO HELP WITH LOSS EXPERIENCES

Experiences of loss are difficult for many people to discuss. Emotions interfere with rational discussion about the loss of a person, an animal, or a place that had special meaning. Verbalization requires thought and a decision about what to say and how to communicate these strong feelings. Often these feelings overshadow talking, and sometimes tears and choked breathing make speaking impossible. When the loss involves a death it can be especially hard to talk, especially for children and adolescents whose understanding about death may be unclear or in the process of formulation. Another reason teens avoid verbalization is because they fear being seen as weak by others, so they avoid crying or showing their emotions in public. This is especially true among males who have been socialized to be strong and told that "big boys don't cry."

Expressive arts therapies can help individuals of all ages express their feelings symbolically and obtain some relief from their stress without necessarily discussing the source of their pain. Arts therapies are especially useful in helping adolescents because the expectation for verbalization is minimal and often discussion is focused on the art project or musical production, rather than on personal issues.

Definition of expressive arts therapies

Expressive arts therapy has been defined as use of the arts and their products to foster awareness, encourage emotional growth, and enhance relationships with others through the creative imagination (Malchiodi, 2003; Lesley College, 1995). The basic premise is that expressive arts such as music, dance, drama, and visual arts permit people to communicate their feelings nonverbally, and to achieve insight and relief from anxiety as a result of this experience. The therapy may occur on an individual, group, or family basis; with adolescents, a group approach may be preferred. Some expressive arts therapies involve writing projects such as poetry and keeping a journal, both which require verbalization. The therapist's choice of activity for a teen or a group takes into account the readiness of the individual(s) to engage in it, based on the preliminary assessment and the youth's openness and ability to try new projects, plus an estimate about the degree of trust and sense of safety that exists among the group members.

Art therapy

Art therapy has been described as "a hybrid discipline based primarily on the fields of art and psychology" (Vick, 2003, p. 5). The purpose of the therapy is to help individuals experience some relief from their anxieties through the creation of an art project. Even people whose art ability is minimal can feel a sense of accomplishment after completing an exercise such as making a mandala, for example. The drawing of mandalas may serve as an initial exercise in adolescent bereavement groups because it requires no drawing ability, verbalization is optional, and it leads to feelings of peace and calm. Typically an art therapy bereavement group is led by a therapist who is trained in both art and bereavement counseling.

Group art therapy

Therapy in a group format may be more appealing than individual treatment for adolescents who have experienced a death or other losses. An initial interview screens the youth for a particular group, provides the opportunity to inform the teen about the group, and offers him or her choice of joining a group of peers who have experienced similar losses. In this initial meeting the therapist explains the structure of the group, typically eight to ten 50-minute sessions, after school, or on weekends, and elicits questions from the teen. The locale of group meetings may be a school, a hospice, a family agency, or in a hospital. Many hospice programs offer both support groups for teens who are anticipating the deaths of a family member or for those who are already bereaved. These groups are led by facilitators who have received special training.

In the first session of a bereavement group the leader explains that everyone present has had a significant loss experience and that the purpose of the group is to offer and receive support during the process of participating in some special art activities. The counselor may introduce an ice-breaking warm-up activity such as The Web, which consists of a playful way to make introductions. The leader holds up a ball of yarn and states that each teen will take a turn holding the ball and introducing him or herself and stating who died and how long ago. The group sits or stands in a circle and the leader begins by showing the group how to hold onto a piece of yarn from the ball before tossing it to someone else across the circle. After each group member has introduced him or herself, everyone will hold up their piece of yarn and a big web will have been created. This provides the opportunity for the leader to point out that they are all connected with one another.

The next phase of the initial group meeting usually includes some kind of introductory statement from the leader such as, 'We're going to continue by coloring some designs and then we will talk about them and how it felt to create them. It will be up to each person to decide whether to make any comments about their personal loss. It's perfectly ok to pass if you do not want to speak."

The mandala drawing exercise

A mandala is "any piece of artwork that is created within a round shape, customarily a circle" (Henderson, Rosen, & Mascaro, 2007, as quoted in Green, Drewes, & Kominski, 2007, p.160). This art activity can be used in a non-directive or a directive (structured) way. The leader begins by providing paper, either white or colored, with a circle already printed on it. The participants then proceed to color in the circle any way they wish. A more directive approach involves suggesting that the teens fill in the drawings, using eight distinct colors that correspond to different feelings they had when they heard about the death (Sourkes, 1991). They can color each segment as wide or as narrow as they wish to depict the corresponding feeling. The feelings might include the following emotions: relief, sadness, anger, guilt, curiosity, surprise, and so forth. These drawings require little or no artistic ability and the process of creating often bring about a cathartic sense of relief without the necessity of extensive talking. Sometimes the leader provides a gentle musical background to further promote relaxation during the drawing exercise. The drawing of mandalas has been cited in the literature as encouraging a meditative state which promotes an inner calmness and sense of relaxation (Beaucaire, 2012; Green, Drewes, & Kominski, 2013; Sourkes, 1991). This can bring welcome relief from the worry and anguish of bereavement.

Subsequent sessions of the bereavement group may include other art activities, such as scribble, "safe-place," and "before/after/future" drawings. All of these art exercises can be created during either individual or group therapy, although most adolescents prefer the group format. The multi-person structure also permits cooperative group art projects, such as the creation of a group mural. If the participants wish to do this it usually is planned toward the end of the group sessions, when people have grown to know one another and when they are open to a cooperative project.

Scribble Drawings

This exercise, which originated with Donald Winnicott (1971), involves two or more individuals taking turns finding pictures or designs in each other's scribbles. The therapist states that there is a picture in every scribble; sometimes the design portrays something from real life, and other times the result is an imaginary figure. Adolescents who say that they cannot draw will be intrigued by the process of trying to create some kind of a picture from the therapist's or other group member's scribble drawing. Once the picture is finished, the therapist may invite the teens to give it a name and, depending on the youths' current degree of verbal communication, to make up a story about the picture. Adolescents really enjoy this activity and often spontaneously ask to repeat it in subsequent sessions. The exercise can serve as a warm-up exercise in beginning contacts when the young people are still developing a sense of safety with the therapist and each other.

The "safe place" drawing

This exercise can be used in individual or group therapy. It is especially helpful for use with individuals whose loss involves a traumatic experience, as a cognitive method that helps teens learn to control their anxiety. The therapist introduces this exercise as a way to instruct the participants about how to calm themselves and subdue their anxious feelings. The therapist might say something like the following as an introduction to the exercise:

> I know that most of us want to feel in control of our own bodies. This method can help you do that. It begins with a mental exercise and then you will draw a picture. So first, please close your eyes and begin thinking of a very, very safe place. It can be either real or imaginary. Think about whether the place is cool or hot; whether there are any smells that you like in the air. Are there any sounds of nature or music, or some other pleasant noises like birds singing, or ocean waves breaking on the shore? Imagine yourself in this place. Are you standing, sitting or lying down? Make yourself very, very comfortable in this special place where no one can ever hurt you and you are completely safe.

After a few minutes of quiet contemplation the therapist instructs the teens to slowly open their eyes and, without saying anything, to begin to draw their safe place. When the drawing is complete the therapist emphasizes that this place belongs to the teen; it is his or her own creation that the youth can think about every night in bed before sleep and during the day at a quiet time. The drawing is a way to escape worries and anxieties, and although it does not change anything in the real world, it can change a person's attitude about the world. Depending on the comfort level of the group, the therapist may invite anyone who wishes to share their drawing with the group.

"Before/after/future" drawings

This exercise is intended to help the adolescent feel a sense of hope about the future. It should be offered after the teen has developed a degree of trust in the therapist and in the group. The exercise involves instructing the teens to recall a specific memory of the deceased person or traumatic experience *before* the actual loss occurred and to draw that memory. Sometimes the therapist instructs the youths to fold a paper in half and write 'before' as the heading of one column and 'after' on the other. Then the therapist suggests that the adolescents recall a happy memory of 'before the loss' and then draw it. After this drawing, the therapist instructs the teens to think about a significant change that has occurred since the loss and draw that. The therapist encourages the teen to talk about both experiences, and then to consider what positive hope the adolescent can now hold for the future. Although it is common for people to believe that "things will never be the same" after a significant loss, and that may be true, the aim is to encourage the youth to consider that despite the loss there still can be positive experiences that will enrich his or her life.

All of these drawing activities serve to engender feelings about the individual's losses. If the youth seems reluctant to draw, and says that he or she has no drawing ability, the therapist can state clearly that the drawings will not be graded; even stick figures are perfectly okay. The drawings may encourage the youth to talk about personal experiences or to view them in a different way. When the exercises are conducted in a group, the youth sees that others have similar feelings; this recognition can prove to be extremely supportive to bereaved teens, who often feel isolated from peers because of their experience

It is notable that the International Society for Traumatic Stress Studies (ISTSS) acknowledges that creative arts therapies (such as these drawing activities) are unique methods of gaining access to traumatic memories and, over time, these approaches can be helpful in the treatment of post-traumatic stress disorder (Steele & Malchiodi, 2012).

Music, movement, and drama as therapy

Music, movement, and drama are other methods for helping teens understand and cope with their loss experiences. As already mentioned, the playing of music can be paired with art activities to provide a relaxing and calming background during the creation of an art project. Combining several creative arts methods together can magnify the effect of each. Music, for example, often stimulates dance or rhythmic movements in listeners. Young people wearing ear buds and bobbing their heads to the sounds of their favorite songs is a familiar image; it is quite natural to include music as part of a therapeutic experience for adolescents experiencing losses. Teens may be invited to bring one of their favorite songs or playlists to share with the group. If other group members wish, they may stand up and move to the music, either shaking or rocking their bodies, or dancing alone or in a circle. Sometimes the choice of music includes selections that have meaning because they were shared with their deceased loved one, or the music may have some special significance related to the loss. It is up to each individual to decide if he or she wants to talk about the reason for the choice of the musical selection.

Music therapy has been defined as "the use of music to restore, improve, or maintain health and well-being" (Loewy & Stewart, 2004, p.192). Research suggests that the listening and playing of music may actually lower stress hormones and enhance immune functioning (Shaller & Smith, 2002). Adolescents who are experiencing losses need to find a way to express their emotions and experience release, and to feel the support of their peers. This can occur in group music therapy through drumming, group singing, dancing, or adapted song-writing (changing the lyrics of a song). Musical ability or experience in playing instruments is not a requirement for participation in a music therapy group. Improvisation occurs when the participants and the therapist together begin a drum beat, a series of chords, or a part of a melody which they then expand upon together, sometimes singing or humming (Tervo, 2001). Some group members can play a drum while others sing or dance. The use of rap, hip-hop, jazz, and country music in teen groups often serves to open up discussion of feelings and serious issues. See Malekoff (in press) for examples of the use of music and song-writing in teen groups.

Music often is combined with drama in expressive therapy groups. Malchiodi (2003) refers to "multimodal approaches" in expressive arts therapy, referring to the use of more than one art form, based on the therapist's judgment about how best to encourage the emotional growth of participants while also enhancing their inter-relationships. Dramatic performances often include music and dance as part of the action. Drama therapy has been defined as "the use of drama/ theater techniques in an intentional, planned way as a specific form of intervention, designed to bring about intra-psychic, interpersonal, or behavioral changes" (Irwin, 2005, p.5). An excellent example from the Dougy Center shows a teen theater troupe in a performance in which seven youths enact several sketches related to their various experiences after the deaths of family members. This presentation includes individual stories about the deaths, their feelings about returning to school after the death, group singing and dancing, and a group review of how they are coping (Leigh & The Dougy Center, 2007). Individual members also talk about how cautious and hesitant they were originally when the group began, and about how important it was for them to gradually realize that the other group members truly understood their losses.

CONCLUSION

Many adults feel intimidated by adolescents who appear to be in their own world and totally disinterested or resistant to interacting with the older generation. When these adolescents are bereaved or suffering losses such as multiple moves, the destruction caused by natural disasters or abuse in the family or among peers, they may deliberately avoid any kind of meaningful contact with adults as they attempt to protect themselves through angry isolation. Well-meaning gestures from adults to express sympathy or offer help are minimized or ignored because the alienated youth do not want to talk about their problems, and if they should decide to do so, their preference would be to share their feelings with a peer, not an adult.

Expressive therapies offer the possibility for connection and help for these youth because these methods do not require extensive verbalization and they bring about relief from anxiety; at the same time, they are enjoyable and provide new ideas and support from other group members. The challenge for the leader or therapist is to introduce these activities to teens in an appealing way, in the form of fun activities that downplays the expectation of talking. Expressive therapies offer numerous ways to express one's thoughts and feelings and obtain relief and new ideas through the creative process. Expressive therapies help bridge the verbal chasm that is so daunting for bereaved teens who do not have the words nor the life experience to verbalize their feelings about death and other serious losses.

When the therapies are provided in a group format adolescents are more inclined to join and participate. They can give vital support to one another in the group at the same time as they receive it. The group removes the feelings of isolation that often accompany a death or other loss experiences, and it becomes a safe haven where bereaved and frightened adolescents find mutual comfort and relief. Through the expression of creative arts all emotions can be expressed and understood and adolescents can discover new and creative ways to deal with their losses (LeVieux, 1999).

Nancy Boyd Webb, DSW, LICSW, RPT-S, is a professor emerita, an author/editor, keynote speaker, and workshop presenter. Her areas of expertise include traumatic bereavement, play therapy, and vicarious traumatization. Her keynote presentations and workshops focus on these topics as they affect children, adolescents and their families. Dr. Webb held the endowed James R. Dumpson Chair in Child Welfare Studies at Fordham University, where she taught in the clinical practice area for 30 years, and was named University Distinguished Professor. In 1985 she founded Fordham's Post-Master's Certificate Program in Child and Adolescent Therapy which continued for 22 years until her retirement. Smith College honored Dr. Webb with its prestigious Day/Garrett award in 2010. In addition to teaching, writing, supervising practitioners, and consulting with schools and agencies, Dr. Webb participates in several interdisciplinary professional organizations.

REFERENCES

Balk, D. (2008). The adolescent's encounter with death. In Doka, K. J., & Tucci, A.S. (Eds.), *Living with grief. Children and adolescents.* Washington, DC: Hospice Foundation of America.

Beaucaire, M. (2012). *The art of mandala meditation.* Avon, MA: Adams Media (A division of F + W Media, Inc.).

Bazelon, E. (2013). *Sticks and stones. Defeating the culture of bullying.* New York: Random House.

CDC: Centers for Disease Control and Prevention. *Suicide Prevention.* Retrieved August 5, 2013.

Doka, K. J. (2002). (Ed.). *Disenfranchised grief. New directions, challenges, and strategies for practice.* Champaign: IL: Research Press.

Erikson, E. H. (1968). *Identity: Youth and crisis.* New York, NY: Norton.

FASTSTATS. (August 5, 2013). *Deaths. Leading causes for 2009, Table 1.*

Green, E. J., Drewes, A. A., & Kominski, J. M. (2013). Use of mandalas in Jungian play therapy with adolescents diagnosed with ADHD. *International Journal of Play Therapy, 22*:3, 159-172.

Green, E. J. (2012). Fostering resiliency in traumatized adolescents: Integrating play and evidenced-based interventions. *Playtherapy, 7*:2, 10-15.

Henderson, P., Rosen, D., & Mascaro, N. (2007). Empirical study on the healing nature of mandalas. *Psychology of Aesthetics, Creativity and the Arts, 1,* 148-154.

Irwin, E. C. (2005). *Facilitating play with non-players. A developmental perspective.* In A. M. Weber, & C. Haen (Eds.), *Clinical applications of drama therapy in child and adolescent therapy* (pp. 3-23). New York, NY: Brunner-Routledge.

Laser, J. A. & Nicotera, N. (2011). *Working with adolescents. A guide for practitioners.* New York, NY: Guilford Press.

Leigh, L. J. & The Dougy Center (2007). *Acting out. The Scarlet D's on their grief trip.* Portland, OR: The Dougy Center.

Lesley College. (1995). *Definition of expressive therapy.* Retrieved from http://www.lesley.edu/faculty/estrella/intermod.htm.

Le Vieux, J. (1999). Group play therapy with grieving children. In Sweeney, D. S. & Homeyer, L. E. *Group play therapy. How to do it. How it works. Whom it's best for* (pp. 375-388). San Francisco, CA: Jossey-Bass.

Loewy, J. V., & Stewart, K. (2004). Music therapy to help traumatized children and caregivers. In N. B. Webb (Ed.), *Mass trauma and violence. Helping children and families cope* (pp. 191-215). New York, NY: Guilford Press.

Malchiodi, C. A. (Ed.). (2003). *Handbook of art therapy.* New York, NY: Guilford Press.

Malekoff, A. (in press). *Group work with adolescents. Principles and practice,* 3rd ed. New York, NY: Guilford Press.

Malekoff, A. (2004). *Group work with adolescents. Principles and practice, 2nd ed.* New York, NY: Guilford Press.

Morrow, D. (2006). Gay, lesbian, bisexual, and transgender adolescents. In *Sexual orientation and gender expression in social work practice. Working with gay, lesbian, bisexual, and transgender people* (pp.177-195). New York, NY: Columbia University Press.

Shaller, J. & Smith, C. R. (2002). Music therapy with adolescents experiencing loss. *The Forum, 28*:5, 1-4.

Sourkes, B. M. (1991). Truth to life: Art therapy with pediatric oncology patients and their siblings. *Journal of Psychosocial Oncology, 9*(2), 81-95.

Steele, W., & Kuban, C. (2013). *Working with grieving and traumatized children and adolescents.* Hoboken, NJ: Wiley.

Steele, W., & Malchiodi, C. A. (2012). *Trauma-informed practices with children and adolescents.* New York, NY: Routledge.

Steinberg, L. (2009, April). *A social neuroscience perspective on adolescent risk-taking.* Paper presented at the biennial meeting of the Society for Research in Child Development, Denver, CO.

Tervo, J. (2001). Music therapy for adolescents. *Clinical Child Psychology and Psychiatry, 6* (1): 79-91.

Vick, R. M. (2003). A brief history of art therapy. In C. A. Malchiodi (Ed.), *Handbook of art therapy,* p. 5-15. New York, NY: Guilford Press.

Webb, N. B. (Ed.). (2007). *Play therapy with children in crisis. Individual, group, and family treatment, 3rd ed.* New York, NY: Guilford Press.

Webb, N. B. (Ed.). (2010). *Helping bereaved children. A handbook for practitioners, 3rd ed.* New York, NY: Guilford Press.

Webb, N. B. (2011). *Social work practice with children.* New York, NY: Guilford Press.

Winnicott, D. W. (1971). *Playing and reality.* New York, NY: Basic Books.

CHAPTER 24

Grief, Adolescence, and the Autism Spectrum

Karla Helbert

Most clinicians, caregivers, and support people in the field of grief and bereavement have long understood that the experience of grief encompasses far more than feelings. Grievers are affected by the pain of bereavement on multiple levels: physical, mental, cognitive, emotional, spiritual and philosophical. Adolescents on the autism spectrum are no different. How grief manifests, what symptoms appear, and how grief is expressed, may differ, but multi-faceted effects are present. On and off the spectrum, grief is a highly individual experience.

Nearly 10 million children in the United States ages 6 to17 were reported by their parents in 2012 as having an Autism Spectrum Disorder (ASD). This number represents a nearly 42% increase from rates of parent-reported ASD in 2007 (Blumberg et al., 2013). Grief professionals need the tools to cultivate knowledge and to feel comfortable and competent to help this growing population and their families when they are in need.

Individuals on the spectrum characteristically display uneven levels of ability in functioning as well as differing levels of progress in various areas of development. It is important to recognize that, on the spectrum, there may exist in any given individual great disparity in cognitive, social, emotional, and physical development and awareness. In general, a person with ASD will experience the same range of symptoms of grief as a typically developing person in the same developmental stage of life (Helbert, 2013). The key is in understanding how and where along the developmental continuum a particular child or adolescent functions as an individual. As a quote popularly attributed to Dr. Stephen Shore, author, professor, advocate and individual with autism, rightly states, "If you've met one person with autism, you've met one person with autism."

Younger children may display regressive behavior, or exhibit behaviors they may previously have "grown out of." They may become more demanding or require extra reassurance and attention. They may become more fearful, have bad dreams, or fear the deaths of others. Much depends on the child, as well as the manner of death of the loved one. Some children can experience self-blame or believe that their thoughts may have caused bad things. Some may withdraw, while others may seem unaffected (Helbert, 2013).

Nearly all young children, and some older children, can have problems understanding the abstract concept of death and its permanence. They can have difficulty with the many abstract ways that grown-ups, and society in general, tend to talk about death. Those on the autism spectrum, including older children and teens, will likely have a more difficult time than neurotypically developing children with this particular aspect of the language surrounding death. Family, friends, caregivers, and professionals should avoid speaking in abstractions or giving confusing information or responses about a loved one's death. Saying things like, "We lost Grandpa," can be confusing. The child may think, or ask, "Why can't we find him? Where did he get lost?" Other common phrases such as, "She has passed away" or "He's in a better place," require further explanation and clarification and may not make sense to a concrete-minded child, tween, or teen. In general, when talking to an individual with ASD, be as concrete as possible. Avoid using euphemisms for death and be sure he or she understands that the person has died and is not "lost," or simply someplace else. Words, phrases, and euphemisms that may make others in society, usually neurotypical others, feel more comfortable about death can create confusion (Helbert, 2013). Letting him or her know that a person has died may include explaining concretely what death means, including the cessation of bodily function, and that the deceased person no longer feels pain or has physical needs. Always tell the truth and be clear, while remaining mindful and judicious about over-sharing.

Teenagers and tweens do not like to be considered children, and don't like to feel different from their peers. Even though a teen with ASD may not behave in a typical teenage manner of her peers, she most likely will fit the teenaged need to be considered an individual who is trusted, respected, and treated as an equal in as many ways as possible. Teens need to be told the facts, want to be allowed to ask questions, and should feel supported in expressing their own thoughts and feelings (Helbert, 2013).

Many clinicians and support people in the field of bereavement routinely help the bereaved by normalizing symptoms of grief and helping them to know that the myriad ways they are affected by grief are overwhelmingly the norm, even when they feel abnormal. It can be extremely helpful and a comfort for the griever to realize that the physical, mental, emotional, cognitive and spiritual effects of grief are indeed typical, and she is not unusual, or abnormal, in her experiences. The same kind of normalization for a person on the autism spectrum can present challenges for the professional or layperson who has not developed the knowledge of how a person with ASD may experience the same symptoms.

Physically, the manifestation of grief for a person with autism can look different than it might for a neurotypically functioning person. A child or adolescent with ASD may express physical symptoms in ways similar to those of a neurotypical child and comparable behavioral changes may occur. How these manifest will be individual. Restlessness or hyperactivity may emerge or increase; he may have difficulty sleeping, or, conversely, may appear more tired or listless, requiring more sleep; he may show a desire to withdraw. These symptoms are not outside the norm for a neurotypical person, but the expression can be very different. Support people may notice no overt physical symptoms at all. Knowing what is the norm for each particular child or adolescent and noticing, and inquiring about, any differences, subtle or overt, is key. Behavioral differences, changes in communication patterns, methods and topics, reactions to environment, sensory stimuli and diet can all give important clues to how an individual on the spectrum may be experiencing and expressing physical symptoms of grief.

Dietary issues are of particular concern for grieving children and adolescents on the spectrum. Very often, these children and adolescents have challenges surrounding feeding issues even at the best of times (Bandini et al., 2010). They may have highly selective diets, ritualistic eating behaviors, sensory or motor issues surrounding eating and foods, as well as difficulty interpreting body signals. Grief can intensify these difficulties. Individuals on the spectrum in grief may also present with increased digestive problems, including constipation, gas, irritable bowel, diarrhea, or nausea. Loss of or increased appetite, or cravings for particular kinds of foods, can occur. Parents and caregivers should take particular care to ensure that children, tweens and teens on the spectrum receive appropriate nutrition and hydration. Some adolescents can remember to eat and drink appropriately by setting alarms or reminders on mobile devices at meal and snack times, or by putting reminders into personal daily schedules. Younger children, or less independent adolescents, can benefit from scheduled meal and snack times as well as support in the form or reminders or incentives to eat and drink. Proper nutrition and hydration can help support the immune system, which can be compromised in times of grief.

Crying is a typical, socially expected physical symptom of grief in children as well as adults. It is important to remember, however, that tears are not a good indicator of emotional response or, depth of feeling for anyone in grief. Neurotypical people may falsely assume that a person on the spectrum who does not cry is not grieving. Support people should understand and remind adolescents on the spectrum that it is okay if they do not express grief though tears; some people may cry a little, some a lot, and some not at all. This can help them to know that their personal expression of grief is theirs alone. It is helpful to remind those who do express grief through tears that crying is okay and can help to relieve stress.

For most people on the spectrum, sensory processing problems are part of life (Kern et al., 2006). It is important to understand that those on the spectrum may experience changes in sensory processing during grief; how each individual's sensory processing difficulties manifest is unique. New or previously unseen sensory difficulties may also emerge during or as a result of grief (Helbert, 2013). This may be due to the stress of the changes brought by grief, disruption in typical routines, schedules, expectations, or other unknown causes.

Professionals, caregivers, and parents should communicate with the child, tween, or teen about sensory processing difficulties and the possibility of increases or changes in sensory issues. Notice the adolescent's behavior, noting particularly any changes that may indicate differences in sensory functioning. Sensory changes can be frightening, and sensory overload can result in increased anxiety, withdrawal, or loss of behavioral control (including at times, loss of safety awareness), often colloquially referred to as a "meltdown."

Families may find it helpful to spend some time thinking about sensory issues that may arise during typical rituals that are part of death and dying. Typical death and grief rituals, such as funerals, memorial services, visitations, and wakes, often include sensory experiences that can be new and potentially difficult for those on the spectrum. These rituals frequently include large gatherings of people with little preparation time. Smells, light, sounds, textures, and other sensory stimuli can all be problematic, whether in a hospital, funeral home, church, or other gathering place. Many on the spectrum suffer from social anxiety, making these situations difficult to navigate emotionally as well. Another issue to bear in mind is the fact that travel may be necessary, or family and friends may come into the individual's home to visit or stay for extended periods. Struggles with symptoms of grief, sensory difficulties, social anxieties, and the disruption to the person's usual schedule and routine can all create serious challenges.

Caregivers can also help teens on the spectrum anticipate hugging and other physical contact as well. Because of tactile, olfactory, or other sensory sensitivities, those on the spectrum may or may not wish to hug. Letting them know that it is okay to say, "No thank you, I would rather not hug," can be helpful. They may choose to shake hands, fist bump, "high five," or explain that they do not want any physical contact.

Any kind of preparation for the event, such as what to expect, what it will be like, who will be there, and what the environment might look like, can be very helpful. Plans or preparations can be verbal or written. For younger children or more concrete thinkers, having photographs or visual representations of what to expect can be useful.

Allowing the adolescent the opportunity to ask questions can be helpful for his or her own preparation as well as in helping others to understand what he or she may be thinking or concerned about, giving clues to the internal experience of grief. Participation in rituals and other events should be allowed and encouraged, with the choice of the individual guiding the decision. Having a plan in place that allows for breaks if needed is helpful. A support person might be identified to assist with leaving or taking breaks. Planning ahead for an exit or calming strategy can help everyone involved have a more tolerable experience in a difficult situation.

Grief for those on the spectrum can be considered a form of disenfranchised grief (Doka, 2002). Some may believe, based on stereotypes, misinformation, or lack of exposure to people on the spectrum, that those with ASD are emotionally incapable, or lack the need, to grieve. These types of beliefs are related to the common misperception that people on the autism spectrum lack empathy, the ability to understand or share in the feelings of another.

Most neurotypically-developed people are generally able to quickly assess the mental states, thoughts, beliefs and intent of others in conversation and social situations. They also instinctually mirror and react to the emotional states, expressions, and affects of others with whom they are interacting. This ability is referred to as "Theory of Mind," a term first used by Cambridge professors Premack and Woodruff in 1978, and owes much to the neural mirroring systems of the brain, in which so-called mirror neurons react and fire when humans (as well as other animals) perform actions or observe the behavior of others. Studies at Stanford University confirming anatomical differences in the cortical substrates of the neural mirroring systems of those on the spectrum may go a long way toward explaining why these individuals have difficulty recognizing emotion and reciprocating in socio-emotional situations. This may also be why they may *appear* to lack empathy, particularly in the midst of social exchanges (Hadjikhani, Robert, Snyder, & Tager-Flusberg, 2006).

This response does not mean that they do not care about others, or that they do not form deep emotional connections with others. Challenges with one's ability to interpret, understand, and mirror the social and emotional responses of another, or being wholly unaware of the internal experience of another in a specific social situation, is not the same as not caring, or not having empathy. Extra time, instruction, support, or reflection is almost always needed for a person with ASD to arrive at a fuller emotional or social picture. When someone important has died, when a known significant relationship has been severed by loss, professionals, caregivers, parents, family members, friends and other support people should choose to assume there is grief. Assume grief, but do not assume you will know how the person with ASD will experience or express grief.

For many adolescents on the spectrum, stress and anxiety are factors of everyday life. Difficulty with change and transitions are hallmarks of ASD. Grief-induced stress and the expected symptomology can create further challenges for those on the autism spectrum. The sorts of challenges adolescents on the spectrum in grief may experience are highly variable and dependent upon each individual, but one aspect of grief which creates difficulty for nearly all those with ASD is the chaotic nature of grief. This chaos, not knowing how one may feel, or what symptoms of grief one might expect to experience from one moment to the next, having one's regular routine, schedule, or one's life disrupted by death and grief, can be highly distressing.

In one case study, Brandon, a 15-year-old boy diagnosed with Asperger's Syndrome, had a strong relationship with his school art teacher. When she died, he became exceedingly distressed that he would not be able to make paintings in the art room. Her students knew only that she had been sick for some time. They had no details of her illness. When she died sooner than expected, the school reported that she had died in a car accident. The confusing nature of the story of what had happened and the lack of concrete information contributed greatly to the difficulties inherent in his resulting grief.

Brandon's distress elevated fairly quickly and turned to anger. The impression his response gave to others was that he was selfish and insensitive, not thinking of the deceased teacher's family, friends, co-workers, or other students who were grieving. It was difficult, if not impossible in the moment, for him to express that his response was very much about deep grief at losing such a caring, supportive person in his life, but also one of deep confusion and high anxiety.

The main activity Brandon and his teacher engaged in was making paintings in the art room. At the time, he was unable to make the emotional connection that his response was linked to her death and to his grief. He was not simply angry that he could not paint in the art room. He was able to make the connection later, through painting portraits of his teacher and through other expressive representations of his various emotions and experiences. It was important for family and support people to recognize that not being able to paint in the art room was, on its own, an incredibly upsetting change in what was his normal routine prior to the teacher's death. Both the disruption of routine and his grief at the loss of his beloved teacher were present.

One exercise that worked well in therapy for Brandon was an exercise called *Color Your Heart* (Helbert, 2013), which asks the grieving individual to think about and identify various feelings experienced in the present moment. He was asked to assign chosen colors to feelings (worry, happiness, fear, hope, etc.) and in so doing was able to practice emotion recognition. He then colored in a blank heart shape with each chosen color representing how much of each feeling he was experiencing at the time. Through inviting him to color, draw or fill in the heart shape any way he choose—with stripes or swirls, a representative picture or abstract shapes—expressive information about his grief or other feelings emerged, giving him more information to help make sense of his experience.

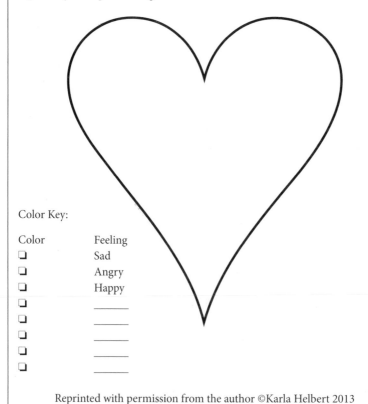

Figure 1:

COLOR YOUR HEART EXERCISE

Choose as many colors as you like from a box of crayons, markers, colored pencils, etc. Allow each color to represent an emotion or feeling you are experiencing in the present moment (e.g., blue might represent sadness, red anger, etc.). Decide what feelings your colors will represent. Create a color key. Color in the heart to show how much of each feeling you are experiencing right now. Your heart might be filled in like a pie, with stripes, with symbols, shading, designs, whatever expresses your experience right now.

Color Key:

Color	Feeling
❑	Sad
❑	Angry
❑	Happy
❑	_____
❑	_____
❑	_____
❑	_____
❑	_____

Reprinted with permission from the author ©Karla Helbert 2013

Brandon also worked on writing down his thoughts in a journal and in letters to his teacher, to his grief, to his family. In therapy sessions, a prompting format was used for letter writing and he revisited Color Your Heart several times. The exercises helped him recognize that many of his feelings and experiences were connected to grief and sadness at missing this important person in his life, and the activities they did together that were so important to him.

Figure 2:

WRITE A LETTER EXERCISE

You can write a letter to your loved one anytime you want. You can write down whatever you are feeling. Tell them how much you love and miss them. Tell them how you are doing. Tell them about what is going on in your life, in your family, at school, whatever you like. If you can't think of what to write, you can use this letter worksheet:

Dear _____,

I always wanted to tell you……

I would have liked to……

I would like……

I hope that…….

Thank you for…..

Love,

_____

Reprinted with permission from the author © Karla Helbert 2013

Brandon's initial response of anger, and similar responses exhibited by others, are likely due to difficulty individuals on the spectrum have with connecting to and understanding their own emotional responses (Samson, Huber, & Gross, 2012). Contrary to a widespread belief that people on the spectrum do not experience deep or complex emotions, people with ASD typically experience extraordinarily strong emotion, but not always with the ability to immediately connect the emotion to a particular event or occurrence. Many people on the spectrum, particularly children and adolescents, can experience extremely profound emotional states yet be consciously unaware of the cause of the emotions, or even what emotions are impacting them. They may lack the ability to verbally describe their own emotions (Samson et al., 2012). The types of exercises described above can help some children and adolescents on the spectrum to identify some of the complex feelings they may be experiencing; in so doing, they may feel some relief of anxiety or have increased insight into their own experience.

Often, intense feelings and the bodily responses that go with them can be incredibly overwhelming for young people on the spectrum. Emotional disconnection can fuel an anxiety response, or the distress can be due specifically to major changes in what is normal. In the example of Brandon, part of his angry reaction focused on the distress experienced due to changes in his normal routine. Families and caregivers should never underestimate the distress created by the change in what was a normal routine in the person's life. The turmoil created by changes in daily routines and expectations alone can cause severe adjustment problems. Even when loss is expected, the actual fact of how a person's life and feelings are impacted once the loss actually occurs cannot be fully planned for.

Disproportionate, socially non-sanctioned, or inappropriate reactions, such as anger, can be very upsetting to others. This kind of disconnect between experienced emotional state and displayed behavior may show up in ways that others perceive as rude, inappropriate, or simply inexplicable. Other examples might include laughter at a funeral; voicing negative or tactless remarks about the deceased or other family members; displays of disproportionate distress, such as excessive crying or having a meltdown over small or seemingly insignificant events. These kinds of reactions overwhelmingly are not meant to be hurtful, but rather are a reflection of the person's lack of coping skills, lack of insight, or disconnection to his or her own overpowering emotional response. The person with ASD can be reminded that it is not acceptable to harm others, or to cause others to feel afraid due to her reactions or behavior, and to work with her to discover what might help.

Such behaviors may be a function of anxiety, an extremely common response in grief. As is true for many neurotypical grievers, anxiety levels of a person on the spectrum can greatly increase during grief. Anxiety may show up as laughter, hyperactivity, fear, meltdowns, irritability, anger, tears, need to withdraw, need for reassurance, increased intensity of focus in special interest areas, and much more. How anxiety manifests depends on the individual.

Anxiety scales can be good tools for adolescents on the spectrum to help them identify the intensity of feeling experiences (whether anxiety, anger, sadness, overstimulation, etc.). Scales can also be helpful for measuring grief in general once the person has identified what grief looks like for him or her. Creating the scale with the participation of the individual helps him to articulate what low-to-high level anxiety feels like for him, what it looks like in his behavior, and what helps most when he is at a low, medium or high level of feeling/experience. The scales should be shared with family and other support people. A good resource for learning how to create personal scales for individuals can be found in *The Incredible 5 Point Scale* by teachers Kari Dunn Buron and Mitzi Curtis (2012).

In times of high stress, young children, adolescents and adults on the spectrum often engage in "stimming:" self-stimulatory behaviors which generally include motor movements, sensory fixations, or vocalizations that help "to counteract an overwhelming sensory environment or alleviate…high levels of anxiety" (Grandin, 2011). Rocking, hand flicking or flapping, humming, or blinking are examples of what stimming may look like. It's important to recognize that stimming behaviors are calming and feel good to the person engaging in them. Allowing the person space and time to engage in these behaviors can be incredibly helpful. Finding balance between supporting a person in escaping the stress of grief to a calm space, and helping them to be focused and present for important activities such as school and other learning opportunities, is paramount. Providing fidget toys, music, opportunities for engagement and physical activity, as well as calming, soothing activities can be helpful. As suggested in Stroebe and Schut's dual process model of coping with bereavement

(2010), active confrontation of grief and loss is not always necessary for positive outcome. In some situations, forms of escape from grief and its related stressors can be essential for helping individuals move through loss. For people on the spectrum who may be easily overwhelmed by anxiety, stress, overstimulation and intense emotion, lessons from this model can be very useful.

Another way to help the adolescent cope with the complexity and chaos of grief is to assist them to engage in rituals designed to bring order to the chaos of grief. It can be helpful to provide a definition of ritual and explain how ritual can help ease the anxiety and, sometimes, the pain of grief. A ritual is an activity or a set of activities that people engage in to help us to feel calmer, more orderly, to help us move through transitions and also to cope with difficult feelings (Helbert, 2013). In grief, ritual can help bring the chaos of our feelings and experiences into a more manageable place. For some adolescents, ritual can help them feel more connected to the deceased; for others, it may serve mainly to decrease anxiety. Not all individuals may need to feel a connection to the deceased. Some may express no interest in ritual. For some individuals on the spectrum, engaging in ritual may be too emotionally trying. They may need time to process the emotional impact of the loss before engaging in ritual; this may mean days, weeks, months, or even years, depending upon the person.

Providing opportunity, support, and the choice to remember a loved one through ritual can always be helpful. When people have choice they are likely to feel a greater sense of control. Opportunities can come through personal or family rituals; observation of special days, such as the loved one's birthday; the anniversary of the death; and remembrances at holidays or other significant times of the year. Whether the person chooses to participate is a personal decision, but supporting and allowing full participation and choice should be encouraged.

Grief is often a spiritual crisis for many. No matter a person's religion or spiritual belief system, the death of someone we love deeply can bring profound changes. Death can spark many questions: *Why did this happen? Why him? Why her? Why me? Why did God let him die? Am I being punished? What did I do to deserve this? Where is she now? Can he see, hear or feel me? Is there a God? Why is life so unfair? What is the meaning of life?*

Some grieving people find that everything they thought they knew or believed in is suddenly called into question after the death of a loved one. Conversely, some grieving people find their spiritual lives become enriched, finding comfort in spiritual or religious practices including prayer, meditation, or other spiritual activities. These responses are true for people on or off the spectrum. Allowing space for spiritual questioning and exploration can be helpful.

A characteristic of ASD is having intensely-focused special interests. Special interest areas may change after the death of a loved one. This may arise from the need to understand the situation, to maintain connection with a loved one, or to help manage stress. New special interests may be adopted having to do with the deceased's interests, hobbies or another subject related in some way to the loved one, or their manner of death. For some, death itself, or aspects of death, may become special interest areas. Examples might include the funeral industry, funerary or memorial rituals of other cultures, wars or aspects of war, the afterlife, the disease process, the paranormal, spiritual or religious topics, ancient Egyptian mummification processes, zombies, vampires or other supernatural creatures, angels, demons, or other mystical topics.

These interest areas may seem peculiar to some, but serve a purpose. Perhaps they are expressions of curiosity, the need to know more; or perhaps they are reflections of struggles with existential questions, or of the need to connect in some concrete way with what was lost. Knowledge is power; in grief, when we can often feel most powerless, learning about things that frighten or mystify us can help reduce confusion and soothe anxiety. This knowledge may also help with understanding or connecting with, in some small way, that which truly is a mystery.

There may be no change in special interests, but questions about spiritual aspects of life, death, or the afterlife may arise, and should be allowed and discussed. If an individual is part of a family that practices a particular religious or spiritual path, these questions can be addressed with family or clergy. When a child or adolescent is curious about spiritual matters in death, the best course is to have as genuine a conversation as possible. If you don't know the answers, say so; there are just some things we don't know. This honesty helps in many ways to ease anxiety, lets them know that their needs are respected by others, and that they are being told the truth, insofar as that is possible to do when speaking of death, dying and the afterlife.

Here is a list of helpful strategies to remember and to share with other support people, including family, friends, caregivers, teachers, and professionals when supporting a child or a teen with ASD who is grieving.

- Be concrete when speaking or answering questions about what has happened.
- Recognize that even if they do not speak, they are grieving.
- Even if they don't appear to understand, assume that they are aware.
- Tell the truth and allow them to make decisions about their own grief process.
- Be as consistent as possible with the person's schedule of activities, including a reliable daily schedule and regular nighttime rituals.
- Ensure plenty of nutritious food and pay attention to food intake and hydration.
- Be aware of sensory processing difficulties and understand that sensory processing difficulties may increase during grief. New or previously unseen sensory difficulties may arise.
- Encourage communication in whatever ways the individual communicates best.
- Encourage learning new activities, new ways of creating and finding ways to direct energy in whatever ways suit the individual.
- Support the adolescent in finding ways to mourn and to remember the person who has died in ways that are authentic to the adolescent and his personality and abilities.
- Be patient with the grief process. There is no time frame for grief.

Observation, sensitivity, and communication are central to understanding and supporting those on the spectrum in grief. If we live long enough and we love people, we will all experience the death of someone we love and the pain of grief. If we can know that others care, that we are supported in learning ways to communicate and to express our unique experiences, we can all go a long way toward finding our way through grief, on or off the spectrum.

Editor's Note: Figures 1 and 2 are adapted from the book Finding Your Own Way to Grieve: A Creative Activity Workbook for Kids and Teens on the Autism Spectrum *(Helbert, 2013).*

Karla Helbert, LPC, operates a private psychotherapy practice in Richmond, VA. With nearly 15 years of experience as a therapist, she currently specializes in grief and bereavement, anxiety disorders, Autism Spectrum Disorders (ASD), and Mindfulness Based Cognitive Behavior Therapy. Ms. Helbert is the author of Finding Your Own Way to Grieve: A Creative Activity Workbook for Kids and Teens on the Autism Spectrum *(2013). She is particularly experienced in helping others with grief due to perinatal loss, death of a child, and traumatic grief. Ms. Helbert facilitates bereavement support groups for local hospices and provides consulting and training on the topics of grief and bereavement, traumatic grief and Autism Spectrum Disorders. She also facilitates a monthly support group for the Richmond Chapter of the MISS Foundation, an international non-profit helping families grieving the death of a child. As a bereaved mother and a trained therapist, she has a deep personal, as well as clinical, understanding of the difficult issues facing those grieving the deaths of loved ones.*

REFERENCES

Bandini, L. G., Anderson, S. E., Curtin, C., Cermak, S., Evans, W.E., Scampini, R., ...Must, A. (2010). Food selectivity in children with autism spectrum disorders and typically developing children. *The Journal of Pediatrics, 157*(2), 259-264.

Blumberg, S. J., Bramlett, M. D., Kogan, M. D., Shieve, L. A., Jones, J. R., & Lu, M. C. (2013). *Changes in prevalence of parent-reported autism spectrum disorder in school aged U.S. children: 2007 to 2011-2012* (DHHS Publication No. 65). Hyattsville, MD: U.S. Dept. of Health and Human Services, Centers for Disease Control, National Center for Health Statistics. Retrieved from http://www.cdc.gov/nchs/data/nhsr/nhsr065.pdf

Buron, K. D. & Curtis, M. (2012). *The incredible 5-point scale: The significantly improved and expanded second edition.* Shawnee Mission, KS: AAPC Publishing.

Doka, K. J. (2002). *Disenfranchised grief: New directions, challenges, and strategies for practice.* Champaign, IL: Research Press.

Grandin, T. (2011 November/December). Why do kids with autism stim? *Autism Asperger's Digest*, 1. Retrieved from: http://autismdigest.com/why-do-kids-with-autism-stim/

Hadjikhani, N., Robert, J. M., Snyder, J., & Tager-Flusberg, H. (2006). Anatomical differences in the mirror neuron system and social cognition network in autism. *Oxford Journal Cerebral Cortex, 16*(9) 1276-1282.

Helbert, K. (2013). *Finding your own way to grieve: A creative activity workbook for kids and teens on the autism spectrum.* London, England: Jessica Kingsley Publishers.

Kern, J. K, Trivedi, M. H., Garver, C. R., Granneman, B. D., Andrews, A. A., Savla, J.S.,...Schroeder, J. L. (2006). The pattern of sensory processing abnormalities in autism. *Sage Publications, 10*(5) 480-494.

Premack, D. & Woodruff, G. (1978). Does the chimpanzee have a theory of mind? *Behavioral and Brain Sciences, 1*(4) 515-526.

Samson, A. C., Huber, O., & Gross, J. J. (2012). Emotion regulation in asperger's syndrome and high functioning autism. *Emotion, 12*(4) 654-655.

Stroebe, M. S., & Schut, H. (2010). The dual process model of coping with bereavement: A decade on. *Omega Journal of Death and Dying, 61*(4) 273-289.

Resources

Listed below are some helpful grief and adolescent-related organizations, many of which are referenced by the authors.

GRIEF AND BEREAVEMENT

The Association for Death Education and Counseling (ADEC)
www.adec.org

The Compassionate Friends
www.thecompassionatefriends.org

The Dougy Center
www.dougy.org

Hello Grief
www.hellogrief.org

Hospice Foundation of America
www.hospicefoundation.org

International Society for Traumatic Stress Studies
www.istss.org

The Mourning Star Center
vnacalifornia.org/outreach/mourning-star

National Alliance for Grieving Children
www.childrengrieve.org

National Center for School Crisis and Bereavement
www.stchristophershospital.com/pediatric-specialties-programs/
specialties/690

The National Child Traumatic Stress Network (NCTSN)
www.nctsn.org

National Students of AMF (Actively Moving Forward)
Support Network [for college students]
www.studentsofamf.org

Scholastic Children and Grief Guidance and Support Resources
www.scholastic.com/childrenandgrief

COPING WITH LIFE-THREATENING ILLNESS

The Make-A-Wish Foundation of America
www.wish.org

SuperSibs!
www.supersibs.org

Voicing My Choices: A Planning Guide for Adolescents and
Young Adults
www.agingwithdignity.org/voicing-my-choices-faqs.php

SUICIDE

American Association of Suicidology
www.suicidology.org

National Suicide Prevention Lifeline
www.suicidepreventionlifeline.org

The Society for the Prevention of Teen Suicide
www.sptsusa.org

MILITARY FAMILIES

Give an Hour
www.giveanhour.org